C0-AOF-713

THE LIBRARY
OF THE
WASHINGTON SCHOOL OF
PSYCHIATRY

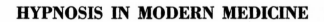

HYPNOSIS IN MODERN MEDICINE

HYPNOSIS IN MODERN MEDICINE
(Third Edition)

Edited by

JEROME M. SCHNECK, A.B., M.D.

Clinical Associate Professor of Psychiatry
State University of New York
Downstate Medical Center
New York City

Founder and Past President
The Society for Clinical and Experimental Hypnosis

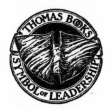

CHARLES C THOMAS • PUBLISHER

Springfield · Illinois · U.S.A.

RC495.S35
1963

Published and Distributed Throughout the World by

CHARLES C THOMAS · PUBLISHER

BANNERSTONE HOUSE

301-327 East Lawrence Avenue, Springfield, Illinois, U.S.A.

This book is protected by copyright. No
part of it may be reproduced in any manner
without written permission from the publisher.

© *1953, 1959 and 1962, by* CHARLES C THOMAS · PUBLISHER

Library of Congress Catalog Card Number: 62-17612

First Edition, 1953
Second Edition, 1959
Third Edition, 1963

*With THOMAS BOOKS careful attention is given to all details of
manufacturing and design. It is the Publisher's desire to present books
that are satisfactory as to their physical qualities and artistic possibilities
and appropriate for their particular use. THOMAS BOOKS will be true
to those laws of quality that assure a good name and good will.*

Printed in the United States of America

CONTRIBUTORS

GORDON AMBROSE, L.M.S.S.A. (London, England): *Late Assistant Psychiatrist and Senior Registrar, Child Guidance Clinic, Prince of Wales Hospital.*

RALPH V. AUGUST, B.S., M.D.: *Chief, Department of Obstetrics, Hackley Hospital, Muskegon, Michigan.*

JOHN PAUL BRADY, B.A., M.D.: *Research Psychiatrist, Institute of Psychiatric Research, Indiana University Medical Center, Indianapolis, Indiana.*

MILTON V. KLINE, M.A., ED.D. (New York City): *President, The Society for Clinical and Experimental Hypnosis.*

EUGENE E. LEVITT, M.A., PH.D.: *Associate Professor of Clinical Psychology, Indiana University Medical Center, Indianapolis, Indiana.*

HOWARD MARCUS, M.D., D.M.D., DR. MED. DENT. (New York City): *Past President, American Hypnodontic Society.*

MILTON J. MARMER, M.D., M.SC. MED. (ANES.): *Assistant Clinical Professor of Surgery (Anesthesiology), University of California School of Medicine, Los Angeles, California.*

AINSLIE MEARES, M.D., B.AGR.SCI., D.P.M. (Melbourne, Australia): *President, International Society for Clinical and Experimental Hypnosis.*

BERNARD B. RAGINSKY, M.D., C.M. (Montreal, Canada): *Past President, Academy of Psychosomatic Medicine.*

GEORGE ROSEN, M.D., PH.D.: *Professor of Health Education, School of Public Health and Administrative Medicine, Columbia University, New York City.*

JEROME M. SCHNECK, A.B., M.D.: *Clinical Associate Professor of Psychiatry, State University of New York, Downstate Medical Center, New York City.*

MICHAEL J. SCOTT, B.S., M.D.: *Instructor in Medicine (Dermatology), University of Washington School of Medicine, Seattle, Washington.*

JOHN G. WATKINS, M.S., PH.D.: *Chief Clinical Psychologist, Veterans Administration Hospital, Portland, Oregon.*

Editor's Dedication

To My Wife

PREFACE TO THE THIRD EDITION

H*ypnosis in Modern Medicine* has been completely revised and rewritten for the Third Edition. Some contributors appear now for the first time. All have special experience and reputations in the areas they have covered. The opening chapter has been changed least from its original form because it contains many facts and fundamental themes generally accepted as basic in the history of hypnosis. An additional historical chapter has been furnished to supply additions and elaborations and to bring the survey up to date. The first clinical chapter now covers General Practice as well as Internal Medicine. It possesses a strong psychosomatic orientation which serves as a desirable preparation for the chapters that follow. The entire text, in fact, has a deeper psychological tone than that of the preceding editions. This conforms to the increasing psychological awareness of forward looking physicians in all specialties and confirms the influence of psychiatric thought on those physicians especially who have developed a scientific interest in hypnosis investigations.

Surgery and Anesthesiology are presented now in one chapter, consistent with developments in recent years. Hypnotherapy for Children is the heading that replaces Hypnosis in Child Psychiatry of previous editions. It implies broader coverage including, for example, the field of Pediatrics. Psychophysiology of Hypnosis has been substituted for the chapter title, Physiologic Aspects of Hypnosis. This heading too is more appropriate, and it reflects the nature of research developments.

In the First Edition, induction issues were included in the chapter on Psychiatry, and in the Second Edition a supplementary section on Induction and Termination was appended. Now a chapter on the Psychodynamics of Hypnotic Induction and Termination is made part of the basic text because of newer insights and understandings regarding their significance in hypnotic behavior and total personality functioning. Clinical Psychology merits a place too as a basic chapter in the text. This conforms to the increasing cooperation among professional psychologists, physicians and dentists in clinical and experimental studies. It points up the search for dynamic elements of personality interplay in hypnotic and associated relationships. A parallel development has been interest in Theory. Whereas this area (as well as some areas just mentioned) was represented in an appended section of the Second Edition, it takes its place as a fundamental chapter in this Third Edition. An increase in practical facilities for Instruction in Hypnosis, the quality of which remains still to be much improved, warrants nevertheless the omission of the chapter on this topic that had appeared in the First Edition.

The changes just noted in the preparation and development of the three editions reflect the steady growth of medical hypnosis and allied disciplines in their scientific aspects. They confirm once again that the study of hypnosis is keeping pace confidently with advances on a broader front in the fields of medicine, psychology, and science in general. There is every reason to feel that the future looks bright for explorations yet to come.

I should like to reemphasize some points made in the Introduction to the First Edition and the Preface to the Second Edition because they are important. Some specialties or areas of study have been omitted because insufficient experience and too few facts are available to warrant their inclusion. For the specialties that are included, contributors to the Third Edition were asked to survey the literature when possible, and in addition to present personal work. Rigid uniformity and consistency have been bypassed to provide for originality and expression of personal points of view. I believe this is desirable and advantageous, and preferable to an unbending editorial conformity. Readers should expect, therefore, to encounter differences in opinion or emphasis. They should anticipate suggestions regarding new paths for exploration in keeping with special concerns of some of the writers.

All chapters are basically autonomous as was the case in the First and Second Editions. Again, however, some overlapping is unavoidable and indeed helpful. It supplies a desirable feeling of unity stemming from the primary investigations that constitute the substance of the text.

It may be stated, finally, that when this volume was presented originally as the first textbook dealing with hypnosis and the medical specialties, the opinion was rendered that it may best be designated as an introduction to hypnosis in modern medicine. The modesty of this assertion is still implied now, but with ten intervening years of fruitful experience it would be fair to point up the presence of a greater feeling of security justified by advances achieved by an ever enlarging group of active clinicians and experimenters.

JEROME M. SCHNECK, M.D.

PREFACE TO THE SECOND EDITION

The initial edition of this volume was issued as the first textbook dealing with hypnosis and the medical specialties. It was made possible by the remarkable growth of medical specialization and the ability of scientific hypnosis to keep pace with this development. Readers received the book generously. In serving their needs and wishes it seems wise in this second edition to retain the original form and content and to supplement the basic structure of the book with the latest significant data. To achieve this aim, a review of the literature has been organized and appended. Emphasis has been placed on clinical advances. The basic chapters on history and instruction have not, therefore, been enlarged. The supplement includes sections on internal medicine, dermatology, obstetrics and gynecology, psychiatry, child psychiatry, and dentistry. It has a section combining surgery and anesthesiology because the new literature integrated these specialties meaningfully and they can be presented best in this way.

Psychophysiology was chosen as the title for the section relating to the chapter on physiologic aspects of hypnosis. The new title is more appropriate to the nature of the data included. The importance of clinical psychology for certain aspects of psychiatry and other medical specialties has warranted a separate section. Pertinent material in this sphere had been included originally in the chapter on psychiatry. Also, researches of clinical psychologists are bringing them into contact more often now with several medical specialties rather than with psychiatry alone. The chapter on psychiatry includes information about hypnotic induction. Recent writings on induction and some new views on termination of hypnosis suggested the desirability of a section for these themes. Finally, as an addendum to the clinical writings, a brief section on theory appeared to be indicated in order to round out the view of research interests in recent years.

The new literature reviewed for this edition covers areas of concern to most clinicians with views and experiences that can serve to stimulate their investigations and thinking. No attempt has been made to incorporate all recent writings. Items have been selected when they have been considered especially important or essentially representative of work in a given field. The sections are basically autonomous but there is some overlapping. Sometimes it is difficult to decide in which sections certain writings should be mentioned. For example, material of interest to the neurologist may be found in several divisions. It would be wise for readers to glance at reference lists for sections other than those relating specifically to their own specialties. The general physician would surely find writings pertinent for him scattered throughout the entire volume.

JEROME M. SCHNECK, M.D.

INTRODUCTION TO THE FIRST EDITION

In an evaluation of the place and need for a volume on hypnosis such as this, it would seem pertinent to outline some ideas that entered into a formulation of purpose and goal. To begin with, investigators in the field of hypnosis are aware of the fact that over the years very many books on hypnosis have been published. While most have just about disappeared from view, some have attained outstanding success and are viewed today as classics. Books such as those by Bernheim (1), Forel (3), Moll (4), and Bramwell (2), have much to offer even today to scientific workers involved with hypnotic techniques. Included in a number of the classic works is material of special interest to medical researchers and practitioners. Setting aside temporarily the specialty of psychiatry, it will be found that many significant items regarding gynecological, surgical, and neurological problems have been mentioned by these writers. There is material pertinent for the internist, the obstetrician and the anesthesiologist. Other specialties have their share too in this early literature.

Over the years, tremendous strides have been made in the development of all specialties. Investigations in hypnosis have, however, continued to be weighted heavily in psychological areas so that in the field of medicine, the applications of hypnosis in psychiatry have received attention exceeding by far the interest in hypnosis as related to other specialties. This remains true today, but in the past few years there has been a reactivation of interest in broader hypnosis investigation, a familiar phenomenon in the history of the subject, and it remains to be seen what the future holds in store. With this reactivation, focus has been centered again on medical areas aside from psychiatry. As these developments have unfolded, books have continued to be published, but consistently a peculiar defect has manifested itself in their mode of preparation. Almost invariably only one or two authors have prepared these volumes, and to varying degrees they have attempted to cover not only the sector of practice most familiar to them, but other areas also in which they very clearly have had little or no experience. Some comments, therefore, regarding the work of others have been presented by them and too frequently experience has been implied regarding fields of practice where no serious practice could have been engaged in unless excursions had been made into areas where experience has not warranted. Medical practice has become too extensive and highly specialized to permit any physician or worker in an allied area to apply his experience with hypnosis to fields beyond that in which he had been especially trained or involved through special interest and attention.

Two issues have become clear. One is that an up to date book on hypnosis in medicine should have its place in current medical literature. The second is that such a volume would best be prepared through the cooperation of a group of workers. In developing this idea further it seemed reasonable to attempt to gather together contributors who are themselves experienced in hypnosis investigations. In addition it appeared reasonable to make a selection of those investigators who, aside from their experience in hypnosis, were directly involved in the specialty to be presented, or who through allied experience are apparently best prepared to discuss the particular specialty insofar as the applications of hypnosis to it is concerned. Thus, an obstetrician and gynecologist was selected to present his field of work, a dentist to discuss his specialty, and so on. Likewise coverage of the historical aspects of hypnosis was sought from a medical historian distinguished in his particular field of study and who has previously contributed also to the literature on the history of hypnosis itself.

In view of the fact that the extent of developments in applications of hypnosis to one specialty has not always paralleled another, some disparity will be evident as these chapters are read. Comment regarding this is directed especially to those professional readers who are not familiar at all with the history of hypnosis. Aside from this, however, other points of difference will be observed. Each contributor had received the suggestion that included in his discussion of the specialty in its broader aspects, some coverage of the pertinent literature be attempted whenever possible. Further, it was indicated that the work of the contributor himself in the area assigned be presented adequately so that his personal experience could be clearly made available to the medical profession at large. In arranging for this, it became evident that the mode of presentation would bear the stamp of the worker himself and to this extent absolute uniformity and consistency in this volume is not possible. If a more rigidly uniform approach were utilized, only the seal of the editor could be apparent. It was felt that the advantages of the former approach would probably outweigh any disadvantages. Any differences of opinion evident in the pages to follow should, therefore, be evaluated with reference to the foregoing remarks.

To imply in any way that this volume represents all there is to be said regarding hypnosis in modern medicine would be both false and presumptuous. It should be most clear that some medical specialties have not been touched at all. Ophthalmology and otolaryngology will be noted immediately by their absence and the reason for incomplete coverage in several fields is based either on data inadequate to warrant separate chapters at this time, or hypnosis workers as yet too inexperienced or not at all available to prepare chapters that would merit inclusion. At most this volume may best be designated as *an introduction to hypnosis in modern medicine,* and if it can be received and regarded as such the efforts of all the contributors would be amply rewarded.

JEROME M. SCHNECK, M.D.

REFERENCES

1. BERNHEIM, H.: *Suggestive Therapeutics.* New York, London Book Company, 1947.
2. BRAMWELL, J. M.: *Hypnotism: Its History, Practice and Theory.* London, Rider, 1921.
3. FOREL, A.: *Hypnotism or Suggestion and Psychotherapy.* New York, Allied Publications, 1949.
4. MOLL, A.: *Hypnotism.* London, Walter Scott, 1890.

CONTENTS

HYPNOSIS IN MODERN MEDICINE

1

HISTORY OF MEDICAL HYPNOSIS: FROM ANIMAL MAGNETISM TO MEDICAL HYPNOSIS

GEORGE ROSEN, M.D., PH.D.

On December 11, 1775, a reader of the *Frankfurt Journal* might have seen the following report from Munich: "Dr. Mesmer, who is famous for his magnet cures, arrived here on his way to Vienna, after having spent some time in his native Schwaban. It is known that he can produce wonderful effects by means of the magnetic force. . . ." Eighteen years later, on December 18, 1793, the *Vossische Zeitung* of Berlin reported from Austria that "Dr. Mesmer has been released from detention. He has prepared an apology and departed for Switzerland."

The man mentioned in these notices was Franz Anton Mesmer, who inaugurated the movement from which modern medical hypnosis eventually developed. Mesmer stumbled upon the phenomenon of hypnosis and offered a theory to explain it. By means of his theory of animal magnetism and its practical applications, Mesmer attracted professional and public attention to the problem so that it could no longer be overlooked and disregarded.

Franz Anton Mesmer was born on May 23, 1734 at Iznang on Lake Constance, where his father served the Prince-Bishop of Constance as game warden. His talents and his father's position helped Mesmer to obtain a good education. Before matriculating in medicine, he had pursued philosophical studies at Dillingen and Ingolstadt and had obtained the doctorate in philosophy. In 1759, Mesmer was in Vienna where he first studied jurisprudence, and then enrolled in the medical faculty. Mesmer graduated in 1766,

presenting a doctoral dissertation entitled *De planetarum influxu*
(On the influence of the planets). While the dissertation is in no
way outstanding, it contains the germ of what later became animal
magnetism or mesmerism. In the course of his medico-astrological
discussion, Mesmer expressed the belief that a peculiar force, which
he termed *gravitas animalis,* animal gravitation, acts on the human
body.

Shortly after graduating, Mesmer began the practice of medicine in Vienna; and on January 10, 1768, he married Marie Anna
von Posch, the well-to-do widow of a lieutenant colonel in the
Imperial Army. He appeared destined to become a prosperous and
successful practitioner, but another fate awaited him. During this
time Mesmer continued to develop his idea that the heavenly
spheres emit influences that penetrate everywhere, and exercise a
direct influence on living organisms, particularly on the nervous
system.

In 1773, Mesmer undertook to test his ideas in the treatment
of Franziska Oesterlin, a young woman, twenty-eight years of age,
who later married Mesmer's stepson, Friederich von Posch. Apparently the young woman suffered from hysteria, which manifested itself in convulsions, pains in the ears, toothache, fainting
spells, retention of urine, furor, delirium, melancholy, dyspnoea,
and paralyses that lasted for several days. Mesmer succeeded in
curing the patient, employing magnets in the course of his treatment. In this he was not original, but followed a practice employed
by a number of his contemporaries; indeed, Mesmer acknowledged
this. What was new was his explanation of the apparent action of
the magnet.

The marvelous cure of Fräulein Oesterlin was reported in the
press, but it was not until 1775 that Mesmer published his first
account of the magnetic cure. In his *Schreiben über die Magnetkur
. . . an einen auswärtigen Arzt* addressed to the Altona physician
Johann Christoph Unzer, he presented the first version of his theory
of animal magnetism. Mesmer held that since the human body is
composed of the same substance as the universe, it is subject to
direct influences, aside from climatic, barometric, and gravitational
forces or the influence of the planets; these influences derive from

forces that fill celestial space and act in the organism by way of the nervous system. Mesmer assumed a subtle fluid that flows about the nerves and in the atmosphere, as well as in the fluids and vessels of the human organism. He employed the term magnetism to characterize a reciprocal relationship between the forces of nature and the human body, and conceived of nature as the harmony of these relations in action. The magnet was only a representation of nature. In space there exist innumerable relations whose totality forms the general fluid in which man as well as the planets float. Through the irritability of nerves and muscles, the human organs are able to receive the vibrations of the fluid. Whenever this irritability is decreased or obstructed, disharmony and disease are produced. There is only one disease, and consequently only one therapy, namely magnetism. Nature endeavors to overcome disease by means of a crisis, and this must be supported and fostered, for if the crisis does not come to a head the condition becomes chronic.

Mesmer's theory of animal magnetism, as outlined above, contains a number of themes and theoretical concepts common to the medical world of the eighteenth century. This is evident, for example, in his interpretation of disease as a disharmony attributable to a functional disturbance of the nervous fluid. This concept is derived from the ancient humoral pathology with its doctrines of dyscrasia and critical days, from the irritability theory of Albrecht von Haller (1708-1777), and from the excitation theory of John Brown (1735-1788). Furthermore, Mesmer presents a physical theory according to which a universal fluid permeates the nervous system of living organisms as well as all manner of inanimate objects. This theory appears to incorporate the metaphysical doctrine of affinity and sympathy as well as the idea which he originally expressed as "gravitation." These diverse ideas and concepts Mesmer combined in a system. Into this combination of ideas he then introduced the claim that it was possible to cure by means of a magnet. In the theory, however, the magnet served only as a means for concentrating, manipulating and directing the magnetic fluid. After awhile, Mesmer recognized that the same effects could be achieved without magnets. This led him to conclude that the magnetizer, in his person, collects and directs the action of this magnetic force.

Mesmer's cures created a sensation in Vienna and aroused attention in various parts of Europe. In July and August 1775, Mesmer travelled to Bavaria, as indicated by the report previously quoted. In Munich he demonstrated magnetic phenomena before the Elector of Bavaria and the Bavarian Academy of Sciences. On this occasion, he was elected a member of the Bavarian Academy, due no doubt to the favor of the Elector who became a convert to animal magnetism. Other medical bodies, however, remained cool to or aloof from Mesmer's activities.

Nevertheless, in Vienna patients streamed to Mesmer for treatment. Hand in hand with public interest and acclaim went professional opposition. The case of Maria Theresia Paradis soon brought the situation to a head. This young woman, whom Mesmer began to treat in 1777, was well-known in Vienna as a singer and pianist. She had suddenly lost her sight at the age of three and a half, and although she had been treated by the best physicians her vision had not been restored. The father of Fräulein Paradis was secretary to the Emperor, and the Empress Maria Theresia, her godmother, had bestowed a pension upon her. Mesmer undertook to cure her blindness, and claimed to have accomplished this. Nevertheless, a number of influential physicians, among them Joseph Barth (1745-1818) and Anton Freiherr von Stoerck (1731-1803) convinced the parents that the "cure" was not real. The father of Fräulein Paradis may also have been concerned about the possible loss of her pension should she recover her vision. At any rate, the patient was removed from Mesmer's care under circumstances which were extremely humiliating.

As a result of the Paradis case, Mesmer found the atmosphere in Vienna intolerable and decided to leave for Paris. Equipped with a recommendation from the Austrian Foreign Minister to the Imperial Embassy, he arrived at Paris early in February 1778. The intellectual climate of Paris was favorable for the implantation of a new medical idea such as Mesmer's animal magnetism. Public interest was aroused promptly, but Mesmer's hope to convince the medical profession of the correctness of his views was destined to be disappointed. The medical faculty was antagonistic and Mesmer could not even gain a hearing. Nevertheless, he established a clinic on the Place Vendôme, and in 1779 published his *Mémoire sur la découverte du magnetisme animal.*

In this work Mesmer presented his doctrine most clearly in the form of twenty-seven propositions. The essence of these propositions is the following: There exists a reciprocal influence between the heavenly bodies, the earth and living bodies. This influence acts by means of a universally distributed fluid of an incomparably rarified nature which is capable of receiving, propagating and communicating movement. The animal body sustains the effects of this agent which affects the nerves by insinuating itself into their substance. In the human body this agent has properties like those of a magnet. This property of the human body has therefore given rise to the term animal magnetism. The action and properties of animal magnetism may be communicated to other animate and inanimate bodies, and this magnetic property may be stored up, concentrated and transported. It has been shown that this agent can cure nervous and other disorders.

Mesmer made use of these principles in his practice. Thus he invented the *baquet,* as a receptacle in which animal magnetism could be stored. The *baquet* was a tub filled with water in which bottles were arranged concentrically. The bottom of the tub was covered with iron filings and pieces of glass, and the tub was closed with a cover from which projected iron rods. The patients grasped these rods in order to receive the magnetic fluid. The clinic was lavishly provided with mirrors and music, for Mesmer believed that these intensified and communicated animal magnetism.

In 1778 Mesmer became acquainted with Charles d'Eslon, physician to the Count d'Artois, the king's youngest brother, who later became Charles X of France. D'Eslon became Mesmer's most prominent supporter and endeavored to gain a hearing for the doctrine of animal magnetism. Between them, Mesmer and d'Eslon roused the opposition of the entire medical faculty. At the same time, friends were not lacking. Some of these subscribed money to help Mesmer publicize his views, and these subscribers organized themselves as a Society of Harmony (Ordre de l'Harmonie), a kind of secret society for the cultivation and propagation of animal magnetism.

Finally, in 1784, the French government appointed a commission to investigate Mesmer's claims. Among its members were Benjamin Franklin (1706-1790), Antoine-Laurent Lavoisier (1713-1794) the famous chemist, Joseph-Ignace Guillotin (1783-1814) who gave his name to the guillotine, and Antoine-Laurent de Jussieu (1748-1836) an outstanding botanist. The commission was easily able to disprove Mesmer's thesis of the existence of an animal magnetic fluid, and there the matter was allowed to rest. In part, at least this was due to Mesmer's theory itself, in that it diverted attention from the phenomena produced by animal magnetism to the agent alleged to produce them. The commission simply ascribed the magnetic cures to imagination, but never bothered to ask how imagination can produce a cure. In fact, this whole sequence of events set a pattern which was to be repeated at intervals during the succeeding decades.

Following the publication of the commission's report, which in effect branded Mesmer a quack, his popularity disappeared and he seems to have left France in 1785. He travelled in England, Italy and Germany and returned for a while to Paris and Versailles. With the outbreak of the Revolution, Mesmer again left France and spent a number of years in Germany and perhaps in Vienna. In 1798 he returned to Paris, and in 1801 entered into negotiations with the Directory to recover some of his fortune. Eventually, Mesmer secured a small annuity as compensation for his previously held government bonds. From 1803 on, he settled in Switzerland, at Frauenfeld, near Lake Constance. Here Mesmer lived a life of retirement enjoying the company of an occasional visitor, treating the poor, and working on his theory. In the summer of 1814, he moved to Meersburg where he died on March 5, 1815.

Mesmer's active historical role came to an end with the publication in 1784 of the report of the French commission. It was left to his followers to develop his discovery further. Most significant among these was the Marquis de Puységur, who observed the sleep-waking state of the hypnotized patient. Puységur called this state of trance, somnambulism. It was this phenomenon which kept alive an interest in animal magnetism, since it was claimed that the magnetized individual was also clairvoyant, with access to extraordinary powers.

Toward the end of his life, while living in retirement at Frauenfeld, in Switzerland, Mesmer must have viewed with considerable satisfaction the interest in animal magnetism that developed in Germany. The introduction of Mesmer's doctrine into Germany was due particularly to Johann Caspar Lavater (1741-1801), who had been converted to Puységur's *somnambulisme magnétique,* which he employed therapeutically in 1785 in the treatment of his wife who was ill. It was Lavater who attracted the attention of the Bremen physicians, George Bicker (1754-1823), H. W. M. Olbers (1758-1840) and Arnold Wienholt (1749-1804) to the new method. Wienholt published his observations in a work entitled *Heilkraft des thierischen Magnetismus nach eigenen Beobachtungen* (Lemgo, 1802-1806). Wienholt believed that the magnetic force was related to electricity, and assumed that magnetism could not cure severe organic illness, particularly when it was chronic. Nevertheless, he reported fifty cases in which favorable results were achieved.

At first the new doctrine met with a cool reception from the German medical and lay public. Although Lavater "magnetized" with the assistance of well-known, reputable physicians, in the opinion of the other medical men his manipulations were morally suspect. Among the opponents was Christoph Wilhelm Hufeland (1762-1836), who, in 1784, severely criticized and rejected animal magnetism, although he was later to accept it. Particularly interesting are the views of Christoph Meiners (1747-1810), professor of philosophy at Göttingen, who also opposed the theory of animal magnetism. In 1788, he analyzed critically the observations of Wienholt, pointing to imagination as the chief cause of the observed phenomena.

Despite all attacks, however, animal magnetism continued to spread in Germany. This was due in large measure to the favorable climate of opinion provided by contemporary philosophical trends. The outstanding German philosophers of this period, Fichte, Hegel and Schelling, all occupied themselves with mesmerism. From Fichte, for example, we have a detailed account of his observations in Wolfart's mesmeric clinic at Berlin, together with theoretical considerations. Hegel discussed somnambulism and clairvoyance in his *Encyklopädie der philosophischen Wissenschaften im Grundrisse* (Heidelberg, 1817). Schelling also discussed mesmeric sleep and made use of this phenomenon in his metaphysical speculations.

A visit which Lorenz Oken (1779-1851), the physician and natural philosopher, made in 1809 to Mesmer at Frauenfeld was important in arousing still further interest in animal magnetism. Even more significant in this regard was Karl Christian Wolfart (1778-1832), who actually rediscovered Mesmer, visited him frequently during his last years, and saw to the publication of his works. Carl Alexander Ferdinand Kluge (1782-1844), likewise contributed greatly to the spread of the magnetic doctrine with the publication in 1811 of his *Versuch einer Darstellung des animalischen Magnetismus als Heilmittel.* In 1812, Kluge sent this book to Mesmer with the request that he correct it for the second edition. It is to Kluge and Wolfart that we owe the term mesmerism. Other important adherents of animal magnetism were the aforementioned C. W. Hufeland, who in 1808 accepted the doctrine (*Journal für praktische Heilkunde,* vol. 29, 1808), and his younger brother Friedrich Hufeland (1774-1839), a representative of romantic natural philosophy who combined animal magnetism with his own theory of polarity and universal sympathy.

The prominence and influence achieved by the doctrine of animal magnetism in Germany during the second, third and fourth decades of the nineteenth century were due also to a very considerable degree to the political influence and machinations of the physician and *littérateur,* David Ferdinand Koreff (1783-1851), the friend of E. T. A. Hoffman, and a member of the Serapion Brotherhood. Koreff was the physician and protege of the Prussian Minister Karl August von Hardenberg (1750-1822), and was also closely associated with Wilhelm von Humboldt. Despite the opposition of the medical faculties, Koreff succeeded through his political connections in having professorships for animal magnetism established at Berlin, Bonn, Halle, Giessen and Jena.

The interest for mesmerism of persons in high places led to various other actions by official bodies. In 1812, a regulation was issued in Prussia that only licensed physicians would be permitted to use animal magnetism therapeutically, and that they would have to report the results of the cures to the authorities. Furthermore, in 1818, the Berlin Academy of Science, despite the opposition of many of its members, offered a prize of 300 ducats for the best thesis on animal magnetism. This prize was not awarded, however, for in 1823 the Academy decided that none of the entries was deserving of this distinction.

At the same time the adherents of mesmerism created a literary forum for their views in the *Archiv für den thierischen Magnetismus* which appeared from 1817 to 1824. This journal contained original papers, clinical observations and reviews. Alongside scientific studies are to be found metaphysical speculations, essays on folklore, and reflections on magic. In 1817, Hufeland also initiated a department in his journal which he called *Medicina magica*, where he published reports on all kinds of male and female wonder workers, including magnetizers.

Although interest in animal magnetism was at its height at this time, critical voices were not absent. In 1814, Johann Stieglitz (1767-1840), Hannoverian physician-in-ordinary, subjected Mesmer, Kluge, Wolfart and Friederich Hufeland to devastating criticism in his detailed and thorough study, *Ueber den thierischen Magnetismus*. He denied the existence of a magnetic fluid that could be transferred from one person to another, but he did recognize the occurrence of mesmeric sleep. However, Stieglitz believed that such phenomena could be due to the psychic influence of the magnetizer. A similar point of view was voiced by C. H. Pfaff in his book, *Ueber und gegen den thierischen Magnetismus* (1817).

The decades from 1820 to 1840 represent the floodtide of animal magnetism on the continent of Europe, whereas in Britain mesmerism did not reach its high water mark until the following decade. During this period the doctrine of animal magnetism in Germany under the influence of the later Romantic Movement took on even more bizarre forms. Although Mesmer cannot be regarded as a forerunner of Romantic thought, and his theory of animal magnetism is clearly and definitely not a mystical, but rather a physical and naturalistic explanation of observed phenomena, it is not surprising that his ideas were integrated with Romantic concepts. The "fluid" which he called animal magnetism could easily be related to the vital principle or "vital force" of the Romantic thinkers. Furthermore, a second point of contact between mesmerism and Romantic thought lay in their common awareness of the "night side" *(Nachtseite)* of the psyche. Mesmerism, somnambulism and clairvoyance all coincided with the ideas of the Romantics who emphasized the role of the subconscious. Mesmeric phenomena were thus called upon to support the Romantic *Weltanschauung*.

Probably the most characteristic representatives of this trend were Dietrich Georg Kieser (1779-1862), professor at Jena, who, in 1822, published an obscure and confused work entitled *System des Tellurismus oder thierischen Magnetismus;* Johann Carl Passavant (1790-1857), who believed that the hand, the eye and the breath can heal because these transmit the nervous force that provides the energy underlying the phenomena of magnetism, and Justinus Kerner (1786-1862), physician and poet, who first described botulism, and who believed that by means of mesmerism he had successfully treated the schizophrenic Seeress of Prévorst.

The development of the mesmeric doctrine in Germany may be said to have culminated in the work of Carl Gustav Carus (1789-1869). This physician and philosopher, who was a friend of Goethe, in 1856 published a treatise entitled *Ueber Lebensmagnetismus und über die magischen Wirkungen überhaupt,* in which he pointed out that the realm of magic is the Unconscious, the "night side" of the soul. Carus's concept of the Unconscious resembles that of psychoanalysis. In his practice Carus employed mesmerism with success, but he selected with great care the cases where he used this method.

In the same year, however, Isidor Bonaventura, another German, clearly expressed his opposition to the fluid theory of mesmerism. In his book, *Die Mysterien des Schlafes und des Magnetismus* (Weimer, 1856), he pointed out that the mesmeric state could be produced in various ways; all that is necessary in any one of them is to divert the attention of the person to be mesmerized from all distractions and to concentrate the attention on some object for an indefinite period.

Around the 'forties, as mechanistic thinking came more and more to dominate German medicine, interest in mesmerism decreased. There was a revival of interest, however, during the 'seventies and 'eighties due to the work chiefly of W. Preyer, professor of physiology at Jena, who first translated some of Braid's work into German, and to the activities of a Danish lay hypnotist named Hansen. A number of physicians were attracted to the subject, among them Heidenhain, Berger, Grutzner and Weinholt. Soon thereafter the work of Liébeault and Bernheim became known in Germany, and this trend merged with the movement emanating from the Nancy School. By this time, however, the fluidist position of Mesmer and his followers had been discarded, and two other theories to explain mesmeric phenomena had been advanced in England and France.

Animal magnetism also occupied the attention of medical and lay groups in other countries. Austria, Italy, Russia, Sweden and United States all had advocates and practitioners of mesmerism. Knowledge of mesmerism was present in the United States throughout the nineteenth century. In 1829, for instance, Joseph Du Commun gave three lectures on animal magnetism at the Hall of Science in New York. However, interest in mesmerism did not become widespread in the United States until the 'forties of the nineteenth century following the activities of Charles Poyen in New England in 1836. In 1842, for example, Charles Caldwell published a discussion of *Facts in Mesmerism, and Thoughts on Its Causes and Uses.* Daniel Drake, in 1844, presented his experiences with mesmeric phenomena in an *Analytical Report of a Series of Experiments in Mesmeric Somniloquism ... With Speculations on the Production of Its Phenomena.* Drake accepted the reality of the mesmeric state, but rejected the idea of a magnetic fluid. "It is quite obvious," he concluded, "that such an effect could only have been produced through the influence of the imagination and feelings." In a letter to her mother dated July 27, 1845, Elizabeth Blackwell related: "I have just performed my first professional cure, and am already dubbed Dr. Blackwell by the household. I mesmerized away a severe headache that afflicted Miss O'Heara. ..." Considerable evidence is also provided by the various reports by American physicians from 1836 onward of surgical operations performed on patients under mesmeric anesthesia. The impact of mesmerism in the United States is also reflected in literature. Edgar Allan Poe employs mesmeric trance in several stories, and Henry James in *The Bostonians,* in the persons of Verena Tarrant and her father, portrays mesmerists in action. Eventually, the influence of mesmerism ramified even further, and at the hands of Mary Baker Eddy produced Christian Science.

More significant for the development of medical hypnosis, however, was the rise in England of a powerful mesmeric movement which began in 1837 under the leadership of John Elliotson (1791-1868), and the circumstance that James Braid (1795-1860) during the same period began the transformation of mesmerism into hypnotism. Although a few publications on animal magnetism appeared in England during the latter part of the eighteenth century, for instance, Bell's *General and Particular Principles of Animal Electricity and Magnetism* (1792), these seem to have had little influence, and it was not until Elliotson became interested in the subject that it received much notice. Elliotson's attention had first been attracted to mesmerism in 1829, but it was not until 1837 that he began seriously to occupy himself with its investigation and practice. Early that year a Frenchman named Dupotet, who had long practiced mesmerism in France, came to London to propagate the doctrine of animal magnetism. Before long he became associated with Elliotson at the North London (or University College) Hospital, where the latter was senior physician. Elliotson began to treat patients with mesmerism, in particular, a housemaid, Elizabeth O'Key, who suffered from epileptic attacks. These demonstrations were soon the talk of London, and the public flocked to see them.

The interest aroused by Elliotson's activities led Thomas Wakley (1795-1862), the crusading editor of the *Lancet,* to undertake a test of his claims. Elliotson believed that animal magnetism was a distinct physical force which could be imparted to non-magnetized bodies, either by a magnetizer or by transfer from magnetized bodies. He also held the firm conviction that the metal nickel possessed unusual powers of inducing the mesmeric state. On August 16, 1838, Wakley put these claims to a critical test at his house. He substituted "non-magnetized" lead for the nickel and showed that the same effects could be produced with the lead. This exposure of Elliotson's claims immediately brought forth an editorial blast by Wakley in the *Lancet,* in which he condemned mesmerism. Thenceforth, he savagely castigated what he termed the "Mesmeric Humbug."

Elliotson continued to lecture on mesmerism and to demonstrate mesmeric phenomena until December 27, 1838, when the practice of animal magnetism within the North London Hospital was prohibited. Thereupon Elliotson immediately resigned. He was now a man with a mission—to demonstrate the truth of mesmerism, and to this end he bent all his energies until his death in 1868.

To present their cause favorably, Elliotson and his supporters in 1843 started a Journal entitled *The Zoist: A Journal of Cerebral Physiology and Mesmerism, and Their Applications to Human Welfare.* This magazine appeared quarterly from April 1843 to December 1855 for complete thirteen volumes. In accordance with the purpose avowed in its title, the *Zoist* presented articles on mesmerism and phrenology. Many papers were contributed by Elliotson who was a constant writer in the journal.

The purpose of the communications published in the *Zoist* was essentially propagandistic. For the most part they comprised reports on patients treated with mesmerism, testimonials and endorsements from physicians and satisfied patients, and polemics with opponents of mesmerism. In addition, the *Zoist* also concerned itself with social problems, such as housing, crime and education. Numerous medical and surgical cases observed by Elliotson and others were reported in the journal. The surgical cases are of considerable interest, for these operations were performed painlessly during mesmeric trance.

The use of mesmerism for surgical anesthesia did not originate with Elliotson. On April 12, 1829, Jules Cloquet, a French surgeon, had performed a mastectomy on a patient in mesmeric sleep. According to Elliotson the first surgical procedure performed under mesmerism in England was the insertion of a seton in the neck of Elizabeth O'Key in 1838. Four years later, a surgeon named Ward performed the first major operation in England on a patient in a mesmeric state; in 1842, in Nottinghamshire, he amputated a leg at the thigh. Before the operation, Ward consulted Elliotson "upon the possibility and safety of operating in the mesmeric state without pain. . . ." This case was reported to the Royal Medical and Chirurgical Society, but the report was received with incredulous hostility. It was asserted that the patient was an imposter who had been trained not to show pain. It was even proposed that no entry be made in the minutes of the Society of the paper having been read.

This hostile reaction aroused Elliotson to defend his associate, and in 1843 he published a pamphlet entitled *Numerous Cases of Surgical Operations Without Pain in the Mesmeric State* . . . in which he gave a full account of Ward's case, and added to it an account of Cloquet's case as well as of numerous dental extractions. At the same time, he continued to collect reports of surgical cases in which mesmerism had been employed. Another group appeared in the second volume of the *Zoist*. In this collection are reports of the use of mesmerism for venesection, dental extraction, the establishment of setons and issues, excision of tumors, amputations, and in a case of labor.

The third volume of the *Zoist* (March 1845 to January 1846) presented three further reports on surgical operations performed on patients under mesmeric anesthesia. Among these are four from America, two describing the removal of tumors from the neck, the third removal of a polyp from the nose, and the fourth amputation of a breast. The same volume also contains the first report on the work of James Esdaile (1808-1859), whose remarkable series of mesmeric operations, performed in India from 1845 to 1851, provided the most significant accomplishment in the application of mesmerism for surgical anesthesia. Up to the time of his departure from India in 1851, Esdaile performed several thousand operations on mesmerized patients; of these about three hundred were major operations, including amputations, lithotomy, removal of scrotal tumors, hydrocele and cataract. These achievements were reported by Esdaile in several publications issued while he was still in India: "Mesmeric Feats," *India Journal of Medical and Physical Science* (1845); *Mesmerism in India, and Its Practical Application in Surgery and Medicine* (1846); *A Record of Cases Treated in the Mesmeric Hospital, from November, 1846, to December, 1847, with Reports of the Official Visitors, Printed by Order of the Government* (1847).

Nevertheless, with the discovery of ether anesthesia, mesmerism and surgery came to a parting of the ways. Unable to compete with the more efficient chemical anesthetics, the use of mesmerism in surgery lost such significance as it had achieved. It may be mentioned in passing that with the revival in England of interest in hypnotism at the end of the nineteenth century, it was once again demonstrated that surgical procedures could be performed on hypnotized patients.

There are two other aspects of the English mesmeric movement that deserve attention. These are the fierce opposition that mesmerism encountered, and related to this phenomenon, the organization of mesmeric hospitals and dispensaries. In part, the origin of the opposition to mesmerism has already been described. But other factors were also involved. Among the hindrances to the progress of animal magnetism, Deleuze reckoned the exaggerations of many magnetizers, which caused even true facts to be scouted without examination. Mesmerism, like various other medical "heresies," attracted to its banner numerous intellectuals and some persons of high social standing. Among these, some were guilty of extravagances, which are not uncommon on the "lunatic fringe" of a medical sect. Furthermore, animal magnetism suffered from being mixed up with matters with which it had no necessary connection, but with whose "sins" it was saddled. A conspicuous instance of this kind was the association of mesmerism with phrenology, which was effected in England chiefly under the influence of Elliotson. Various phrenological items are scattered through the *Zoist*. For example, the first two volumes contain several phrenological articles by Herbert Spencer. In 1846, the use of phrenology in choosing members of parliament was proposed. This association of mesmerism with phrenology only intensified opposition to the former. There was considerable feeling against phrenology, mainly because it was regarded as "atheistic," belief in this doctrine being considered by many people to lead infallibly to materialism.

The exclusion of the practice of mesmerism from the regular hospitals made it necessary for the medical mesmerists to have their own institutions. The first steps to create such an institution were taken in July, 1846, but it was not until March 1850, however, that the London Mesmeric Infirmary was finally established. At about the same time a Mesmeric Institute was opened in Bristol and another at Exeter. The Bristol Institute did not last very long, for in 1852 the *Zoist* reported that it had ceased to exist. The same year, however, saw the appearance of the Dublin Mesmeric Infirmary. None of these establishments was long-lived. When the Scottish Curative Mesmeric Association was formed in 1854, Elliotson advised its supporters to "remember that similar attempts in Dublin, Bristol and Exeter have failed."

The London Mesmeric Infirmary had four paid mesmerizers, who worked from 10 A.M. to 4 P.M. daily, except Sunday, and were "allowed each, but not all at the same time, an hour in the middle of the day for dinner." The cost of treatment was apparently quite considerable—"half a guinea a week at least, and a guinea or more if much above half an hour is occupied in it or the mesmerizer lives at some distance." Because many patients were unable to pay half a guinea a week, and did not want to receive charity, a reduced price of five shillings a week was established in 1854.

The nature of the ailments treated in this and other mesmeric institutions may be seen from the following list: severe headache, loss of voice, tic douloureux, stiff knee, chronic rheumatism, inflammation of the face, erysipelas, acute rheumatism, chlorotic anemia with anasarca, hysteria with violent convulsions and delirium, deafness of seven years duration, wry neck, strumous ophthalmia with ulcers of the cornea, and St. Vitus dance.

Nor can one overlook the attempts during this period to use mesmerism therapeutically in cases of mental illness. Esquirol, in 1813 and again in 1816, in collaboration with the Abbé Faria, an early magnetizer, tried the effects of animal magnetism on eleven insane women. Only one patient responded at all, but her condition remained unchanged. Guislain another French psychiatrist of this period concluded that the results obtained with animal magnetism were unsatisfactory. Elliotson claimed to have cured periodic insanity by mesmerism. However, in 1842, Amariah Brigham, in his annual report for the Hartford Retreat, stated that "animal magnetism had been tried during the past year (1841) on five patients unavailingly." Similarly, John W. Galt, in his *Treatment of Insanity* (1846) expressed doubt as to the efficacy of mesmerism in the treatment of mental illness. Generally, American psychiatrists of this period agree that psychotic patients were accessible to suggestion only to a limited degree.

According to another American physician, J. K. Mitchell, mesmerism could be employed temporarily to relieve nervous conditions. The French psychiatrist B. A. Morel, was much more definite, citing a number of cases where hysterics had been cured by means of animal magnetism, and stating that it could be therapeutically useful in stubborn cases of hysteria.

There can be little doubt that in addition to well-delineated organic ailments, the mesmerizers treated numerous cases of neurosis. Furthermore, the dramatic results of the procedure were highly impressive, and its therapeutic intent too clear for mesmerism to be pushed aside lightly. This, indeed, is the historical significance of the English mesmeric movement. It focused attention on the treatment of certain conditions, which we now call neuroses, through the agency of an effective therapy; eventually, it helped to make mesmerism respectable by providing it with another name and explanation; and finally, it provided a bridge for the transmission of this new approach to France where the next stage in the development of medical hypnosis occurred.

While Elliotson was fighting the battle of animal magnetism with a stubborn courage that was as gallant as it was futile, there were those who accepted the reality of mesmeric phenomena, but rejected the theory of animal magnetism with its idea of a magnetic fluid. The most important of these was James Braid (1795-1860), a surgeon who was educated at Edinburgh and practiced at Manchester for most of his life. Braid became interested in mesmerism in 1841 when he attended a seance given by Lafontaine, a travelling mesmerist. Although at first Braid regarded the performance as a fraud, he later undertook to investigate the mesmeric state, and in 1843 published his conclusions in his *Neurypnology, or the Rationale of Nervous Sleep*. It is to Braid that we owe the terms hypnosis and hypnotism, which he used in place of mesmerism. Braid gave mesmerism a respectable physiological foundation, attributing the phenomena to suggestion. However, he considered suggestion only as the device used to excite the phenomena, but not as an explanation of the process underlying them.

The *Zoist* completely ignored Braid for years, and the few references to him that do occur are hostile. Elliotson contemptuously referred to hypnotism as "that coarse method practiced by Mr. Braid," yet it was the latter who made it possible for mesmeric phenomena to achieve medical respectability. Braid died in 1860, but though Elliotson outlived him by eight years, dying in 1868 at the age of 80, he never accepted the non-existence of animal magnetism as originally postulated.

The further development of mesmerism, or hypnotism, as it was now called, was connected not with England, but with France. Interest in hypnotic phenomena had persisted in France since the time of Mesmer. Some among Mesmer's followers reported new clinical facts, thus contributing to an extension of the problem. Perhaps the most important of these was Armand-Marc-Jacques Chastenet, Marquis de Puységur (1751-1825) who in 1784 discovered the state that became known as somnambulism. Puységur rejected as unnecessary Mesmer's baquet, and all the rest of his ceremonialism. While he was a fluidist, Puységur believed that the most important factor in producing the magnetic state was the magnetizer himself. As he conceived the process, the will of the magnetizer could direct the fluid to the spot where it would act, and that this could even occur at a distance. Puységur also believed that in the somnambulistic state the subject was clairvoyant.

Joseph-Philippe-François Deleuze (1753-1835), a follower of Puységur, whose *Histoire critique du magnetisme animal* (1813) is an important source for the history of animal magnetism, also maintained that mesmerism was produced by a fluid transmitted from the magnetizer to the subject, but that this fluid was directed by the will, the faith and the confidence of the magnetizer in himself.

It is interesting to note that both Puységur and Deleuze, while remaining fluidists, tended to regard the process of mesmerism less from Mesmer's mechanistic viewpoint, and to emphasize its psychological character. In contrast to modern views, however, they looked to the magnetizer, rather than to the subject as the source of the process involved.

Another approach to a psychological interpretation of animal magnetism was provided by Abbé Faria. Joseph Custodi di Faria (1756-1819), who came to Europe from Goa (Portuguese India), may rightly be regarded as a forerunner of Braid's suggestion theory of hypnosis. In 1819, there appeared his book, *De la cause du sommeil lucide ou étude sur la nature de l'homme,* containing his views. Most important of all, Faria pointed out, is the disposition of the subject; mesmerism will not be successful with a refractory subject. His influence was very slight, however, and his views were soon forgotten.

By the third decade of the nineteenth century, animal magnetism in France had in large measure been freed of Mesmer's ceremonial. Physicians continued to show interest in the subject, among them Etienne-Jean Georget (1795-1828) and Jacques-François-Alexander Bertrand (1795-1831). Bertrand began to lecture on animal magnetism in 1819. Originally a follower of Deleuze, in the course of time he began to depart more and more from the view of his teacher, and in his books, *Traité du somnambulisme* (1823), and *Du magnétisme animal en France* (1826), vigorously opposed the fluid theory of mesmerism. Bertrand occupied a middle ground between the two opposing camps of the mesmerists and the anti-mesmerists. He recognized the occurrence of mesmeric phenomena, but rejected the fluidist explanation. Instead, Bertrand expressed the conviction that these facts are the result of imagination and a firm belief on the part of the subject. Here, too, there is an intimation of the later suggestion theory of hypnosis. Precisely because of its mediating position, however, Bertrand's work made very little impression on his contemporaries. He died in 1831 at the age of thirty-six, and was soon forgotten.

Nevertheless, several other physicians who were active in the cause of mesmerism at this time did succeed in getting a hearing for their views. In August 1825, Pierre Foissac addressed to the Academy of Medicine and the Academy of Science a small pamphlet entitled *Mémoire sur le Magnétisme animal.* On October 11, 1825, he again addressed himself to the Paris Academy of Medicine and demanded that it undertake a serious examination of animal magnetism. After a good deal of discussion, the Academy appointed a commission to study the problem. Beginning in 1826, the commission studied various aspects of the problem, examined subjects presented to them by Foissac, and five years later, in 1831, presented a report written largely by Henri-Marie Husson (1772-1853). According to this report, the fact of somnambulism could not be doubted. In a certain number of cases the alleged effects of animal magnetism were not observed; in others they could be ascribed to the subject's imagination or boredom. Nevertheless, Husson concluded by urging the Academy to foster further study of animal magnetism, "one of the most remarkable branches of physiology and natural history." In view of the fact, however, that the tests carried out in the course of the investigation had not been strictly controlled, the conclusions were not too convincing, and Husson's report was simply ignored.

Nevertheless, the matter could not be disposed of so easily. At the end of 1836, Jean-Victor Oudet (1788-1868), a physician who was also a member of the Academy, painlessly extracted the tooth of a patient whom he had mesmerized. The case was discussed in a stormy session, but no agreement was reached. Shortly thereafter a magnetizer named Berna offered to give the Academy striking proof of the truth of mesmerism. In February, 1837, a new commission was appointed which concluded its investigations in June of the same year. Its conclusions as presented by Frédéric Dubois d'Amiens (1798-1873) were diametrically opposed to those of Husson. One of the points at issue was the alleged clairvoyance of subjects in a hypnotic trance. To test this claim, the physician Claude Burdin (1777-1858) offered a prize of 3000 francs to any person who within two years would actually prove that one could read without the aid of the eyes and of light. The tests were strictly controlled by a seven-man commission chosen from among the members of the Academy. Finally, in 1840, the Academy of Medicine decided not to occupy itself any further with animal magnetism.

As far as scientific circles were concerned, the matter was closed. Nevertheless, mesmerism remained alive in France during the 'forties and 'fifties chiefly through the activities of such lay mesmerists as Baron Dupotet, who had introduced Elliotson to animal magnetism. One need only consult Dureau's bibliography to realize that hypnotism was practiced and discussed (A. Dureau: *Notes Bibliographiques pour servir à l'histoire du magnétisme animal* . . . Paris, 1869, pp. 121-167).

It was not until the end of the 'fifties, however, that scientific interest in hypnosis revived. In 1859, Azam, a surgeon of Bordeaux, became acquainted with Braid's work, and began to study the subject. His attention had been attracted to hypnotism by an article on "Sleep" in Todd's *Cyclopaedia of Anatomy and Physiology*. An account of Azam's experiments appeared in 1860 in the *Archives de médecine*. About the same time, at the end of 1859, Paul Broca (1824-1880) read a paper on hypnotic surgical anesthesia before the Academy of Sciences, and A. A. Velpeau (1795-1861) presented to that body a copy of Braid's *Neurypnology*.

It is noteworthy that this reawakening of interest in hypnosis was due to a report on hypnotic anesthesia by two surgeons who treated the whole matter as if it were something radically new. As a result of these events, however, a number of physicians again began to experiment with hypnosis. Among these were Demarquay and Giraud-Teulon who treated a number of patients in a municipal hospital of Paris with hypnosis. In 1860, they published the results of their work, and expressed the opinion that hypnosis was useful not only for surgery, "but even more so for the relief of certain neuralgias." These authors felt that hypnosis should not be practiced outside the medical field.

In the same year, 1860, the man who was to influence the future development of hypnosis most significantly began to study mesmerism. This was A. A. Liébeault (1823-1904), a hardworking country doctor, who in 1864 settled at Nancy, where he practiced among the poor and applied the methods of mesmeric therapy. Two years later, in 1866, Liébeault published his results in a volume entitled *Du sommeil et des états analogues, considérés surtout au point de vue de l'action de la morale sur le physique.* He rejected the fluid-ist explanation of hypnosis and ascribed the observed hypnotic phe-nomena to psychological rather than to physical forces. According to Liébeault, hypnotic effects were produced by suggestion. The hypnotized subject, he claimed, grasps the suggestions communi-cated to him by the operator. According to Milne Bramwell, only one copy of Liébeault's book was sold when it first appeared. Nevertheless, he continued his work, and after 1882 was joined by Hippolyte Bernheim (1837-1919). For a time Bernheim was pro-fessor of medicine at Strasbourg, but after becoming interested in hypnotism he moved to Nancy.

In 1884, Bernheim published the first part of his book, *De la suggestion,* and in 1886 issued the second part entitled *La thérapeu-tique suggestive.* These publications made Liébeault's work widely known. Together, Liébeault, Bernheim and their students consti-tuted the so-called school of Nancy.

Liébeault and Bernheim were essentially therapeutically ori-ented; their interest was focused chiefly on the cure of the patient. As a result a large amount of carefully recorded clinical informa-tion was obtained. In the first four years after Bernheim began to hypnotize patients under his care, 5,000 cases were recorded; and in 75 per cent hypnosis was obtained. A few years later the number had increased to 10,000, with success in 85 per cent. Despite a com-parative lack of interest in theory, Bernheim's work was carefully watched by Beaunis, a physiologist, and Liégeois, an expert in legal medicine.

It is clear that Braid had anticipated many of the observations of the Nancy group. In fact, Braid's researches were the stimulus leading to the revival in France of interest in hypnosis. Neverthe-less, it is equally clear that Liébeault arrived independently at the view that hypnotic phenomena were purely subjective in origin, and to Liébeault we owe the development of modern hypnotism.

While Liébeault's work was still largely unknown, however, other French workers interested themselves in hypnotism. For example, in 1878, Charles Richet (1850-1935) pointed out that the phenomena of hypnotism were genuine. In the same year, Jean Martin Charcot (1825-1893) also drew attention to hypnotism. The activities of Charcot and the Salpêtrière school, as he and his associates were called, occupy a significant place in the development of hypnosis.

For some ten years the Charcot school opposed the views of the Nancy group. The issue between them was *physical action versus psychological suggestion*. Charcot, trained in neurology and thinking in terms of objective structure and physical effect, developed the following theory: The phenomena observed in hypnosis are pathological, since these are found only in people suffering from hysteria. Hypnosis could be produced by physical means, and certain hypnotic phenomena could be induced and terminated by means of magnets and metals. Hypnosis was not of much therapeutic value. Charcot was not unaware that psychological elements were involved, and he recognized autosuggestion in hysteria.

Liébeault and Bernheim criticized these views, basing their stand on the experience derived from their much larger clinical material. Bernheim put his emphasis on the nub of the problem— the need for studying the characteristics of suggestibility and the dynamics of the process of suggestion. This basic problem must be studied because suggestion is not restricted to hysterical individuals but is found in most people. Eventually, the controversy was settled in favor of the Nancy group.

Thus, by the last decades of the 19th century there was no longer any question of the reality of hypnosis. While its place in medicine might still be disputed, medical hypnosis was now a subject for research and study.

REFERENCES

1. Académie De Médecine, Paris: *Rapports et discussions de l'Académie royale de médicine sur le magnetisme animal,* recueillis par un stenographe, et publiés avec des notes explicatives par P. Foissac. Paris, 1833.

2. *Archiv für den thierischen Magnetismus,* vols. I-XII. Leipzig and Halle, 1817-1824.

3. AZAM: *Hypnotisme, double conscience et altérations de la personnalité,* préface par le prof. J. M. Charcot. Paris, 1887.

4. BERJOT, A.: *Manuel historique élémentaire et pratique de magnetisme animal.* Paris, 1858.

5. BERNOULLI, CHRISTOPH and KERN, HANS (editors): *Romantische Naturphilosophie.* Jena, 1926.

6. BERNHEIM, HIPPOLYTE: *Hypnotisme, suggestion, psychothérapie.* Études nouvelles, Paris, 1891.

7. BERSOT, ERNEST: *Mesmer et le magnétisme animal.* Paris, 1853.

8. BJORNSTROM, FRIEDRICH: *Hypnotism, Its History and Present Development.* Translated by Baron Nils Posse [Humboldt Library No. 113], New York, 1889.

9. BONNEFOY, J. B.: *Analyse raisonnée des rapports des commissaires chargés par le roi de l' examen du magnetisme animal,* [n.p.], 1784.

10. BRAID, JAMES: *Neurypnology, or, the Rationale of Nervous Sleep, considered in Relation with Animal Magnetism.* London, 1843.

11. BRAMWELL, J. MILNE: *Hypnotism, Its History, Practice and Theory.* Philadelphia, 1903.

12. BURDIN, C. and DUBOIS, FRÉDÉRIC D'AMIENS: *Histoire académique du magnétisme animal: accompagnée de notes et de rémarques critiques sur toutes les observations et expériences faites jusqu' à ce jour.* Paris, 1841.

13. CALDWELL, CHARLES: *Facts in Mesmerism, and Thoughts on its Causes and Uses.* Louisville, Ky., 1842.

14. CARUS, CARL GUSTAV: *Ueber Lebensmagnetismus und über die magischen Wirkungen uberhaupt.* Leipzig, 1857.

15. DELEUZE, J. P. F.: *Histoire critique du magnétisme animal.* Paris, 1819.

16. DEMARQUAY and GIRAUD-TEULON: *Recherches sur l'hypnotisme ou sommeil nerveux, comprenant une série d'experiences instituées à la maison municipale de santé.* Paris, 1860.

17. D'ESLON, CHARLES: *Observations sur le magnetisme animal.* London, 1780.

18. DRAKE, DANIEL: *Analytical report of a series of experiments in mesmeric somniloquism, performed by an association of gentlemen with speculations on the production of its phenomena.* Louisville, 1844.

19. DU COMMUN, JOSEPH: *Three lectures on animal magnetism, as delivered in New York, at the Hall of Science, on the 26th of July, 2d and 9th of August.* New York, 1829.

20. DURAND, JOSEPH PIERRE: *Cours theorique et pratique de Braidisme.* Paris, 1860.

21. EGAS MONIZ, ANTONIO CAETANO DE ABREU FRIERE: *O padre Faria na historia do hipnotismo* [Universidade de Lisboa. Faculdade de medicina. Primeiro centenário da fundação da (R.) Escola de cirurgia de Lisboa. 1825-1925]. Lisboa, 1925.

22. ELLIOTSON, JOHN: *Numerous Cases of Surgical Operations without Pain in the Mesmeric State.* London, 1843.

23. ELLIOTSON, JOHN: *The Harveian Oration, delivered before the Royal College of Physicians, London, June 27, 1846.* London, 1846.

24. *Entretiens sur le magnétisme animal et le sommeil magnétique dit somnambulisme, dévoilant cette double doctrine, et pouvant servir a en porter un jugement raisonné.* Paris, 1823.

25. ERMAN, WILHELM: *Der tierische Magnetismus in Preussen vor und nach den Freiheitskriegen* [Historische Zeitschrift, Beiheft IV]. Munchen, 1925.

26. ESDAILE, JAMES: *Mesmerism in India and its Practical Application in Surgery and Medicine.* London, 1846.

27. FOREL, AUGUST: *Der Hypnotismus, seine Bedentung und seine Handhabung.* Stuttgart, 1889.

28. GALDSTON, IAGO: Hypnosis and modern psychiatry. *Ciba Symposia, 9*:845-856, 1948.

29. GAUTHIER, AUBIN: *Traité pratique du magnétisme et du somnambulisme, ou résumé de tous les principes et procédés de magnétisme, avec la theorie et la definition du somnambulisme.* Paris, 1845.

30. HARTE, RICHARD: *Hypnotism and the Doctors, 2 vols.* London, 1902-1903.

31. KERNER, JUSTINUS: *Franz Anton Mesmer aus Schwaben, Entdecker des thierischen Magnetismus.* Frankfurt, 1856.

32. KIESEWETTER, CARL: *Franz Anton Mesmers Leben und Lehre. Nebst einer Vorgeschichte des Mesmerismus, Hypnotismus und Somnambulismus.* Leipzig, 1893.

33. MESMER, FRANZ ANTON: *Schreiben über die Magnetkur an einen auswärtigen Arzt.* Wien, 1775.

34. MESMER, FRANZ ANTON: *Précis historique des faits relatifs au magnétisme animal jusques en avril 1781.* London, 1781.

35. MESMER, FRANZ ANTON: *Mesmerismus oder System der Wechselwirkungen, Theorie und Anwendung des thierischen Magnetismus als die allgemeine Heilkunde zur Erhaltung des Menschen.* Berlin, 1814.

36. PODMORE, FRANK: *Mesmerism and Christian Science, A Short History of Mental Healing.* London, 1909.

37. *Rapport des commissaires chargés par le roi de l'examen du magnétisme animal* (1784), in F. M. von Grimm and D. Diderot: *Correspondance littéraire,* pt. 3, vol. 3. Paris, 1813, pp. 10-20.

38. ROSEN, GEORGE: Mesmerism and surgery. A strange chapter in the history of anesthesia. *J. Hist. Med., 1:*527-550, 1946.

39. ROSEN, GEORGE: John Elliotson, physician and hypnotist. *Bull. Hist. Med., 4:*600-603, 1936.

40. SCHÜRER-WALDHEIM, FRITZ: *Anton Mesmer, Ein Naturforscher ersten Ranges.* Vienna, 1930.

41. TISCHNER, RUDOLF: *Franz Anton Mesmer, Leben, Werk und Wirkungen* [Münchn. Beitr. z. Gesch. u. Lit. d. Naturwissenschft. u. Medizin, Heft 9-10]. Munchen, 1928.

42. TOURNIER, CLEMENT: *Le Mesmérisme à Toulouse, suivi de lettres inédites sur le XVIII siècle.* Toulouse, 1911.

2

HYPNOSIS IN INTERNAL MEDICINE
AND GENERAL PRACTICE

Bernard B. Raginsky, M.D., C.M.

The psychologic approach to medical problems has been accepted by internists only within the past two decades. In contrast, the generalist, because of his unique relationship to his patients, has always been aware of the importance of this approach. In a recent editorial in the *Journal of the American Medical Association* (24), the writer states: "It is noteworthy that at least fifty per cent of a physician's practice may involve patients with functional disorders. I would increase this percentage to include functional problems related to organic disease as well as functional problems with a recognized organic basis. In previous years, when I was concerned with specific types of metabolic disorders and problems in arthritis and rheumatism, I found that the art of medicine was as rewarding in treating the patient as was the administration of specific therapeutic agents." Hypnotic procedures have much to do with the art of medicine. Just as the patient's attitudes and emotions depend upon his constitutional make-up and experience, so the attitudes and emotions of a physician depend upon his natural endowments and cultural exposure during his formal years of education and professional experiences in the practice of medicine.

It is imperative that the physician exploit to the maximum the technical advances in medicine. This is possible without excluding a sympathetic understanding of the organic and functional problems of the afflicted. There need not be a conflict between the practice of scientific medicine and the sympathetic understanding of the patient.

At the start of World War II, the formation of the Society for the Study of Psychosomatic Problems, later to be known as the American Psychosomatic Society, brought into focus the need to re-evaluate the psychologic elements in disease entities. This group was able to demonstrate the intimate relation between emotional disturbances and physical disease. It soon became apparent that the findings could not be used easily by the average non-psychiatrist. As a result, about ten years ago the Academy of Psychosomatic Medicine was formed with the stated objective of bringing to the average physician the findings of the investigators in a form and language that he could make use of in his everyday practice of treating the "total patient." The Journals of these two Societies reflect the growing knowledge of the role that emotions play in the production and extension of disease states.

In order to use hypnosis safely and effectively for diagnosis and treatment, the physician must be well grounded in the general principles of psychosomatic medicine. We published these views in 1948 (95) and note that the findings of the Committee on Therapy of the American Psychiatric Association published in 1961 are similar (7). It is essential that the student of hypnosis be well grounded in the knowledge of psychodynamics and psychiatry if he is to make good use of this modality in medical practice. If these prerequisites are met, he will find that as he uses hypnosis in a passive and non-authoritarian way, there will be a feedback of knowledge about human behaviour not easily learned in the ordinary patient-physician relationship. In our practice we have very little use for the aggressive, authoritarian approach, either for the induction of hypnosis or in its use for therapy. This approach appears to be assaultive and while it may on occasion produce spectacular results, these results are rarely fundamental or lasting. For good results with hypnosis there should be no need to use this technique for demonstrating the physician's "power."

Kline (53) recognizes that the values and limitations of hypnosis in psychotherapy have much more to do with the values and limitations of particular psychotherapeutic approaches. The selective value of hypnosis in itself is almost completely dependent upon these factors rather than upon anything unique in hypnosis alone. We deem it proper to deal with the psychodynamics of illness at much greater length than was thought to be prudent when the first edition of this book was published in 1953. Physicians are now better trained in this field and therefore more ready to accept this essential aspect of the use of hypnosis in medical problems. Dorfman's (19) pungent description of the situation emphasizes the point well. He writes that: "In a truly comprehensive medical setting, the presystolic rumble of mitral stenosis, or the deleterious effects of a one-celled, invisible filtrable virus are not necessarily more or less important than the rumpus that can be created by a multicellular mother-in-law, who is not only visible and audible, but has infiltrated the entire household and shows suspicious signs of metastasis to the master's bedroom."

Since the selective value of hypnosis is dependent upon the psychotherapeutic approach in general, it is of interest to discuss the emotional aspects of disease in general. The central nervous system has both the function of the regulation of the internal vegetative processes of the organism and also the regulation of its external affairs, its relation to the environment. It is assumed that the complex neurophysiology of mood, instinct and intellect differs from other physiology in degree of complexity but not in quality. Whereas physiology approaches the functions of the central nervous system in terms of space and time, psychology approaches it in terms of the subjective phenomena which we call psychologic and they are the subjective reflections of the physiologic processes. The functions of the ductless glands ultimately are also subject to the functions of the highest centres of the brain, that is to say, the psychic life (74).

The fact that the mind rules over the body, no matter how much it was neglected by biology and medicine, is the most fundamental fact which we observe continuously throughout our lives. All our emotions are expressed through physiologic processes: sorrow by weeping, amusement by laughing, shame or hostility by blushing (79), fear by palpitation, anger by increased heart activity, elevation of blood pressure and a change in the carbohydrate and cholesterol metabolism, and despair by sighing. Because these processes belong to our normal life and have no ill effects if the stimuli are not prolonged or repeated too often, medicine, until recently, paid little attention to their finer investigation.

These changes in the body as reactions to acute emotions are of a passing nature. When the emotion stops, the corresponding physiologic changes also stop. The study of neurotic patients shows that under the influence of more permanent disturbances, chronic dysfunctions of the body develop. At first these chronic bodily changes were observed in hysterics. Emotionally conditioned disturbances of the internal vegetative organs which are not under voluntary control, such as the heart and the stomach, have also been observed. In such cases the anatomic structure of the organ is unchanged, only the co-ordination and the intensity of the organ function are disturbed. They are reversible. Since these functional disturbances are caused by emotional factors, psychotherapy has gained a legitimate entrance into medicine proper and can no longer be restricted to the field of psychiatry. Indeed, the modern psychiatrist is becoming more interested in medical problems as a whole.

Psychogenic factors in disease represent the production of physical symptoms by the powerful biologic urges which motivate our lives: fear, hate, love and the forces which drive men and women to heights of accomplishment and heroism but unfortunately also to the depths of despair, to neurosis or psychosis, to murder or to suicide. It is the latter group the physician has to deal with. These motivations can best be understood by studying their manifestations in thought, phantasy, dreams and behaviour. Under certain conditions, particularly the intensification of these drives without adequate expression, they can affect the physiology sufficiently to produce symptoms in the psychologic, the muscular or the vegetative spheres. Using hypnosis, Yekimi and his collaborators (48) were able to show the influence of the emotions on the physiologic functions of the digestive system. In experimentally designed situations, they demonstrated the role of hyperventilation in the production of psychoneurotic symptoms in the digestive tract and showed how important a role the emotions play in stimulating infections of the digestive system.

More and more clinicians are beginning to understand that the functional disorders of long duration may lead slowly to genuine organic disorders based on visible organic changes. Thus, the hyperactivity of the heart due to long-standing emotional turmoil may lead to hypertrophy of the heart muscle. Hysterical paralysis of a limb may lead to certain degenerative changes in the muscles due to inactivity. Certain types of arthritis follow periods of emotional strain and are relieved when the pressure subsides. In all these cases the pathologic-anatomic changes are secondary results of a disturbed function and the disturbed function itself is a result of chronic emotional conflict. Thus we have pathologic function as a cause of pathologic structure. If hypnotherapy is to be effective instead of producing transitory results simulating a "cure," the causes of the disturbance must be dealt with. Combinations of therapeutic modalities flexibly employed as indicated by the total clinical condition is necessary and dependence upon hypnosis alone is to be avoided in most cases.

The increasing knowledge of the relations of the emotions to normal and disturbed function requires that for the modern physician, emotional conflicts should become just as real and tangible issues as visible micro-organisms. Menninger (66) emphasizes this point more dramatically by saying that this knowledge will bring an awareness of man's daily struggles as having as much or more to do with the way he may feel than bacteria or bullets. This psychologic approach to the problems of life and disease brings the internal body processes into a synthetic unit with the individual's external relations to the social environment. It gives a scientific basis to such empirical everyday observations as that a patient often shows remarkable recovery if he is removed from his family environment (93), or if he interrupts his everyday occupation and is relieved from those emotional conflicts which arise from family life or professional activity. The detailed knowledge of the relation of emotional life and body processes extends the function of the physician. Hypnosis gives much valuable aid in evaluating these elements and also in reorganizing them.

It is well for the physician to be aware of the fact that depression is one of the commonest conditions met with which produces physical symptoms requiring medical aid. Depression in its milder transient form as seen in most people from time to time, is a mood which cannot be called abnormal or morbid. It is more appropriately termed sadness or dejection. It is used in this chapter as a psychiatric disorder where the saddened mood is the fundamental and important pathologic change. In a physiologic context, depression implies a decrease in function. In the psychiatric sense it implies an increase in certain autonomic and other activities. It is a response of the human organism usually characterized by sadness and despair, but in which a physical symptom or symptoms may be the only indication of the unexpressed depressive affect. Depression becomes the concern of the physician when it is pathological and manifests either physical or psychic changes, or both combined. Some victims only exhibit complaints which are predominantly physical and are accompanied by anxiety. They may be regarded as "masked depressions" or "depressive equivalents." They may complain of anorexia, abdominal discomfort, weight loss or constipation.

Working in a general hospital without a psychiatric ward, Sloane (90) found that out of one hundred case reports of adults referred to him, 61 per cent were found to be suffering from depression. Two-thirds of these were primary depressions and 75 per cent of these had primary somatic symptoms which were usually aches and pains. He found that there was frequently a persistent hypochondriacal preoccupation and anxious self-scrutiny with the fixed belief of severe heart, intestinal or lung disease. The secondary depressions were most commonly found after operations or severe illnesses such as coronary occlusion, encephalitis and arthritis. The next largest group was found to be that of anxiety phobic hysterical conditions. Hysterical is used to imply somatic conversion embracing a variety of predominantly painful conditions such as backache, headache, urinary and menstrual symptoms, abdominal pain, convulsions and vertigo. These are usually associated with long-standing character disturbances as will be demonstrated in the cases treated under hypnosis and reported later in this chapter.

It would seem important for the physician to understand depression and its manifestations. The newer drugs may help but do not clear up the underlying problem. The high incidence of presenting physical symptoms leads doctors to suspect organic disease and accounts for the high percentage of negative findings in diagnostic laboratory tests. The number of negative findings in the radiology and other laboratories are higher than they should be and certainly would be less if the emotional elements of the presenting symptoms were evaluated correctly at the clinical level. One should be on the lookout for evidence of guilt, exhaustion, loss of interest, failure to concentrate and inability to cope. These may give a clue to the diagnosis which can then be explored further on the hypnotic level both for diagnosis and therapy.

General fatigue is the predominating complaint of the patient with a psychogenic asthenic reaction. It may be associated with visceral complaints but it may also include mixed visceral organ symptoms and complaints. Present weakness and fatigue may indicate a physiologic neuro-endocrine residue of previous anxiety and not necessarily an active psychologic conflict. Man, feeling threatened, may use for long-term purposes, devices designed for short-term needs. Costly protective activities are essential and life-saving. They are devised for fleeting emergencies so that they may destroy those forces that threaten his survival. But they are not designed to be used as life-long patterns. When so utilized they may damage structures they were devised to protect (120). To prevent these disorders, more knowledge concerning the origin of these patterns in childhood is necessary. To interrupt them once they have become well established requires a vigorous and fresh approach to methods and means. To deal with these disturbances it is necessary to study the functions of organs widely separated in the body. Because the methods require cutting across the lines which usually separate the various medical skills, the horizon of the physician must be broadened (120). It is for these reasons that physicians in all specialties have become more interested in psychodynamics and psychiatry.

Hypnosis may be used here to delve into the earlier patterns of the individual and to give him some insight into his behaviour and help him work through some of his conflicts. Post-hypnotic suggestion may be given to help him use this newly acquired insight. The general improvement and the better understanding of the causes of his behaviour combine to give him greater freedom of choice in meeting frustrating situations. He may learn that it is not necessary for him to develop dyspnea neurosis when the emotional load he is carrying becomes too heavy. He is taught to use more rewarding methods in handling his emotional problems.

He may find that he need not become exhausted when things are not going the way he wants them to go.

A middle aged male who became easily exhausted when he had to shovel snow in front of his garage but who was able to portage for miles in the woods carrying heavy fishing gear with a sense of power instead of exhaustion, was found to have marked hostility to his wife. With the help of hypnosis he was found to be sexually impotent with his wife but not with other women. After shovelling some snow he would have to lie down in a cold sweat with the implication that he was on the verge of a heart attack. On further investigation it was determined that he also found much simpler tasks, such as hanging pictures on the wall for his spouse, more than he could do. These dynamics suggest the direction of treatment as compared to the organic approach with its repeated electrocardiograms, investigations and attempting to reassure both the wife and husband that all was well physically. We have reported another such case of extreme exhaustion in which the dynamics were revealed under hypnosis and suitable treatment instituted (105).

Those who have used hypnosis in the treatment of this psychogenic asthenic reaction know how productive it can be. Since results obtained in this particular field do not lend themselves to easy and simple reporting in the literature, the frequency of satisfactory results obtained should not be underestimated. As medical men learn to use this approach with due regard to the fundamental issues involved, much may be expected from it.

The mere removal of a symptom through the use of the authoritative hypnotic command is fraught with some danger. The hypnotic suppression of symptoms can result in the appearance of substitute symptoms of equivalent psychological value. In this way nothing helpful is accomplished for the patient except for a redistribution of the stress focus and possible proof that the symptoms were of emotional origin. Meldman (63) reported a psychotic episode resulting from hypnotic suppression of a symptom. Without trying to find the cause of an airplane phobia, a colleague removed it under hypnosis. The patient was then able to take a plane trip, though he did suffer from a mild generalized anxiety prior to and during the trip. When the trip was over he suffered from a profound decompensation of the entire organization of his personality, developing multiple physical and psychologic symptoms. These were so severe that it was found necessary to hospitalize him. It would seem that in taking the airplane trip he had violated a taboo and he thought of his subsequent difficulties as punishment for wrong doing.

The use of suppressive hypnotherapy as compared to supportive hypnotherapy in managing a patient's problems may not take into consideration its significance for him. Some of the symptoms met with may be more than just a conditioned response. There may be other unconscious or internal reasons. For example, two patients presenting almost identical symptoms tangential to their main complaint, were found to require diametrically opposite dynamics for their treatment. Both complained that they could not touch or wash dirty dishes, remove garbage or handle soiled clothing. Using hypnoplasty (107), it was found during a single interview that one patient equated dirt and decaying food with stool and found it distasteful. It also explained why he was a finicky eater, avoiding all ripe fruit, smelly cheeses, mustard and sausages. The other patient equated her symptoms in the hypnoplastic interview with the *secret love* of stool. Since this was a secret, unconscious love, she would not remove the soiled dishes, clothes and garbage until forced to by her husband or others. She took secret pleasure in having it around her as long as possible as treasured objects.

The first patient was allowed to handle brown plasticine under hypnosis until he lost his aversion to it and until he came to his underlying love of stool. During spontaneous hypnotic regression he began to "love" his stool. Within two weeks time he had lost the secondary symptoms which were only incidental to his major problem. The second patient was allowed to "enjoy" the brown plasticine which she equated with stool and within a comparatively short period of time did not need to treasure soiled objects. Her secret love was secret no longer. In both these patients the removal of what appeared to be minor complaints resulted in better family functioning and improved interpersonal relationships.

It appears to be self-evident that it is safest for the hypnotherapist to use an etiologically oriented therapy. It is taken for granted too that not all physicians are trained in this particular area. The pressure of doing a comprehensive medical evaluation in as short a time as possible with sufficient emphasis on the medical and psychiatric aspects of the illness has led Winn (116) to formulate a practical way for the clinician to measure the degree of neurosis, its influence on the illness and the possible need for psychiatric referral. If the physician plans to use hypnosis for differential diagnosis or therapy, he should find out:

1. *What the Disease Means to the Patient:* All patients have some anxiety about their discomforts. One must determine if the anxiety is related normally to the presenting symptoms or if it is out of all proportion to the discomfort. The patient's phantasies about the meaning of the symptom are often determined by his personality structure and life's experiences. For example, if the patient's friends or relatives suffered from gastric haemorrhage or coronary occlusion, any sign of hyperacidity, dyspepsia, extrasystoles or tachycardia in himself may throw him into a panic. He may condense his thinking and see only the tragic end results as observed in some of his friends or relatives. If the meaning of the complaint cannot be made out in an ordinary interview, it often helps to clarify it at the hypnotic level. Under these conditions it may be possible to bring to consciousness forgotten memories and associations related to the condition and as a result help relieve the associated anxiety.

2. *How the Patient Uses His Symptoms, Even a Specific Abnormality, in the Service of His Neurosis:* Would the patient's life pattern return to normal if the symptoms of the disease were removed or do the symptoms help him avoid facing situations too difficult for him? In an emotionally healthy person, the illness does not markedly change his way of life or thinking. In a neurotic whose symptoms serve a defensive need, the removal of symptoms would increase anxiety or produce other symptoms to replace the one which was "cured." Using hypnosis it may be possible to determine the value of the symptom to the patient.

3. *How the Patient Responds to the Treatment Situation:*
Does he communicate well? Is he able to listen to the physician?
Does he co-operate with him? If any or all of these questions are
answered in the negative, we may be certain that the illness has a
high emotional content for the patient. The physician must decide
at this point whether he is capable of handling the emotional elements of the illness or whether it is better to refer the patient to
a psychiatrist. If the physician decides that he is capable of handling the problem he may use hypnosis to get under the patient's
defenses. In this hypnotic relationship with the therapist the patient gives up a degree of control over what determines reality for
him. In this new situation, reality is being filtered through the
ego of the doctor. He may now permit reality to assume any range
of dimension that the doctor can organize. As such, the patient is
attached to him in a retrogressive relationship. Thus the nature
of reality to be experienced by the patient is determined to a large
extent by what he does and at times by what he does not do. While
such changes in reality situation may be produced by certain drugs,
the similarities to hypnotic effects are only superficial and are far
removed from the benefits observed through hypnosis (52).

With these three rules in mind, one can see how hypnosis may
be used in doubtful cases to separate functional from true organic
states or to determine the degree and extent of the functional
overlay in an organic disease. It may be used to suppress symptoms
temporarily in order to observe where and how the energy is discharged. The patient may be made to visualize all sorts of situations or relationships in order for the physician to see how he reacts
emotionally and physiologically to these experimentally induced
situations.

The ways in which hypnosis may be used in the practice of
medicine depends upon the ability, imagination and the resourcefulness of the physician. For example, hypnosis may be used to
improve motivation. It is not uncommon for some patients to
reach a plateau in their convalescence far removed from the level
normally expected. In such cases one or two hypnotic interviews
may change the course of events and increase the rate of improvement. This method may be used when the patient appears to "dry
up," does not communicate or appears to lose interest in himself

and others. Of course, hypnosis is not the only method open to the physician in such situations. It is well known that improvement obtained by this means can be attained also at times by changing doctors or even by changing medicines from one innocuous drug to another innocuous drug. However, it would seem that with hypnosis one can get closer to the cause of the arrested improvement than by other means.

In the rehabilitation of patients who have used organic illness for secondary gain, hypnosis may be used with caution. This type of secondary gain is seen occasionally in patients who make unexplained poor or slow recovery after an illness or operation. The orthopedist is familiar with the patient who hates to give up his cast, his crutches or his insurance benefits. This type is easily diagnosed. There are other cases where the mechanism involved is not seen as easily but where free association in the hypnotic state may point out the cause. Muscular paralysis and speech difficulties following cerebral accidents have been helped with hypnosis used in such a way as to help the patient to reorganize his body image and to motivate him to get well to take his place once again in society (88).

Rehabilitation has a wider connotation than is usually recognized. It includes not only the restoration and extension of the physical and psychological capacities of the patient who has suffered the loss of function through trauma of various sorts, but also the habilitation problem itself (121). As Wright (122) states in his well documented paper, "Hypnosis, as a psychological investigatory and clinical tool, is of importance to rehabilitation because of its potentials for initiating and facilitating various kinds of psychological change." He believes that psychotherapy under hypnosis can often be used with much better therapeutic effectiveness because of: (a) the heightened intensity of the interpersonal relationship between the patient and physician; (b) the greater readiness on the part of the patient to utilize the therapeutic offerings; and (c) the characteristics of the hypnotic experience which may enhance the patient's feelings of control and accomplishment.

The following case is described in some detail to demonstrate how flexibly hypnosis can be used within the framework of total therapy over a prolonged period of time. It is a report on the habilitation of a youth of seventeen. Habilitation implies helping patients who, because of heredity, congenital or early traumatic events, never had the opportunity to acquire certain skills and functions. This case has been chosen because the early trauma is clear cut and his subsequent inability to handle life in any area is easily demonstrable and also because he showed the many somatic symptoms so commonly observed in an inadequate personality make-up.

The patient was born in Europe at the start of World War II and within a short time he and his family were placed in a German Concentration Camp for the duration. They were never separated from each other during that time but were exposed to all the rigors of such a Camp. Following release from this Camp at the end of the war, he could not adjust physically or emotionally to any children, any school, nor even to his parents and sister who was two years older than he. Many schools were tried but after a short period of time he would have to drop out because of various physical illnesses and inability to learn. This occurred many times and in many places. The parents were kind and intelligent. They consulted various physicians in many cities but the patient continued to deteriorate.

A tonsillectomy did not help his persistent sore throat, the newer drugs did not stop his tantrums, his depression or his exhaustion. Four months in Switzerland did not help him in any way. On his return, he was still emaciated, pale and weak. Because of tenderness over his spleen he was referred to us for investigation and treatment. His complaints on his first visit were: 1) Pain and tenderness over the splenic area for several months. 2) Physical weakness as long as he could remember. 3) Inability to concentrate (very marked). 4)Constant sore throat. 5) Severe headaches since childhood. 6) Pain in both feet for years with no relief from corrective shoes or supports. 7) Lack of appetite and fullness after eating even small quantities of food since infancy.

When first examined he was found to be emaciated. His extreme pallor was not the result of anaemia since his haemogram was normal. His liver and spleen were palpable and tender. The musculature was flaccid. He had difficulty in keeping his arms raised over his head for more than half a minute at a time due to weakness. He found it difficult to hold a pencil for writing for the same reason.

His inability to communicate verbally was so marked that it was impossible to carry out the usual psychological tests. For example, when asked to solve an arithmetic problem set for the age of nine, he could not solve it but went into panic instead. Similar results were obtained when he was asked to place a few coloured blocks in sequence. All forms of testing were given up for the time being. We had to rely on his previous record of accomplishment. In a private school in England which he attended from the age of thirteen to fifteen, his scholastic average was thirty per cent. He was excused from all sports and gym work which were a prerequisite for all other pupils. In view of all these observations and negative physical findings except as reported above, the following working diagnosis was made: 1) Generalized stress disease. 2) Negative transference to all people including his family.

Our impression was that he did not suffer from a congenital condition but that his symptoms were basically due to his poor start in life. The goals of treatment were to provide him with a much more sheltered environment, a re-education of his parents as to how to handle the situation, and to start his scholastic training as if he were in the first grade of the elementary school even though he was seventeen years old at the time.

We assumed the role of a very benign foster parent and protector from all forms of pressure. For many months in this setting he spoke no more than four or five sentences during an interview. He was then gently and almost imperceptibly conditioned to hypnosis at irregular times to avoid excessive regression and dependency. In the hypnotic interviews he was trained to verbalize instead of having headaches, aches and pains and weakness. After many months, he volunteered in the waking state that in the past he had brought on his headaches purposefully in order to gain sympathy, attention and to avoid meeting his problems of living. From this point on he soon began to understand that he had been misusing his body in an attempt to withdraw from the world in order to remain a dependent infant.

Since at this point he did not have a single friend and his world was limited to his home and our office, he was enrolled as a private pupil in a business college to learn typing and shorthand for one or two hours daily. This sheltered arrangement worked fairly well in that he obtained marks ranging from 90 per cent to 100 per cent in his weekly tests, an accomplishment he had never experienced before. In a few months, however, the work became more complicated and his symptoms returned. As a result, this aspect of his re-education was terminated and he was given the confidence that he would not be pressured when he found himself to be in an untenable position.

By this time the use of hypnosis was out in the open and at the hypnotic level it was found possible to determine the limits of his current abilities. Under hypnosis he was able to accept the idea of having a tutor to help him start the studies for his eventual admission to the University. This seemed somewhat unrealistic at the time and matriculation extremely distant, but the idea appealed to him as a sort of phantasy of accomplishment. A very able, understanding, patient and capable tutor was found for him. After a very slow and painful start, he accepted his role as a student with very gradual decreasing evidence of tantrums, headaches, sore throats, weak spells and withdrawal.

After eighteen months and many hypnotic sessions he was able to take half of the prescribed matriculation examinations at the University. This was his very first experience at taking examinations in a non-sheltered climate. The results were encouraging for him. He passed the five subjects with an average grade of 75 per cent with a top percentage of ninety in trigonometry. Making use of his improved status he was guided into doing photography, taking dancing lessons, public speaking classes and a rapid reading course, all with the purpose of helping him to communicate with his peer group. At the same time he learned to drive a car and was able to take a trip to Washington, D. C., by himself.

During the bleak periods of struggling, he was helped to collect rare books, which gave him considerable pleasure and excursions not only in the local book stores but also in the auction rooms of rare book dealers in other cities. He developed a deep interest in the subject and this brought him into contact with serious book lovers who, as a group, are passive and permissive. He began to identify himself with his excellent collection of books. His pride in them stimulated him to invite a few people to his home to see them. This was his very first experience of being a host and it became the focal point for further adventures in living.

At the present writing he is about to take the last half of his matriculation examinations with a good chance of passing them well. He has gained twenty-two pounds, is able to eat in restaurants and elsewhere, rarely has headaches and feels considerably stronger. There has also been a psychosexual growth. He attends sorority dances, pairs off in courtship behaviour and is found to be an interesting friend by members of both sexes.

Although still under "treatment" for guidance and support, he has lost all the symptoms for which he came. The liver and spleen are normal, his colour, appetite and strength have improved. This is a case of *habilitation* where treatment had to be very flexible and groping. There were many setbacks and periods of discouragement both for the patient and the therapist. Hypnosis was used here in many ways and for various objectives. At first it was used to get closer to the patient emotionally. Later it was used to relax him and to improve interpersonal relationships. It was used analytically to determine why he could not touch any soiled dishes, even his own. He equated them unknowingly with stool. Hypnoanalysis revealed the cause of his restlessness at meal time. He could not relax until the dishes in front of him were removed because of the fact that since the days of the Concentration Camp he was trained by his father to finish everything on his plate. He had not realized on a conscious level that he felt guilty, tense, restless and irritable if there was the smallest trace of food left on his plate. At the start of treatment this state of affairs made him try to avoid eating altogether.

He was made to abreact to many traumatic situations which occurred early in his life and during his stay at the boarding school in England when he was completely unable to express or defend himself. These hypnotically induced abreactions were considered to be a type of conditioned response and as such should follow the general rules which apply to conditioning and extinction (55). He was made to abreact many times over a period of a year to the same traumatic incidents in his earlier life until he found that his anxieties and phobias to the old, as well as to new situations which resembled the older ones, disappeared. For example, it was found that the mere mention of the fact that he would have to study Shakespeare and Dickens as part of his matriculation requirements, would throw him into a panic and depression. Under hypnosis it was determined that these subjects had been taught him in England when he was at the breaking point, by severe, demanding and occasionally disturbed teachers. He was determined that he would rather die than go through it again. His frequent hypnotically induced abreactions allowed him to reach the point where he is enjoying these subjects.

Posthypnotic suggestion was used to help him talk before the public speaking class. It worked well enough for him to win the first prize in a group of thirty adults. All these small victories helped to strengthen his ego, making him less afraid of people as he became better able to defend himself. It would seem that in the field of *habilitation* every known technique used in hypnotic therapy can be used to advantage. Not described in reporting this case because of lack of space was the use of the intensification of emotions during his "barren" period, positive and negative hallucinations to overcome current difficulties and suggestions leading to dissociation when such a state was thought to be helpful. At the present time of treatment, hypnosis is used only very occasionally in this patient. Gentle guidance, support, understanding and protection are all that seem necessary at the moment.

In a broad sense, the anxiety involved in so-called psychosomatic diseases is relieved by channeling the original impulses through the autonomic nervous system into visceral organ symptoms and complaints. These reactions represent the visceral expression of anxiety which is thereby prevented from becoming conscious. The symptoms are due to a chronic and exaggerated state of the normal physiology of the emotion with the feeling or subjective part repressed (33). Gorton's (35) review of the physiologic aspects of hypnosis and the excellent and comprehensive review since 1948 by Crasilneck and Hall (15) help the student to understand the mechanisms involved. Since the gastrointestinal system is most sensitive to changes in the emotional state a brief discussion of the topic follows.

The scientific literature on digestive malfunction and its relationship to emotions has been covered by the exhaustive works of Dunbar (21), Wolf and Wolff (118) and Alexander (2). Mittle- mann and Wolff (72) have described the peptic ulcer conflict as developing from an unconcious longing for a dependent relation- ship and a reactive striving for assertive independence. These patients have a passive-receptive fundamental personality structure (110). Hypnotherapy can be effective in selected cases of psycho- genic gastrointestinal reactions typified by peptic ulcers, chronic gastritis, constipation, pylorospasm, "irritable colon" and anorexia nervosa (26, 25). We use hypnosis in these cases either as a method of choice or the method which produces results more quickly or because no other method seems to work.

The writer has described in some detail the use of hypnosis in the treatment of a patient suffering from a post-gastrectomy syndrome which had not responded to medical treatment usually used for this condition (105). The reason for this lack of response to routine medical therapy became evident when, under hypnosis, it was found to be related to the patient's sexual impotence with his wife and the guilt feelings resulting from his extra-marital rela- tionships. His symptoms disappeared when his problems were worked out with him and his wife. A recent communication from him many years after therapy indicated that all is well.

Because emotions play such an important role in the produc- tion of peptic ulcers it is not surprising that, following subtotal gastrectomy, some of the patients develop the "dumping syn- drome." This consists of symptoms of anorexia, nausea, vomiting, vertigo, sweating, cardiac palpitation, fatigue and loss of weight. Some of these symptoms may disappear in a few months after operation, but they may become chronic and require intensive treatment. Since these symptoms are linked with anxiety and neuroticism, Dorcus and Goodwin (17) were able to clear up this condition in their series of patients through hypnotherapy.

In a series of eighteen cases of intractable hiccoughs where medical therapy was unsuccessful, Dorcus and Kirkner (18) were able to stop the hiccoughs in fourteen of the patients by producing muscular relaxation through hypnosis and by relieving them of the anxiety concerning the spasms and the physical disorder asso- ciated with it.

Unless the physician is particularly well trained in psycho-dynamics it would seem prudent not to undertake the hypnotic treatment of some of the gastrointestinal disorders such as peptic ulcers and the "irritable colon." Those who are well trained, report good results in selected cases. Moody (73) evaluated the effect of hypnotic versus conventional therapy on two well matched groups of duodenal ulcer patients. The group treated by hypnotherapy alone showed greater clinical improvement. It does not seem to us that it is too difficult to ameliorate peptic ulcer symptoms in the average patient with hypnosis by providing a more protective and relaxing programme for him. But to treat the condition in depth, to produce a "cure," is altogether another matter.

In a number of peptic ulcer patients we have treated with hypnosis, it was found that the symptoms subsided rather quickly, but in the process one could observe deep behavioural and character abnormalities that one would have to contend with for final resolution of the problem. For example, a patient under hypnotherapy whose x-rays showed complete healing of the ulcer, started to drink heavily. As a result, he accumulated many domestic, professional and financial problems which all ended up in the recurrence of the ulcer. A prolonged treatment of his basic problems aided by hypnosis resulted in a more permanent improvement, not only in the ulcer but in his total personality as well. This sequence of events following superficial therapy for peptic ulcers occurs frequently enough to make us treat any patient with gastrointestinal complaints as a major problem.

This is true especially in cases of non-specific ulcerative colitis. The onset or recurrence of the disease is preceded usually by an emotional trauma which produces an internal conflict associated with acute love loss combined with humiliation. This makes these patients feel their inferiority as men or women (40, 5, 115, 56, 77). Such patients may be helped occasionally through hypnotherapy, but a word of caution is necessary here since some of these patients border on the fringe of psychosis. Cases are on record to show that in some instances where the symptoms were removed (suppressed), the patient later developed a psychotic reaction, which in turn disappeared when the bowel symptoms returned.

More amenable to hypnotherapy is the syndrome of anorexia

nervosa. Nearly all the investigators interested in this subject emphasize the factor of the child-parent relationship, especially the mother-child relationship, as the most important factor in the disease. Ferenczi's view of the hypnotic relationship as a reactivation of the oedipus complex and his description of the "maternal" and "paternal" forms of hypnotic induction is of interest here (30). The promise of success in treatment increases when a combined hormonal and psychiatric approach is used. The general overall clinical improvement produced by the steroids, greatly facilitates psychiatric management. The following case report antedates the use of steroids.

The patient, a sixteen year old boy, was being discharged from a general hospital as incurable after a stay of several months for the treatment of anorexia nervosa. His weight was down to seventy-eight pounds, and his father, a physician, was desperate. He was seen for the first time the day he was discharged from the hospital. While the appearance of the patient was shocking enough, the family constellation in which he was seen was even more of a shock. The mother, a former head operating room nurse in a large hospital, was cold, rigid, and against the idea of using hypnosis to help her son. She was cold and harsh to her husband who had asked for this consultation without her knowledge—a rare occurence in that household. It soon became obvious too that an older son, the only other sibling, was her favourite.

This was the climate of the first interview. It seemed urgent to accomplish something at once, not only for the patient but also for the whole family if a second interview was to be possible. Discussion of the aims and technique of hypnosis was aimed primarily at the mother with the objective of draining off some of her hostility. It was directed also to reassure the patient that he would not have to contend with her anger nor to feel guilty for being the cause of an argument between his parents. Permission to treat her son was finally obtained from the mother.

An acceptable hypnotic state was induced and non-specific suggestions for relaxation, comfort and hope were given. After forty-five minutes in this state, he appeared to be more cheerful and the drooling from the side of the mouth stopped. An encouraging report was given to the family and their favourable response to the new situation was relayed to the patient. At this point he volunteered the suggestion that he would try to eat something "if his mother would prepare it for him." This was done, and the patient finished a very modest portion of the food placed before him. We stayed on with him for another hour to make certain that he would not bring up what he had eaten at this first session.

He was seen again eight times in a period of two months. Supportive suggestions were given under deeper stages of hypnosis, though it did not seem that the depth of hypnosis helped to make the suggestions more acceptable. Post-hypnotic suggestions of the same order were given during the last four visits. No probing of relationships were carried out. The patient did volunteer material relating to earlier episodes in his life which were meaningful to him but no effort was made to interpret or synthesize them for him. At the end of two months he was doing quite well. He was able to go for walks and to eat in a friend's home.

As the danger of dying diminished, the mother's fear and resentment of the use of hypnosis became more marked. The discord between husband and wife appeared to be increasing. In view of this we informed the family that it was unnecessary to see the patient again. If treatment would be necessary in the future it could be handled by their regular physician. This decision was received quite cheerfully by the mother, though some ambivalence about it was noticeable. He was not seen again until he introduced himself to us eighteen years later following a lecture given to a medical specialty group of which he was a member. There was no opportunity to discuss his subsequent history except to note that he had reached the status of specialist, while his father was a generalist. A random remark made by his mother at the time of treatment that general practitioners were not appreciated became more meaningful to us in this setting. It would have been interesting to learn if he was married and if he was, was his wife a nurse!

After taking a careful history, it is wise at times to refuse to use hypnotic symptom removal or suppression, even if pressed to do so by the patient. In some instances it is better to advise the patient to live with his relatively mild symptom or inconvenience, or to seek out an etiologically oriented therapy rather than the quick treatment the patient usually asks for. From time to time we are consulted by some of our colleagues because of their "second hypnotic session failures." It would seem that these physicians were able to remove the presenting symptom hypnotically during the first interview but could not understand the patient's resentment, hostility and unco-operativeness on the second visit, in spite of the absence of the symptom. Most commonly this is due to the fact that the patient was not quite ready to have the symptom removed—nor removed so easily.

Symptom removal or suppression is carried out successfully often enough to know that it works well in selected cases. When symptom removal is carried out through chemotherapy, untoward results may be laid to the "side effects" of the drug (101, 103). Untoward results following hypnotic symptom removal should not be regarded as side effects. In an experimental situation, Seitz (86) showed that suppression of symptoms can result in the appearance of substitute symptoms of equivalent psychological value. The newer symptoms were found to occur either at the same level of psychosexual development (arm paralysis substituting for torticollis) or at a more regressive level (vomiting, gagging and upset stomach substituting for arm paralysis). The new symptom could be shown to have an equivalent value in the patient's value system (an ugly facial rash substituting for obesity as a means for the patient to "show off" in an unattractive way). Thus, nothing helpful is accomplished for the patient except for a redistribution of the stress focus and possible proof that the symptoms were of emotional origin.

Some symptoms disappear while the patient is under hypnosis without any direct suggestion having been made for its removal. When the patient awakes, the symptom returns. This should indicate to the patient, even without verbal communication, that the symptom complained of is emotionally determined and appears to be lost in the hypnotic state. The severity of the symptom to be removed has less to do with a successful result than the duration of it. Severe symptoms but of short duration have a better chance of removal under hypnosis than those of a milder nature but of long duration. It is important for the clinician to grade his therapeutic suggestions, starting with the most simple ones in order to see how they are being accepted by the patient. It is unwise to proceed further if these simple therapeutic hypnotic suggestions meet with resistance. If the simple ones are well received he can then proceed with more difficult ones.

Following a successful interview of this kind, there may be a generalized feeling of well being which allows the patient to work better and to have a better relationship with those about him. This type of feed-back may allow self-healing to take place without too much "interference" by the physician. The patient is allowed to improve at his own pace. In any event, theoretically at least, an attempt should be made to resolve the underlying conflict if that is possible. It is unwise to give post-hypnotic suggestions unless one is certain that the patient will be able to carry them out completely. If the post-hypnotic suggestion is not carried out as suggested, there is usually a resulting anxiety, restlessness, tension and somatic symptoms usually referable to the gastrointestinal or cardiovascular systems.

All suggestions, whether post-hypnotic or not, should have a clear meaning for the patient and be acceptable to him. This implies that the physician knows the patient well and is sensitive to his needs. If he has had considerable experience with hypnotherapy or has had the patient under observation for some time, it may be possible to put suggestions to him which allow him a choice. In this instance the choice the patient takes gives the therapist a clue to the dynamics and the course he should take from that point on to the next step of treatment. It should be clear, however, that when one uses suggestive therapy, his chances of success are less if there is an active psychological conflict going on. As Meares states, (62) this is so because in the face of an active psychological conflict the removed symptom which is the expression of the conflict will tend to recur or result in the formation of a substitutive symptom, and in any event one can anticipate subjective anxiety in the patient.

Most physicians using hypnosis have had the occasional patient who appears to be too frightened to take a hypodermic injection and asks to have it done under hypnosis. Usually this request is granted without a second thought and almost always it works out well. One must be on the watchout for the occasional patient who makes this request for ulterior motives. The following case report may serve as an example.

A new patient expressed her great fear of any type of injection and requested that a series be done under hypnosis. She was about to take a cruise with her husband and another couple and the inocculations were required for immigration purposes. Brief questioning on the subject revealed the fact that she had had many injections at various times in her life without apprehension or ill effects afterwards. Further gentle questioning exposed the real reason for her fear of this particular series of injections. It was simply that she was afraid to go on this particular trip as she was in love with the husband of the couple they were to travel with. She had tried to dissuade her husband from taking the trip but could give no reason acceptable to him. As a final desperate measure for self-protection, she was determined to avoid taking the injections and in this way avoid meeting immigration requirements. She readily admitted that she would have resisted any attempt to hypnotize her. One week prior to this visit she had asked her own physician for the inocculations. As soon as he had removed the syringe and needle from the sterilizer she went into a hysterical faint. Her physician wisely did not go through with the injections. By asking for hypnosis as a last resort, she felt that it would convince her husband to abandon the trip. An interview with her husband was arranged and he was told that it would be most unwise for his wife to take the trip. It was not possible to tell him the whole story, but he accepted the decision. The final outcome of the basic problem remains a mystery as the patient was not seen again.

Since pain is one of the most common complaints the physician has to deal with, it is important for him to assess it psychiatrically if he intends to relieve it under hypnosis (94, 96-98). It is well known that there are two elements to the pain which brings the patient to the doctor. One is the pain sensation itself. The other is the distress arising from the pain and its significance to him. It is common to hear a patient say that he could stand the pain in the chest if it were only located somewhere else—in the foot, for instance. Some types of pain, epigastric for example, are often accompanied by the distress resulting from depression associated with this type of pain. Hypnotic suggestions should be directed at relieving the distress. When this is done, the pain itself seems more bearable. If it is found that the pain is functional in origin, an attempt should be made to help the patient develop some insight into its origin providing it is not too deeply rooted. Organic pain almost always has a large functional overlay associated with it. It is unnecessary to evaluate the percentage of each, since it varies from moment to moment. For best results one should try to find the cause of the pain, to be aware of the secondary distress resulting from it and to understand the significance which the patient places on it. Russian physiologists have been interested in the complexity of an organism's reaction to pain. They have tried to differentiate between reflexes that may be harmful and reflexes that have a useful defense function. Tonkikh (111) has made significant contributions to the understanding of some of the physiological mechanisms which take part in the complex reaction of the patient to stimuli that are followed by the subjective feeling of pain.

Hypnotherapy of insomnia follows the same general rules as for the treatment of pain. Some patients who suffer from insomnia do not seem to mind it much. They may tell you that they sleep only four to five hours a night but feel well enough during the day. In contrast to this type there are some patients who are very distressed when they are unable to sleep for an hour or two during the entire night. They turn and toss. Some may even go into panic. Hypnotic therapy is directed here at relieving the distress and restlessness. Amelioration of these symptoms helps them to tolerate the insomnia better, which in turn helps them to sleep better. Where organic pain is present, some patients may be taught autohypnosis to induce sleep and overcome some of the pain. Success in this field depends upon the selection of the patient. A passive, dependent individual will more likely seek the help of increasingly strong analgesics and hypnotics rather than try to help himself with the assistance of the physician.

It is common for patients suffering from unresolved current reality problems to find it hard to fall asleep, but once they do they sleep quite well. Hypnotic suggestions directed for relaxation often help such patients. If, however, the patient is able to fall asleep quite quickly but awakens after a few hours and cannot fall asleep again, we may be dealing with an anxiety resulting from repressed material. This may show up by recurrent nightmares, which in turn prevent him from allowing himself to fall asleep again. For the psychiatrically trained physician, insight therapy under hypnosis often leads to better sleeping habits.

Every physician has seen patients who suffer from severe insomnia which responds neither to chemotherapy nor hypnotherapy. These are the patients who, if they are not actually in a psychotic episode, are bordering on it. They may be found to be suffering from an agitated depression, a recurrent depression, paranoidal reactions or hypomania. They are best served by referring them to a psychiatrist for treatment of the underlying condition.

Hypnosis may be used to advantage in another condition more commonly seen by the general practitioner than the internist. This is sterility in the woman. The psychological elements in this condition are well known, especially by those who are interested in the emotional aspects of the subject. There is no overall method of approach to psychogenic sterility, but some aspects are common to most of them. The anxiety resulting from sterility makes the woman tense and spasm of the fallopian tubes may occur just as spasms occur elsewhere in the body under tension. The anxiety in these patients is increased further by iatrogenic factors. Being told to take their temperatures daily to determine the time of ovulation, to use certain positions in coitus, to douche before the act, to take hormones and injections, all increase the patient's anxiety and tension, and usually leads to frigidity as well as sterility. Hypnotic relaxation and non-specific suggestive therapy is the method of choice to start with.

The following case of psychogenic sterility is reported because it reveals most of the mechanisms seen in this problem and the good results obtained by the use of simple hypnotic suggestion for support and relaxation. Hypnosis was used also analytically to determine the reason for her recurrent spontaneous abortions once she did become pregnant.

The couple had been married for five years. Two years prior to their first visit, both had been examined and the husband was found to be adequate both in performance and sperm count. For these two years the wife had been taking her temperature twice daily, assumed various positions during coitus as directed by her physician, and had many hormonal assays during this period. The situation between husband and wife had become intolerable and the reason for their visit was to determine whether they should divorce or if the adoption of a child would hold them together.

The husband was passive and dependent. The wife was aggressive, dominant and abusive. Verbal communication between them was almost nil for several years. The first interview was taken up with quieting the wife and reassuring the husband. The suggestion was made that the wife would have to be seen several times for a month and the husband once or twice during that time. It was implied that the problem would be resolved one way or another in that time. In other words, their anxiety, anguish and indecision would have a terminal point.

Under hypnosis it was found that the wife preferred to use the masculine position for coitus but had accepted her previous physician's suggestion to assume the feminine position. She did this with great resentment and without enjoyment. Hypnotic suggestions were given that she could assume any position she desired *without guilt* and that she would enjoy the act again as she used to when first married. The husband was informed of this and accepted it. She was asked to destroy her temperature charts, to stop taking her temperature and all medication and douches. She was much relieved and became easier to live with. In three weeks time she was pregnant.

Unhappily, this is not the end of the case report. She aborted spontaneously at the end of the third month. It surprised us to observe that the loss disturbed the husband much more than it did the wife, but we were not perceptive enough to determine the reason at that time. After three months she was told that she could try to conceive again. She became pregnant quite easily during that month. She appeared to be happy and her husband reported that their home life was better than ever before. It seemed a little strange that she began to wear maternity clothes after the first month, but it was put down to the fact that she was anxious to show her friends through non-verbal communication that she was pregnant again.

By the end of the second month she began to be afraid of falling, as she believed this was the cause of the first abortion. She became very meticulous in climbing stairs and in walking on the street but finally slipped and fell. At two and a half months she had her second spontaneous abortion. Her obstetrician and endocrinologist could find no reason for these two abortions. Once again the wife did not appear to be too disturbed by this event. Hypnoanalysis was then used to try to find out if there was a psychological reason for these untoward events.

In the sixth hypnoanalytic interview she revealed the fact that it was satisfactory enough for her to show that she could be pregnant whenever she wanted to, but that she was in great fear of giving birth to a live child as she felt too immature and too inadequate to bring up a child. The idea frightened her and she felt relieved when she aborted. The situation was reviewed again with both of them and the problem resolved itself into the question of either getting a divorce or being treated so that she could go through the pregnancy to fulfillment. The latter solution was chosen and treatment was started.

Once again she became pregnant without difficulty, but this time she was asked not to wear maternity clothes until it became necessary. This idea was reinforced under hypnosis with the implication that no one would know that she was pregnant until her own figure would disclose the fact. Since she was so proud of being pregnant but was afraid to have a child, it was hoped to see her through the first four months of "silent" pregnancy before her friends would realize it and satisfy her need for their approbation. By this time it was hoped that she would be able to go through the rest of her pregnancy without trouble. She was seen weekly and given supportive and encouraging suggestions under hypnosis. All went well up until the middle of the ninth month.

It was at this time that hypnotic therapy made its greatest contribution. The patient had been making her routine visits to her obstetrician with a very close friend who was also pregnant and expected her baby about the same time. They arranged their obstetrical visits so that they would be seen one after the other and then spend the rest of the day together. Her friend started labour two weeks ahead of her expected time and was delivered of a normal child but died suddenly two days later from an embolism. One day later our patient was informed by the obstetrician's secretary that he was in no condition to deliver her and recommended a colleague.

As expected, the patient's identification with her friend set up a sort of folie à deux. She was inconsolable and became quite disturbed. Hypnotic suggestions, direct and indirect, were used to tide her over the next two weeks and to help her form some type of trust in her new obstetrician. It was also used to relieve her of her ambivalent feelings towards her original obstetrician whom she trusted until the tragedy occurred. The therapist had to move in closer to give her more support. She was delivered with the help of very little chemoanesthesia as she had been conditioned under hypnosis to withstand her contractions and be as awake as possible for the whole procedure so that it would fit in with her aggressive dominant personality needs. It also helped her to understand that if she remained active there would be less chance for an embolism to develop.

She made an uneventful recovery and surprised everyone by not developing a postpartum depression. It was felt that she had drained off much of her anxiety during her pregnancy, especially in the last two weeks of her pregnancy (102). She was reassured also of her husband's co-operation in looking after the infant, and actually for the first two years of the child's life, he was more of a mother to her than a father. This has resolved itself gradually. The child is now at school and doing well emotionally, intellectually and in her interpersonal relationships.

Because of its many ramifications, this case represents the variety of changing situations in a patient's life which can be handled through the flexible use of hypnotherapy and hypnoanalysis. It is readily admitted that if the problem had been investigated more carefully from the beginning, the dynamics would have been revealed much earlier and perhaps some of the subsequent difficulties could have been minimized or eliminated. The practice of medicine, however, is far from theoretical and the urgency of immediate help needed by both husband and wife as revealed in their first interview set the tone and direction of therapy. When more time is available it might be wiser to make a more detailed survey of the problem first before outlining a course of treatment.

Treatment under hypnosis can be of considerable help in psychogenic cardiovascular reactions. This holds true whether the emotional disturbance is a factor in the production of the illness or is merely the result of organic distress. Thus, some cases of neuroses with cardiac manifestations respond to hypnotic therapy directed at the underlying neurosis, while in other patients the anxiety and emotional distress resulting from organic heart disease may be ameliorated by the same use of hypnosis, but in this instance it is directed primarily towards reducing the fear and emotional turmoil which results from the impaired cardiac function and consequent fear of death. In patients in the lower income bracket who suffer from an acute heart attack, the anxiety about providing for the family should be recognized and supportive therapy used within the limits of the reality situation. In any event, some improvement in the general sense of well being, as well as in the circulatory function, can be expected in all the cases mentioned through the judicious use of hypnotherapy. Best results may be anticipated in cases where the symptoms are primarily emotionally determined and less where the organic components predominate.

Perhaps in no other system of the body is the iatrogenic factor as important as in the cardiovascular system. Functional disorders of the heart or blood pressure apparatus induced in the patient by the physician during his examination of the heart and blood pressure occur more frequently than they should. Doubt in the patient's mind as to the integrity of the heart or blood pressure is a very frequent cause of chronic incapacity that is sometimes difficult to alleviate in a neurotic patient (8, 20). Kline (51) reports on the successful treatment of one such case by means of hypnotherapy. His case illustrates how situational experiences can, on the basis of their relationship to a primary psychological function (perceptual), give rise to physical symptomatology which becomes easily reinforced. In his opinion, psychosomatic reactions involving psychopathology can make best use of hypnosis as an integral part of the psychotherapeutic approach to personality reorganization and adjustment.

The writer has had occasion to see a few patients in the course of the years within an hour of the onset of coronary occlusion, paroxysmal tachycardia, heart block or the onset of frequent extrasystoles. Electrocardiograms taken on arrival as compared with electrocardiograms done a half to one hour later, following immediate hypnotherapy directed at reducing anxiety and shock, are indicative of what can be accomplished by a so-called "hypnotic leucotomy" (83). More recently we were privileged to be present at a patient's home when, during a discussion, he developed a massive cardiac infarct. He was hypnotized immediately and rushed to the hospital by ambulance. The marked progressively deteriorating changes in the electrocardiograms taken at the hospital during the next two days were not accompanied by the shock usually associated with such massive damage. He was not restless in the oxygen tent and did not complain of claustrophobia which he suffered from time to time in the past. Since no other measures were taken at the time, it is possible that the "hypnotic leucotomy" helped to prevent further damage and perhaps avoided a fatal outcome of the cardiac accident.

In a less acute situation, Schneck (80) reported his findings in a hypnoanalytic study of a patient with extrasystoles. Some cardiovascular symptoms are learned responses and can be brought about by certain stimuli to which the patient has become sensitive. Raginsky (104) reported a case of temporary cardiac arrest induced under hypnosis. This was an experiment done on a sixty-five year old male who had suffered from a severe form of a Stokes-Adams syndrome. At his worst, he fainted from six to seven times within a period of a few hours. The symptoms were cleared up after a bilateral sinu-carotid neurectomy. Here was an ideal set of circumstances for an experiment to show, if possible, that one could have a patient in the hypnotic state re-enact a previously emotionally charged situation with all the intensity of the original fainting episodes. While his hospital records showed that he had had fainting attacks with loss of consciousness for six years prior to the experiment, he had no such episodes following the bilateral sinu-carotid neurectomy one and a half years prior to the experiment. The following investigation was carried out with his permission and full co-operation.

Under hypnosis he was asked to visualize earlier experiences of all kinds. Random pleasant memories were brought to the surface and the patient appeared to go into a deeper hypnotic level. He was then asked to discuss some of his experiences with doctors, nurses and orderlies during his many stays in hospitals. He started out with emotionally neutral memories but soon brought up unpleasant experiences with some apprehension and anxiety. At this point he was asked to visualize with all the clarity possible his worst attacks of faintness. He became restless and agitated but did not go into a faint. After a little rest and relaxation under hypnosis he was asked to see the same scene as before but even more vividly. The suggestion was given in a tone of considerable urgency. This time he suddenly turned pale, limp, and a cold perspiration appeared on his forehead. His pulse was unobtainable. The electrocardiogram showed a complete auricular and ventricular standstill for four and four-fifths seconds.

In a few minutes time his colour, respiration and pulse returned to normal and he was allowed to rest for another ten minutes. At the end of this rest period the same experiment was tried again and similar results were recorded with a complete auricular and ventricular standstill of five seconds duration. The experiment was stopped at this point and the patient showed no ill effects from the experience. He had four subsequent hospital admissions up to the time of his death from uraemia following a prostatectomy at the age of eighty-one.

Alexander (3, 4) believes that the early fluctuating phase of essential hypertension is the manifestation of a psychoneurotic condition. This is based on excessive and inhibited hostile impulses. We have had hypertensives abreact under hypnosis, resulting in a rather remarkable drop in the systolic pressure. It was found to be more effective if the patient was given some old magazines to be held in the hands while emoting. More recently we have used hard plasticine as described later under hypnoplasty. More often than not the patient would tear the magazine into shreds with a strength transcending his normal capacity. The salutary effect on the blood pressure would last for several days. In those patients who were treated over a period of months, the response was more lasting.

The most impressive result obtained by this method was in a

forty-nine year old physician whose blood pressure was 270/130 when first examined. He had been found unfit to undergo a sympathectomy. After six months of hypnotherapy during which he was allowed to abreact violently his pressure levelled off in the range of 160/100 to 180/120. It is now more than twelve years since his treatment was carried out and he remains in good health. Instead of semi-retirement he was urged to carry on a full practice. This gave him the opportunity of getting rid of aggression. He enjoyed going out on night calls. It made him feel needed and wanted, and he was praised for his exceptional devotion to his patients. Apparently this was a reversible process in which a more optimistic prognosis, together with a chance of giving in to his compulsive needs, gave him a better chance to meet his problems.

Dunbar (22) and Wolfe (119) call attention to the increased tension and occasional spasm of smooth or voluntary muscle, either or both of which may be alleviated as unconscious conflicts become conscious. They believe that this tension is part of the whole defense mechanism, psychologically and physiologically a general attitude of being on guard. Hypnotherapy directed at reducing these factors has met with encouraging results in selected cases (13). Binger and his co-workers (9) came to the conclusion that "What appears to differentiate this from other neurotic disorders is that after prolonged unresolved struggle between dependent strivings and compensatory aggressive drives, there is finally submission on the part of the patient to the hostility of the parent figure and acceptance of defeat of his own aggressive drives. When this occurs, anxiety, depression and temporary disorganization of the adaptive functions of the personality manifest themselves. Such acute decompensations coincide with the discovery of hypertension."

Stevenson *et al.* (91) and Duncan *et al.* (23) demonstrated in their series of unselected patients with extrasystoles that the life situation and emotional state of the patients were found to be relevant to the occurrence of the arrhythmias in each patient. The excitability of the heart may be significantly altered by prolonged hyperactivity of the cardiac muscle during anxiety with tachycardia and increased stroke volume. Structurally diseased hearts are less able to stand the strain of such hyperactivity and more readily develop an altered excitability than normal hearts. Extrasystoles are therefore particularly common in patients with structural heart disease who exhibit prolonged anxiety and the associated reaction of cardiac mobilization. The treatment of subjects with extrasystoles should include attention to the life situation and the patient's adjustment to it, not only for its effect on the arrhythmia but also in relieving the stress on the heart, of which the extrasystoles are an indication.

In a case of psychogenic cardiovascular reaction incurred in combat, Schneck (81) was able, by means of hypnosis, to produce a revivification of a combat scene resulting in abreaction of an affect-charged experience. This abreaction, together with an interpretation of the psychosomatic symptomatology resulted in recovery. In this communication, Schneck makes mention of the fact that in World War II the technique described by Grinker and Spiegel (39) of inducing abreaction by means of narcosynthesis had largely supplanted the use of hypnosis for the same purpose. It is our impression that while this was so during the war and for several years afterwards, this method was not as effective as hypnotherapy and hypnoanalysis for civilian problems. In civilian patients, the cause and effect are not as easily demonstrated as in soldiers under acute battle or war conditions where the precipitating factor is not too difficult to demonstrate. The emotional trauma in civilian life is usually less intense, less circumscribed and induced more slowly. It is of interest here to record Menninger's (67) observation that: "Hypnosis, while a relatively simple procedure, is not widely used by American psychiatrists. Its efficacy in war neuroses seems to have been well demonstrated in the last war by both American and German psychiatrists and it is therefore surprising that more use of it was not made. The security and ease of the drug sedation and the widespread lack of experience with, and the medical acceptance of, hypnosis seem to be the logical explanations."

In the broad field of immunology there have been instances of apparent allergic responses, including hives and angioneurotic edema which appear to have had a major emotional element in their production. The literature on the psychogenic factors in asthma has been well summarized by Dunbar (21) and Wittkower (117). Mitchell, Curran and Myers (71) found that the group of patients with negative skin reactions are also the multiple complaint group. They express a variety of illnesses and complaints indicating a strong content of factors characteristic of emotional maladjustment. Abramson (1) in his discussion of pseudoallergic schizophrenia as a new clinical entity brings attention to the important findings of Hoch (46). Some patients heretofore considered neurotic may show clinical symptomatology very similar to that seen in schizophrenia. A number of such patients have short psychotic episodes but do not deteriorate as schizophrenics usually do. He classifies them as pseudoneurotic schizophrenics. They are the multiple complaint group and because of their personality structure do not respond well to the usual measures carried out by allergists. Hypnotherapy in these patients produces brilliant results at times, but it should be clear that hypnotherapy for such patients should be reserved for those clinicians well trained in psychiatry.

Of the fifty unselected cases of bronchial asthma taken from the allergy clinic by McDermott and Cobb (57), 72 per cent seemed to have an emotional component in their asthmatic attacks. In summarizing the literature on the subject, French and Alexander (32) state: "The impression gained is that attacks of bronchial asthma seem to be associated with a very considerable variety of emotional conflicts. Outstanding among these are the suppression of any sort of intense emotion, threats to dependent relationships and to the security based upon them, and sexual conflicts. The outstanding personality traits of the asthmatic children seem to be over-anxiety, lack of self-confidence and a clinging dependence on parents which appear to be a reaction to a tendency to over-solicitude upon the part of the parents."

We have treated a fair number of such asthmatic children and adults with hypnosis. In some, non-specific suggestions for relaxation and normal breathing repeated in interviews over a period of weeks helped to reduce the frequency and intensity of the attacks. In others it was necessary to resort to etiologically oriented hypnotherapy. In a twelve year old boy who showed extremely marked dependent needs for his mother which he satisfied by having many asthmatic attacks day and night for years, it was thought wise to separate the boy from his mother as a first step in treatment. As soon as this was attempted, the boy became much worse. He was able, however, to accept this idea under hypnosis and his dependence was transferred to an aunt in another city. He remained with that aunt for several months and the dependence was transferred again to another group of boys where it was arranged for him to be their mascot. He enjoyed this attention and was better able to contend with his younger brother when he returned home after another few months time. Though he had already developed the barrel-shaped chest so typical of these asthmatics, he became free from asthma after two years of manipulating his environment and strengthening his ego structure. It is obvious that it is essential to have the complete co-operation of the parents in order to carry out such a program. During the subsequent years of college and professional life, he has had occasional need for help and guidance but did not have a return of his asthma.

It is not uncommon to attain similar results in adults in the fifty to sixty-five year age group. The group referred to is made up of men and women who have had no history of asthma in their earlier life but who now develop asthma following upper respiratory infections. They may or may not show positive skin reactions and usually have had all the help the allergists can give them before resorting to hypnotherapy. By this time the asthma is present almost constantly and is no longer immediately related to an upper respiratory infection. In reviewing the life situation of these patients it is common to observe that in some way they have managed to place themselves in an apparently non-reversible dependent relationship in their household or place of work or both. They have exhausted the effects of chemotherapy and drained the emotional and financial resources of their colleagues and relatives. It is in such cases that the use of hypnosis makes the difference between success and failure in relieving the symptoms.

Hypnosis is used at first to make them more comfortable and as a result they begin to have a little more confidence in the physician and in themselves. The next step is to persuade them to go away. It does not matter where. One patient decided to go to a city considered to be the worst place for asthma, especially during the winter season. Though he could afford it, he refused to go south or to a drier climate. This was due partly to the fact that he knew some people in that city but did not know anyone in the warmer or drier climate areas. The other factor was the fear of getting well and having to face reality. Thus, getting him to go away at all was a small victory. It so happened that a few days after his arrival there, the city had the worst snow storms and blizzards in many decades. Being a Canadian and used to this type of weather, he was impressed with the inability of the municipal authorities to contend with what they considered a disaster, and felt superior to the people who were afraid to venture out in the snow. During the first week of his stay there he showed little if any improvement, but by the end of three weeks, when he returned home, he was completely free from asthma and not taking any medication for the first time in two years. This improvement has continued not only in the form of absence of symptoms but in a remarkable general improvement in his sense of well-being and ability to sleep. He had defrosted himself from the "cold-freeze" in which he had been living for the past few years. In spite of positive skin tests he remains free of all allergic symptoms.

The principles of therapy in asthma, as in other conditions with a high neurotic content, are to treat the patient as a hurt *child,* no matter how intelligent he may be, and to realize that a hurt child is apt to hurt others and usually succeeds; to give somatic and psychic comfort as quickly as possible; and to understand that the neurotic fears to get well too quickly since he is afraid to give up his *excessive* need for protection, comfort and guidance. The physician who uses hypnosis in his therapy and who takes these factors into consideration is not so likely to "assault" his patient with commands to get well, but instead will use the patient-oriented approach where the patient's real and unconscious wishes are taken into consideration in outlining the total psychotherapy, of which hypnosis is only one aspect. One should not strive for brilliant results as evidence of the doctor's "power" or his ability in the use of hypnosis. There are too many neurotic patients who do not appreciate a sudden return to health for several reasons. Such a result may make them appear foolish in the eyes of those close to them. In others, it makes them lose confidence in themselves. In still others, there develops a feeling that "now that I am cured, I still cannot face the problems ahead of me," and they must find other neurotic means of avoidance.

Van Pelt (113) and Marchesi (60) report cases of bronchial asthma which have remained cured following hypnotherapy. Hansen was able to eliminate a sensitivity to horse dander by means of several sessions of hypnotherapy. Many workers in this field have found that abreaction under hypnosis may occasionally terminate status asthmaticus. We have trained interns and residents who were able to arrest attacks of asthma in patients on the medical wards by hypnotherapy when ordinary medical measures failed. In cases of chronic asthma with a strong emotional component, it it usually necessary to resort to a longer re-educational program in order to attain more lasting results. In some cases of status asthmaticus the use of ACTH or cortisone for the acute phase followed by sessions of hypnotherapy appears to work well.

While the treatment of urticaria lies within the province of the dermatologist, it is not unusual for the general physician to come in contact with this condition either as a presenting complaint or as a complication. While the following short discussion is based on the internist's viewpoint, a more comprehensive outline will be found elsewhere in this book.

The association of urticaria with stressful life situations has been observed by many authors (37, 47, 78, 92). It is well recognized that the skin may react to normal emotional situations by flushing, pallor or sweating and that the degree of this reaction depends upon the individual. Fenichel (29) indicated that the tendency of the skin to be influenced by vasomotor reactions, which in turn are evoked by unconscious impulses, has to be understood from the point of view of the general physiologic functions of the skin. It displays four characteristics whereby it represents a boundary between the organism and the external world (1). In its protective function, the skin treats internal and external stimuli alike and uses vasomotor functions as an armour (2). The skin is an important erogenous zone. In addition to the stimuli of touch and temperature, pain too may be the source of erogenous cutaneous pleasures (3). Being visible, the skin is a site for expressions of conflicts centered around exhibitionism. These conflicts concern not only fear and shame, but also various narcissistic needs for reassurance (4). Anxiety is physiologically a sympathicotonic state, and sympathicotonic reactions of vessels in the skin may represent anxiety. Making use of this knowledge of the physiologic functions of the skin, hypnotherapists have reported excellent results in all types of skin lesions. They are able to increase and decrease the supply of blood to the parts involved by suggesting situations where it would be natural for the patient to feel warmth or cold in the selected area. The patient may be taught how to do this for himself several times a day between treatment sessions, and it is remarkable what results can be obtained in some cases. Similar approaches may be made using different dynamics for lesions having to do with the erogenous, narcissistic and exhibitionistic needs of the patient.

It is well recognized that the skin may react to normal situations by flushing, pallor or sweating, and that the degree of this reaction depends upon the individual. Davis and Bick (16) suggest that in the same manner anxiety is a quantitative exaggeration of mild skin reactions. This is an additional symptom of an anxiety state occurring in a sensitive individual whose anxiety is reflected through the skin rather than through the gastrointestinal tract or the cardiovascular system.

Some people can become just as sensitive to certain ideas or situations as others are to pollens. Menninger and Kemp (65) report on a case of urticaria in a young man caused by his inability to "be a man" in a love affair. Others have suggested the possibility of a relationship between certain states of allergic sensitivity and states of intense frustrated longing. These emotions can often be elicited during free association under hypnosis and help reduce or even eliminate the urticaria.

There are certain differences between acute and chronic urticaria. Chief of these is the fact that while certain specific allergens are usually found in acute urticaria, it is exceptional to find this etiology in chronic cases. Kaywin (50) came to the conclusion that his patients with chronic urticaria were shy, easily embarrassed, prone to blushing, relatively passive-dependent and immature, with perhaps a tendency towards exhibitionism. We have been able to help a number of such patients, since they are the ones who are so easily hypnotized and accept the psychologic manipulation under these conditions with comparative ease. Graham (36), in his excellent article, observed that traumatic life situations responsible for attacks of urticaria were almost exclusively those in which the patient developed resentment because he saw himself as the victim of unjust treatment about which he could do nothing. In such cases we have allowed the patient to abreact, usually violently, while under hypnosis where resentment is not only expressed by the patient, but also accepted by the therapist. It is not uncommon to see the weepy type of eczema dry up after one or two such sessions. Recurrences are treated palliatively by repeated sessions of abreaction under hypnosis, but a more permanent result can only be expected when the conflicts are dealt with at a more dynamic level.

Where once it was hoped to remove symptoms and to cure patients by simple procedures, we now know that we must creep up slowly upon their many secrets and that we must use to the utmost all our diagnostic and therapeutic resources. Throughout this chapter the reader is reminded directly and indirectly that hypnosis should always be used within this framework. This holds true especially in the treatment of compulsive smoking, eating and alcoholism. The more cases of stammering and stuttering we have seen, the more apt we are to start treatment in areas far removed from the presenting symptom.

It has taken the writer many years to fully realize what anguish even a mild stammerer goes through almost daily and the many devious and subtle defenses he must put up to protect himself daily from those around him. This was brought to out attention by a patient who complained of mild stammering, but who during a forty-five minute interview did not show any such symptoms in spite of attempts to bring it on by upsetting him. If it were not for the fact that he had been referred by a colleague and had travelled more than three thousand miles (with his wife) for this consultation we would have told him to forget the whole matter. He had been treated under hypnosis many times by several physicians but obviously not to his satisfaction. It was decided to attempt to find out what was really bothering him. At is turned out, the patient was quite right—he did stammer, but did it silently and had developed a technique of covering it up by speaking in a deliberate and apparently cultured manner so that the hiatus between certain words was not apparent to anyone but himself.

He was regressed to earlier periods of life and brought up incidents which were very frightening to him up to the age of six.

He brought them up so easily and with so much affect that it appeared to be only what had been brought out by other therapists or had been suggested to him indirectly. It was not until he was brought up to the age of thirteen, a time that he remembered consciously as being his worst period of stammering, that hypnotherapy became fruitful. He was asked to relive one of his worst experiences of stammering and he did it with great gusto. It was in a "public" school in England where his teacher thought he would help the patient get over his stammering by having him order the school supplies over the telephone. At is happened, he was at his worst on the telephone and more so in the school setting. At this point of his investigation he stammered and stuttered very badly. He was awakened with the suggestion that this condition would continue after he awakened and it did. Since he did not seem at all upset by the new situation, the interview was ended without removing the post-hypnotic suggestion. It was gratifying for him to know that he did really stammer and that it was not an hallucination.

On his next interview two days later he was still stammering but appeared to be very bright and cheerful. A clue to the reason for this sense of well-being was found in his report under hypnosis of what had transpired since the previous visit. His wife was shocked to hear him stammering so badly and asked him not to return for treatment. He became very angry and told her that in the past no one, not even she, believed how much he had suffered from his "silent" stammering and how he had become increasingly annoyed at his friends and doctors who told him not to worry about it since it didn't show when he spoke in public. The stammering and the anger towards his wife continued for about a week. Both diminished gradually by the end of the second week. When seen at the end of this period, his speech was less deliberate and perhaps less "cultured" or artificial. He appeared content and it was his decision to stop therapy and return home. Two letters from him received several months after he returned to England were interesting and instructive. He visited the therapists who had told him to forget about his stammering because it was so minimal and he once again reacted in the same way as he did to his wife on the occasion when his stammering returned following the post-hypnotic suggestion. "He let them have it" one after the other until he vented all his pent-up anger at not having been understood and helped. In view of the dynamics involved, it was not surprising to learn that he did not get angry or stammer when he contacted the referring physician.

This experience helped the writer treat with more assurance and direction another patient with the same symptoms. Here again there were no outward manifestations of stammering or stuttering, though the patient complained bitterly of it. He was relieved considerably by having the symptoms brought out under hypnosis after the first few visits. He felt he was understood and appreciated the writer's concern over the amount of energy and effort used to keep up the facade of apparently speaking normally. Over a period of months, he was able to relive some of the most traumatic experiences in connection with stammering while under hypnosis. When this phase wore off he began to gain insight into his intense hostility towards his mother. Apparently the outward anger he showed her was not enough to get rid of the hate and tension. Some of his hostility was discharged by spending unreasonable amounts of money through her charge accounts while demanding still more in cash. He rarely spent any of his own money. He showed his resentment also by refusing to be awakened in the morning to attend classes, and as a consequence failed his year at college. When first seen he had failed his year in two different faculties in succession.

As soon as his stammering was brought to the surface and was quite audible to the therapist, there was a distinct improvement in his general behaviour, at first towards his scholastic work at a new college, then to his friends, and finally to his family. In time his "silent" stammer disappeared almost altogether and he was able to graduate without difficulty. In spite of the disappearance of the symptoms he was still obsessed with the idea that the cause of the stammer was organic in nature. This idea had been implanted by his mother and re-enforced by a speech therapist in his youth. It was removed by the following method.

In the hypnotic state, he was made to stammer badly. While in this condition he was asked to read out loud. This he did with obvious difficulty and embarrassment. By prearrangement we were called out of the consulting room, but requested him to continue reading out loud until our return. He was aware that the tape recorder was not turned off during our absence. On our return within a few minutes, he volunteered the fact that he did not stammer at all while he was alone. The tape was replayed from the beginning of the interview and it verified his observation that he had stammered in the interview at command but was able to read freely and normally when left alone. This experiment removed the last vestige of doubt in his mind about the functional nature of the condition.

Patients with chronic headaches present a considerable problem to the physician, both because of their numbers and because of the stubbornness with which their symptoms often persist despite every effort of treatment. The great majority of all patients with chronic headache fall into one of three groups—migrainous, post-traumatic, or psychogenic. Regardless of the precise mechanism of the production of pain, there is abundant clinical experience to prove that all three types of headache are readily precipitated and made worse by emotional stress and inner conflict. In a truly comprehensive approach to the subject of headaches it is necessary to deal with the repressed psychic conflicts and their corresponding emotions which produce the painful sensations. The frequent complaints of patients who consider their headaches as produced by a brain tumor or swelling inside the head suggests the foreign-body-like quality of the repressed conflicts and their damaging effect.

We have been able to help some of these patients by allowing them to ventilate repressed anger while under hypnosis. Where this method had been found helpful, the patients were then helped to understand the causes of the repressed affect. Additionally, they were trained to meet stressful or conflictual situations in a more adult fashion. Where masochism was found to underly the feelings of hostility and the head used as the organ of expression, a much deeper psychological approach was necessary. For example, it is well known that patients suffering from the disabling type of migraine headaches also suffer from deep emotional isolation though it is often masked by an acceptable superficial contact. Tension, insecurity, sensitivity, perfectionism and intolerance are some of their "trademarks." They are scrupulous, hard workers, stubborn and politely obstinate. In such patients we have found the use of hypnoplasty of considerable help.

Meares' (61) pioneering work with plaster of paris led him to the conclusion that modelling under hypnosis (hypnoplasty) is of particular value. The suppressed or repressed ideas can be given expression in modelling and this is accompanied by the expression of a good deal of emotion. The idea in modelling arouses the appropriate emotion and soon brings the patient to express himself in words in a manner which might be achieved only after many hours of orthodox verbal hypnoanalysis. Hypnoplasty demands motor activity in the patient and this in itself makes it easy for him to use his behaviour as a means of communicating with the therapist. Hypnoplasty shortens the time of psychotherapy through the initiation, intensification and acceleration of the effective psychodynamic processes in treatment. It prevents him from using his everyday patterns of defense or at least minimizes them. Not only is the therapeutic process more quickly initiated, but it is also intensified in the patient's emotional relationship to the therapist, in abreaction and insight. The model tends to prolong the process of insight so that it remains longer with the patient.

Using Meares' basic concepts, we have experimented with various media for hypnoplasty in office practice (107). We have found that by using soft, warm (heated) flesh-coloured plasticine we were able to initiate associations dealing with interpersonal relationships in a few minutes time. In the same way, moist, warm, brown plasticine brings out memories of stool and bowel training. Semi-solid, moist, warm red plasticine brings out associations dealing with menses, injuries, wounds, etc. Hard green plasticine brings to the surface many repressed phobias and fears. It was found that the incorporation of faint traces of various body odours into the plasticine readily brings out unconscious material in the patient not usually possible in our past experience.

With this method it is possible to get under the migrainous patient's rigid resistances. Within the framework of total psychotherapy the hypnoplasty sessions are so structured as to bring out the material required. We start first with the warm, sticky, flesh-coloured plasticine and before the patient learns to line up his defenses he has exposed many of his conflicts, enough to start him off in many troubled areas he would otherwise have avoided. The other colours, temperature, consistency, degree of moisture and odour are used as needed to explore the problem and resolve the conflicts. This method is not only useful in the migraine patient but in any patient who finds it difficult to express himself under hypnosis. It is particularly useful in patients suffering from anxiety neuroses and in compulsive-obsessive patients who find it difficult to enter into the treatment situation.

Erickson (27) uses the technique of time distortion to help the patient with periodic headaches. He allows the patient to have the headache but through hypnotic suggestion makes the patient believe that the headache has gone through its usual duration, while in reality it lasts but for a few minutes. Simons *et al.* (89) showed the correlation between the occurrence of headache and the strong and continued contraction of the scalp and neck muscles. When hypnosis is used to relieve these headaches by direct symptom-removal, suggestions should be directed towards relaxation of the scalp and neck muscles. Much better results can be expected from this approach than when it is suggested that the headache itself disappear. Tucker (112) reports that most headaches are associated with anxiety states, though they may also occur quite frequently during the menopausal reaction and in agitated depressions. The psychiatric condition in these patients is often mild with headache as the outstanding symptom, for all that is needed as a background is chronic muscular tension.

The secondary reaction to the headache is usually an important part of such disorders, and sometimes the most important part. Thus, the sufferer may withdraw from his usual recreations and activities, tends to shun contact with others and, because of fatigue, avoids physical exercise and tries to obtain more rest. Since these measures do not relieve tension, and since rest is interfered with by insomnia, the patient may go downhill. The more symptoms, the more anxiety, and the more anxiety, the more symptoms. Chemotherapy does not get rid of the cause of the disorder and accounts for the poor results attained by this method of therapy. As with any medical condition, neither the psychologic nor the physical aspect of the headache may be neglected with impunity. Anyone who has had experience with cerebral neoplasms will understand the significance of this statement.

When hypnosis is used to help these patients develop insight, much can be accomplished in a few sessions. If recognition of the conflict does not of itself remove the symptoms, hypnotherapy is directed towards helping the patient realize the significance of the conflicts and attitudes brought to the surface, and then is guided to modify them in order to make a better adjustment. Patients whose symptoms are of long standing, with a history and present symptoms of constitutional emotional instability and inadequacy, are poor subjects for insight therapy which may serve only to bring out their inadequacy. Should hypnosis be used in these cases, it is deemed advisable to make use of direct suggestions only. Harding (44) treated twenty-three patients with migraine headaches by hypnosis. Six had complete relief. Six experienced reduction in severity or frequency of attacks. Eleven were not helped.

The large group of patients who complain of general aches and pains without demonstrable organic cause are susceptible to hypnotherapy. Patients with rheumatoid arthritis were found by Halliday (42, 43) to have an air of detachment and a lack of exteriorized tension. They show a quiet friendliness and a comparative absence of depression. In his opinion it remains to be seen whether further research will uncover a more specific rheumatoid personality type. Towards this end, many observers have contributed important observations on the relationship of psychologic mechanisms. Johnson, Shapiro and Alexander (49) found that these patients express and discharge unconscious emotional tendencies through the voluntary muscles, just as in hysterical conversion. They assume that these muscle spasms and increased muscle tonus may, under certain conditions, precipitate an arthritic attack. Menninger (66) reports that in World War II there were many cases of psychogenic disorders characterized by joint or musculoskeletal pain resembling myositis or fibrositis.

We have reported a case of rheumatoid arthritis in a married woman which responded rapidly to psychotherapy in which the use of hypnosis was an important element in diagnosis and treatment (105). The condition was a progressive one lasting for several years with two periods of hospitalization, one of five weeks and another of four months. Diet, physiotherapy, vaccine therapy and hyper-pyrexia were ineffective, as was a rest in Florida. She showed marked improvement within two weeks as a result of the psychiatric approach. The focal point of her difficulty as determined at the hypnotic level was a difficult marital relationship. She, a frigid, cultured woman, resented the primitive sexual approaches of her coarse and uneducated husband. The more she became incapaci-tated, the less call for sexual contact was made by her partner. She soon learned to use her illness not only to avoid sexual relation-ships, but also to harass her husband and to make him spend as much money as possible on consultations, hospitalizations, nursing care and trips to a warmer climate. The husband was given some insight into his role as the causative agent, and he promised to make no sexual demands for six months. She made a complete recovery in two months time and her husband divorced her at the end of six months. She remarried and has had no recurrence of her arthritis.

Many years ago we demonstrated that some uric acid is ex-creted through the bowel (82) and since it is well recognized that the function of the gastrointestinal tract is especially vulnerable to emotional conflicts, it is not surprising that we have had several patients with gout under observation for years, in whom attacks of gout could be predicted accurately. These attacks occurred when the proper emotional stimulus presented itself. This stimulus was found to be almost specific for the individual involved. As a result he would become embroiled in a conflict which resulted in this specific symptom formation. What is of importance and interest here is that once the attack of rheumatism or gout developed in these patients, the attacks could be shortened measurably through hypnotherapy directed at the cause of the conflict.

The occurrence of neurotic manifestations in and around the spinal column has been receiving attention in recent years. Inves-tigators have described the "neurotic spine," "hysterical spine," "railroad spine" and the tired back of the over-worked and neurotic housewife. These have been found to be susceptible to hypnother-apy in varying degrees, depending on the condition, the suscepti-bility of the patient to hypnosis, and the skill of the therapist in evaluating the components of the problem. We agree with Rosen (109) that unless the clinician is trained in psychodynamics it is unwise for him to use uncovering techniques in these patients. At times it is even imprudent to remove the symptoms which may be the patient's last stand against emotional decompensation.

Schwartz (85) treated a patient suffering from disabling pain as a result of a dislocated disc which was not relieved by three surgical procedures. He used hypnosis to produce regression, hallucinations and body image dissociation. As a result of some improvement after the first two sessions, the patient made up his mind to "let loose" and give hypnosis every chance. He remained symptom-free after the third session. This is an example of an organic condition helped psychologically through hypnosis.

The literature on the treatment of obesity with the aid of hypnosis is becoming voluminous. For more permanent results than is usually reported it seems necessary to pay more attention to the fundamental needs of these patients. This holds true of compulsive smoking and drinking. The emotional elements in the production of obesity are described very clearly by Mirsky (58). He explains that the over-eating usually is the result of some disturbance in the emotional development of the individual, so that he reacts to frustration in the present by withdrawing to a behaviour which was more gratifying in the past. This can be traced back to the time when the infant was dependent upon being fed by some other person in order to satisfy his psychologic requirement for food. The satisfaction of this requirement relieved the tension of hunger so that food, or being fed, became associated with a pleasurable sensation such as warmth, odours and the soothing aspects of the person who was providing the food. As a result of this experience, eating came to mean something which is inseparable from the relief of tension, affection and other pleasurable feelings. This is an association which is never completely abandoned but remains to some degree in all individuals.

He goes on to say that if an infant has been overindulged with respect to food, or has been given excessive satisfaction in consequence of the parents' attitude towards food and its significance, he may become reluctant to relinquish this early phase of his development for a more mature one. Thereafter, he automatically returns to it whenever he encounters a situation which is unpleasant, anxiety-producing, or frustrating. In such an individual the tension induced by the need of affection, for prestige or by loneliness, may be relieved only by withdrawing to that infantile phase when eating was a satisfactory solution. Alternatively, if an infant's earliest tensions were not relieved adequately, he may never outgrow his insatiable need for food or for being given things, and will persist in his attempts to receive that satiation of which he was deprived. Thereafter, such individuals may relieve their anger, envy and the frustration of their desires by eating. Irrespective of the genetic background, it appears that overeating is the obese person's habitual response to the necessity for solving such difficulties as are encountered in adult life by everyone.

We have drawn attention to the fact that for each individual, very early in life, foods become associated with diverse emotional meanings, so that for any given person there is scarcely a food which can be considered to be emotionally neutral (99). In our way of life, such foods as chocolate, hot dogs, candy and ice-cream have come to be regarded as reward foods. Parental insistence that foods such as spinach, carrots and milk must be eaten by the child often calls forth resistance on the child's part. This is retained even in adulthood as a symbolic rejection of parental authority. On the other hand, forbidden foods usually have a great appeal for the child. This is particularly true when he is told that he can have coffee, tea, beer, etc., only when he is "grown-up." Occasionally over-indulgence in these foods in later adult life is over-determined by the individual's desire to make up for earlier deprivations of childhood and to assert adultness. A person's patterns of choosing and eating foods thus become psychologically highly structured, conditioned responses. Foods have emotional values for an individual over and above the hunger satisfying capacity of all foods. Some foods are "gustatory pleasure" foods, "pleasure associated" foods, "security" foods, "reward" foods, "texture" foods, "fetish" foods, and so on. The patient's urgent need for ingesting foods in the above categories in times of stress may be so great that the emotional support derived from eating them far outweighs the consequences of obesity.

Inadequate as it may be, obesity is the result of a person's attempt to adapt to the emotional stresses to which he is exposed. With an understanding of the conflicts involved, the intelligent use of hypnotherapy has assisted many obese patients to reduce. Using the time distortion technique and regressing the patient to earlier periods in his life, one can "fill in" some of his emotional needs for the time being which makes dieting for that patient relatively easy. For some patients, the close personal interrelationship involved in hypnotherapy satisfies their emotional needs for this kind of relationship. As a consequence they find it quite easy to follow a restricted diet. In others, the suggestion of symptoms of anorexia appear to accomplish the same purpose. In still others, the authoritarian command to restrict both the intake and the type of food meets with success. Using the latter technique, a woman, thirty-nine years of age, weighing 286 pounds, was able to lose eighty-six pounds in one year without much hardship. Her past attempts in this direction without the use of hypnosis never exceeded the loss of eighteen pounds. It is wise to re-enforce the suggestions at intervals after the desired weight has been reached. In this way the patient may be kept under observation until a new habit of eating has been developed and other satisfactions substituted for food.

The physician should be on the lookout for those patients whose obesity has a more serious defensive purpose. An example of this is the adolescent girl or woman in her twenties or thirties who weighs about 200 and wants to reduce. One may find that this marked obesity is her defense against having to have a boy friend, husband or other social relationships. In truth, they have deep anxieties about sex and are afraid of facing aggression and social contacts. It is wise to treat the underlying neurosis in these patients while treating the obesity, otherwise they eventually put on more weight than when treatment was started. In other obese patients whose main problem is repressed rage and aggression, we have found that abreaction under hypnosis, to the point of tearing thick magazines and throwing objects about, makes for easy dieting until the next similar session. As these patients are allowed to express their aggressions without retaliation on the doctor's part, they are capable of maintaining themselves on a dietary regime without need for much help from the physician.

"Emotional glycosuria" has been demonstrated in man and experimental animals (12, 31, 34). There has also been recorded the occurrence of diabetes in a setting of emotional conflict and, furthermore, fluctuations in the disorder have been correlated with the emotional state in some patients (68-70). Rosen and Lidz (108) studied twelve patients in diabetic acidosis who revealed features of the immature, poorly integrated personality structure. These patients utilized their diabetes as a means of escape, either into the shelter of the hospital or by way of suicide. We have seen a fifteen year old girl who did both. Hinkle and Wolf (45) report their experimental findings in an anxious, maladjusted and severely diabetic fifteen year old girl, in which they show that stressful life situations which aroused the emotions of fear and rage were accompanied by alterations in the metabolism. Ketonuria appeared within approximately twelve hours of the onset of the stressful situation. With the continuation of the stress under experimental conditions the ketosis was observed to continue to the point of clinical acidosis. Without change in diet or additional insulin, the acidosis disappeared when the subject regained confidence and security.

Much more can usually be done for the diabetic than just keeping his urine sugar-free by means of diet and insulin. An appreciation of the patient's personality make-up, his strivings and frustrations, the home constellation and current stresses, allows a wider scope for the physician in the treatment of this condition. Aside from using hypnosis to differentiate borderline diabetic from non-diabetics, it can be used in selected cases to reduce the quantity of insulin needed to keep the urine sugar-free and so reduce the frequency of attacks of ketosis. Hypnotherapy often induces an easier acceptance of the restricted dietary regime. Similar methods can be used for patients who find it difficult to stay on a low fat, low salt or low carbohydrate regime.

The treatment of tinnitus taxes the physician's ability and resourcefulness. Schwartz (84) uses hypnosis to regress the patient and suggests deafness for the wavelength at which the tinnitus appears. These suggestions are repeated until new patterns are set up. As Guild (41) observes, "Whatever the origin of tinnitus, psychophysiological or pathophysiological, the role it has come to play in the patient's life and social adaptation must be considered of central importance in planning hypnotherapy." His approach in the treatment of tinnitus can be considered a classic method of the way in which hypnosis should be used to treat any condition for which hypnosis is indicated. Since various personality conflicts and anxieties can come to be secondarily expressed by a tinnitus once established, whatever its origin, these factors must be assessed by a full psychiatric history. If therapy is to be constructive and effective and reduce to a minimum the possibility of substitutive symptom formation, hypnosis must be used within the framework of such a psychologic evaluation and form part of a new balance in the total personality readjustment.

Tangential to this problem is the study of hypnotic deafness by Malmo, Boag and Raginsky (100, 101). The study was undertaken to investigate the question of similarities and differences between hysterical deafness and hypnotically induced deafness. Similarities between hysterical deafness and hypnotic deafness were listed as follows: (a) Significantly reduced motor reaction (exclusive of blink) to strong auditory stimulation in the deaf state. (b) Complete hearing loss in the hysteric and in one of the hypnotic subjects, even with strong auditory stimulation (i.e., denial of any auditory sensation). (c) With elicitation of strong startle reaction to the first stimulus in the deaf state, much smaller reaction to the next stimulus than would have been predicted on the basis of habituation. (d) Suggestion of substitution of somesthetic for auditory sensations in all subjects (although this was much less definite in the hypnotic subjects than the hysteric). The most outstanding dissimilarity lay in the absence of emotional reaction when "hypnotic defense against sound" was broken through, in contrast to marked affective reaction in the hysterical subject under these conditions. The usefulness of these findings lies mainly in the formulation of questions for further experimental attack on these problems.

Hypnosis has been used as a tool for the differential diagnosis and treatment of psychomotor epilepsy. A patient suffering from organic epilepsy may be made to have a convulsion while under hypnosis. Once started, however, the convulsion cannot be stopped by suggestion but must complete its cycle. Psychogenic epilepsy may be induced through hypnotic techniques but is differentiated from the organic type by the observation that the convulsion can be stopped at will by suggestion while the patient is still hypnotized. Much can be done to reduce the frequency of this type of convulsion and at times it is possible to stop it altogether.

The results at times appear to be inexplicable with our present knowledge. For example, we treated a thirteen year old boy who had been having from one to four epileptiform seizures daily for several months prior to his first visit. He had a history of occasional seizures for years, which the neurologists diagnosed as organic with electroencephalographic proof. Anticonvulsants helped but did not control the seizures altogether. Hypnotherapy was tried because of the increasing frequency and severity of the attacks. After three forty-five minute sessions of hypnotherapy, he remained completely free from these attacks up to the present time, which is a matter of nineteen years. This result was completely unexpected, as the only goal set for the interviews was to relax the patient and to set the stage for him to express himself without fear of reprisal. Other clinicians have observed similar results and have become interested in investigating this problem (75).

An interesting and unusual use of hypnosis has been reported by Cohen (13) in connection with the Ridley operation for cataract. This operation consists of an extracapsular cataract extraction followed by the insertion of an acrylic lens through the pupil into a position between the posterior lens capsule and the iris. The lens is more easily inserted through a relatively small pupil, yet it should be fairly large for the capsulectomy. Should the pupils dilate markedly, the lense cannot be inserted and the more orthodox operation is substituted at this moment. The patient was hypnotically conditioned for complete relaxation and at the right moment it was suggested that he imagine himself to be in a dark room. When he responded to this suggestion, he was told to watch the eye of a cat and that his pupil would become as large as that of the cat. The pupil dilated at once and the damaged lens was removed with ease. In order to insert the acrylic lens it was now necessary to contract the pupil and this was accomplished by suggesting to the patient that he was now out in the bright sunshine. The pupil contracted and the new lens was inserted without difficulty.

Mellor (64) believes that psychotherapy with the aid of hypnosis can be very effective in juvenile delinquents. It is his opinion that since the family physician is usually the first one consulted by the parents, he is the one who can and should initiate the proper treatment. As a generalist trained in dynamic psychotherapy, he used hypnotherapy in a pilot study of fourteen patients. He reports thirteen good results, with an average total treatment of six hours per patient. All patients were referred through a city police agency or county probation department and were on a long-term follow-up. It is of interest to record that written permission from the parents and the court was obtained before hypnosis was used. The technique was patient-centered. The answers to both diagnosis and treatment-oriented questions came from the patient, thus emphasizing statements that his problems are his and his alone, and that he can learn about them and how to overcome them. The patient develops his own insight and relieves his own tension. He learns a better way of feeling and responding. He cures himself.

Our own results in treating these patients psychotherapeutically with the aid of hypnosis falls short of those obtained by Mellor. This may be due in part to the fact that our patients had not yet become seriously involved with the law, and so the motivation and drive to get well may have been different. In our experience the distrust of parents and parental figures, the depression, the poorly formed ego structure which lead to their antisocial behaviour have deep roots and are not easily changed. Perhaps with more experience and with a better selected group of patients we will obtain better results.

Not infrequently the physician is consulted by parents or students themselves for help in correcting poor study habits or to help reduce the panic some students suffer from before and during examinations. More and more educators, both civilian and military, are becoming interested in the use of hypnosis to facilitate learning and to aid recall of material already learned. Farina (28) working in a university setting with groups of eight students of relatively similar age, aptitude and education found that hypnotic suggestion improved their capacity to learn more quickly. The suggestions were directed toward helping concentration and memory. He observed improvement in all but one case. As far as he could judge, beneficial results could not be correlated with the depth of hypnosis which had been induced, nor was the improvement persistent in every case.

Over the years we have helped many students at the university level to pass their examinations and in some cases to win the top graduating awards. This was done almost without exception through the use of hypnosis, not alone but within the framework of the total therapy. The more one uses this method in pedagogy the more one is impressed with the many ramifications involved in the process of helping these students. One student who comes to mind told us that the therapy was working very well and that he was passing his final medical examinations very well but was rather afraid of the last one. He asked if it would not be wise for him to spend the night before his last examination in a local hotel to get a good night's rest as there were too many distractions in his own home. We agreed, but were disturbed to learn later the next day that he had slept right through the morning and missed this last important examination for his medical degree. It was, of course, necessary to work through this apparent accident and find the cause. Under hypnosis it was found that on getting his degree it was arranged that he would announce his engagement to a young lady he had been going out with for a number of years. He was quite ambivalent about her and this was the real reason he sought help in the first place to help him pass his examinations. As he admitted later, he thought hypnosis would not help and that in the end he would find a way to break his engagement. When the therapy did help him pass his tests, he unconsciously manipulated the situation so that he would fail his last one in order to avoid becoming engaged. Further therapy resolved the problem. He graduated after taking the supplemental examination, then married the same girl. When last heard from several years ago, he was doing well.

In chronic and hopeless diseases such as disseminated sclerosis and cancer, the physician's ability to carry these patients through their travail taxes not only his therapeutic resourcefulness but also his general ability to deal with human suffering. Hypnosis has been used as a tool of general psychotherapy in some of these cases with gratifying results (106).

We have reported in some detail such treatments in two cases of carcinoma which may be considered as representative of this group of patients (105). Hypnosis may contribute to the patient's comfort, not only in the terminal stages of the disease but also during any time starting at the point when the patient is informed of his malignancy. Morphis (76) assists the patient in accepting the diagnosis through the use of hypnosis. As a radiologist and radium therapist he helps his patients to tolerate better the radium needles inserted in the malignant area through the use of the same modality. Finally, he uses it to help control the nausea and vomiting associated with radiation therapy. Butler (11), in his detailed study of the subject, finds hypnosis very helpful in the care of the cancer patient. Conn (14), using this method, reports that this type of patient is relieved from distress for varying periods of time. In his experience, hypnotherapy substantially reduces the need for narcotics and keeps the patient comfortable and free from anxiety.

Shapiro and Kline (87) have used hypnosis in evaluating the physiologic and psychologic components in the functional impairment of the patient with disseminated sclerosis. Psychologic data were used to formulate a mechanism whereby the patient's hypnotically altered perception and conception of his damaged body image served as a means of reducing anxiety and depression and in this way improved his performance. Ambrose (6) treated six such patients under hypnosis with a resulting marked subjective improvement. His aim is to put the patient more in control of his organism. He believes that while the nature of the illness prevents the clinician from "feeling scientific in his approach to these cases," nevertheless, much subjective improvement is possible with the use of hypnosis.

We are in accord with the findings of these investigators. In a series of eleven cases of disseminated sclerosis treated with hypnosis as a part of the total therapy in private practice, the results were somewhat impressive but hardly consistent. A married woman, twenty-two years of age with one child aged two, had been confined to her bed for seven months with disseminated sclerosis when we were first asked to see her.   She was treated at the hypnotic level weekly for the next sixteen years, during which time, though bed-ridden, she gave birth to two healthy children.   She died nineteen years from the time of the first consultation.

A young executive committed suicide a little short of five years from the time we made the original diagnosis of disseminated sclerosis.   It seemed as if hypnotherapy was helpful in allowing this patient to carry on his business duties from his bedside during these years, but the suicide note revealed that while hypnotic sessions were "helpful" in enabling him to carry on, nevertheless he could see that he was "deteriorating" organically and could carry on no longer.   Another young man suffering from this disease requested hypnotherapy.   He was convinced from his reading on the subject that he could be cured through hypnosis.   He was intelligent and determined to succeed.   Unhappily, he could not be hypnotized, at least not by us, and after six attempts during a period of a month, he did not return.   The impression gained in this instance was that the patient was intent and desperate in helping himself, which allowed for very little outside help.

In contrast to the others, a bright young business man aged twenty-seven, who suffered from the most acute and fulminating type of disseminated sclerosis we have seen, appears to be doing very well indeed.   When first seen one and a half years after the onset of partial blindness, deafness, ataxia, with motor and sensory changes of a marked order, he responded so well to hypnotherapy that the diagnosis of disseminated sclerosis was suspect.   However, the diagnosis was made and confirmed on several occasions at two of the best Neurological Institutes on the continent and appears to be borne out in that five years after his hypnotherapy, while he has no subjective symptoms of any kind, physical examination still reveals the presence of nystagmus, migrating sensory changes, weak-ness in various muscle groups and altered superficial reflexes.   Dur-ing these seven years, up to the present time, he has been working full time and has had no return of the symptoms experienced dur-ing the first year and a half of his illness before hypnosis was used. The prognosis for a patient with this type of onset, as recorded in various neurological textbooks, is from two to three years.

To us, the important factor in making this patient comfortable was the use of hypnosis to allow him to ventilate his fear of the situation and its probable outcome. We have never seen a patient so able to hide his overwhelming fear with such an outward attitude of nonchalance. This attitude impressed his physicians in the hospitals as well as his relatives and friends. Under hypnosis, with his defenses down, his fear was of remarkable intensity. Surely it must have affected the functioning of the total organism. By means of dissociation, reassurance, allowing a marked degree of dependence in the hypnotic relationship which would have been intolerable in the waking state, he was able to reorganize himself within the first month of treatment. In the subsequent years he received no therapy. It would seem that what had been done for him within the first month allowed the condition to become "self-healing." The problem of helping these patients with hypnosis is worth further investigation.

The physician is called upon occasionally to help the patient recall amnesic material. Hypnosis, at times, may be the only tool capable of recovering this material. For example, a pilot who crashed with many passengers aboard his plane could not remember anything that happened for a moment or two before the crash. The Board of Inquiry ruled that the accident was the result of human error and his commercial license was suspended. He was sorely troubled not only by the loss of his license but also by his inability to remember just what had happened to cause the crash. Innumerable visits to numerous physicians and psychiatrists were unsuccessful and only helped to confuse his memory of what really occurred. Intravenous sodium amytal and sodium pentothal gave no additional information.

He was first seen two years after the accident. By this time his license was reinstated and he was working for a secondary type of carrier, as he put it, "hardly the cream of a job for a first class pilot." Using hypnosis, the cause of the accident was found on the first visit. The second visit was used to check on the findings and the third and last visit was on a non-hypnotic level to share with him what his future work should be.

On his first visit he was asked to hallucinate a frightening situation. This he did by visualizing a giraffe. Another more alarming situation was hypnotically suggested and this time he was able to see a man on an old fashioned bicycle with a very large front wheel. When asked what was so frightening about the man on the bicycle he answered, "Hell, it's so easy for him to fall off." When similarly questioned about the giraffe he said that the head of the animal was so high up in the air it made him dizzy. He was then asked to relive the last few minutes prior to the accident with all the attending emotions. This was unsuccessful as he was able to relive the experience only up to the point of his amnesic period. This is what had happened in all his previous interviews. It was then suggested that he could dissociate himself into two people, one the man piloting the plane and the other an observer to see what the pilot was doing wrong. This technique was successful. At first he, as the observer, could not see what the pilot was doing as he was too far back of him. He was apparently afraid to see what was happening. An urgent, authoritative command was then given to move quickly into a position which would give him a full view of the operation. He broke out into a sweat, not only all over his face and chin but also on the back of his hands. A hand was placed gently and reassuringly on his shoulder and he was told that it was perfectly all right for him to report what he saw. "He's going down too low! He doesn't know how to read the altimeter!" By this time the patient was very upset. Suggestions for relaxation and reorganization of the "two" individuals was given and then he was awakened and asked to report for the second interview. No comment was made of what had been revealed at the interview. He was allowed to handle the material as he wished; to forget it, deny it, or to synthesize it.

The second interview showed that he had decided to synthe-size it and the session was used to find out why he had chosen to forget the cause of the accident in the past. It became clear that he had no intention of "forgetting the cause" but a series of events immediately following the crash initiated by well-meaning col-leagues at the scene and at the hospital led him to believe that he was not responsible. Their leading questions and suggestions directed at absolving him from blame acted like hypnotic suggestions while he was in a state of shock and vulnerable to a non-critical acceptance of suggestions which would make life easier for him. It was this conflict which made him seek out so many doctors to relieve him from his guilts.

The third session consisted of a heart-to-heart talk about what had happened and why. It was pointed out to him that since the accident he had fears, unconscious at least, of height differentials as brought out by his hallucination of a giraffe and a man on an old-fashioned bicycle which would not be cause for alarm in an ordinary individual. He admitted this concern but thought he would get over it as time went on. "We are proud bastards," he said. "Flying a desk" held no interest for him. It is most difficult to reorient such an individual in such circumstances. Perhaps it could have been done with ordinary psychotherapy over a period of time, but here again, one would need his co-operation and acceptance of the goal, which we were unable to do.

Another case of amnesia which a generalist may be confronted with in one of his regular patients may serve as an example. This business man, aged sixty, whom we had treated on and off for many years for ordinary medical conditions, came to the office in a state of emergency. He had been to another city in charge of a sales promotion project. In a morning session he had instructed his men what they were to do that day, and outlined his own plans for the day. At the evening meeting his men brought in their reports, but he could not remember what he had done all that day. His men reminded him of what he had planned to do. That he had done what he had planned was verified by telephone calls, but in spite of them he could not remember that he partook in any of them.

Review of his service in the war as a Colonel in the Army revealed no trauma which could account for the present lapse of memory. All avenues of questioning were non-productive. Under hypnosis he was asked to relive his experiences of the day in question and through time distortion it could be done quickly. It was with considerable embarrassment that he revealed the cause of his upset. He was driving through the countryside with a prospective customer when suddenly the scenery brought to mind a traumatic incident of his early adolescence. A farmer's son with very few friends, he had often experimented sexually with the animals on the farm. Though he was now a grandfather and relatively impotent, he began to have a strong urge to re-enact his youthful explorations. He got out of the car and told his friend he would like to walk the rest of the way and that he would meet him again that evening. He apparently carried out his explorations, and in the attempt to hide them from the others in the group he was unable to be selective in his suppression and as a result suppressed everything he had done that day. Aside from his embarrassment as a result of bringing up this material, he was quite relieved to fill in the amnesic period and left the office feeling considerably better. It is not intended to suggest that hypnotherapy alters the ego structure of these individuals. Hypnosis was used here for limited goals only.

The era in which problems related to the integration of psychiatry with other disciplines of medicine were largely confined to psychiatric consultation is on the wane. In the development of the emphasis on comprehensive medicine, the psychiatric approach has infiltrated into the working environment of all disciplines of medicine, extending the frontiers of issues which theretofore were given fewer opportunities for testing and solution (38). With the new psychosomatic orientation, it is conceivable that with added training, the physician may understand better the broad patterns of human motivation and personality development, its adaptations and its maladaptations. He will be able to recognize anxiety and frustration, depression and agitation in their many forms of expression and become as familiar with the neuroses as he is with bacteria. In this way he may be in a better position to use psychotherapy adequately, basing it on the emotional conflicts underlying the disorders he treats.

Where applicable, he may use hypnosis as a psychologic scalpel to cut through the patient's emotional resistances while probing for causative factors. He may then use hypnosis as a psychologic microscope to bring into brilliant focus material which might otherwise appear hazy and confused. And finally, hypnosis may be used as a psychologic suture to hold together the interpretations and suggestions made for the personality reorganization and adjustment. Posthypnotic suggestions given to the patient so that he may carry on what had been started in the hypnotic state can be compared to the prescription for medicine which the patient takes home with him. It must be emphasized, however, that the physician who uses hypnosis in this way must be no less trained in the use of the psychologic scalpel than in the use of the surgical scalpel, no less experienced in the use of the psychologic microscope than in the use of the optical microscope and no less dextrous in handling the psychologic suture than the surgical suture. Used in this way, hypnosis may be a valuable multi-functional instrument in the kit of the generalist and internist. With it, they may add speed and directness to their therapy.

The excellent controlled studies of Borland and Epstein (10) point up the paradox which exists at the present time for those who use hypnosis in fields other than psychiatry and psychology. While their work involved dentists only, their findings are applicable to a degree to physicians. They studied the personality characteristics of seventeen dentists who employed hypnosis in their practice and used a similar number and equivalent grouping of dentists who did not use hypnosis. They came to the conclusion that "dentists who are well adjusted, who are relatively satisfied with themselves, and who obtain satisfaction from the conventional practice of their profession, do not tend to use hypnosis or to become interested in its use. It is as if they do not need such an additional and unusual source of gratification." They go on to say that: "There is a place for hypnosis in dentistry in carefully selected instances. Our concern, like that of medicine, is for well-trained, qualified dentists who have a knowledge of psychodynamics to use hypnosis only in performance of dental treatment, and who are qualified to recognize patients whose personality is such as to make them unsafe subjects for hypnosis."

The paradox lies in the situation as determined by these authors that dentists who are not well adjusted and self-accepting seem to require some extraordinary activity or interest to satisfy their own personal needs. Since hypnosis has been found valid and useful by the British Medical Association, by the American Medical

Association, by the Committee on Therapy of the American Psychiatric Association, as well as other responsible groups, it seems strange but true, that some physicians use it as an "extraordinary activity." The authors came to the conclusion that it was not hypnosis per se that was at fault, but rather: "Perhaps it would be more useful to look at the ways hypnosis was learned by the people who use it. The hypnosis users in general, learned hypnosis in a commercial one-to-three day seminar which had no university sanction." This seems to be the crux of the matter. The vast majority of dentists included in the study had taken one or more of these short commercial courses. This would immediately separate them out from the type of physician who is more stable and mature and who prefers to receive his training in hypnosis under university or hospital auspices, just as he had received his original medical education.

There is good reason to believe that the paradoxical situation described above will peter out as more universities and hospitals teach the use of hypnosis at the post-graduate level. At the time of this writing, seven American Universities are giving year-round post-doctoral courses in hypnosis in a clinical setting. Additionally, such a continuous course is also being given by the Society for Clinical and Experimental Hypnosis through its Institute For Research in Hypnosis under an absolute Charter granted by the Board of Regents of the University of the State of New York.

In our opinion, the statement made by the Committee on Therapy of the American Psychiatric Association that "hypnosis is a specialized psychiatric procedure," needs some clarification. As Kline (54) and Watkins (114) point out, hypnosis is not a psychiatric technique, in fact it is not a technique at all, but a psychological condition which is both state and relationship. Under such a state it is often possible to apply various psychotherapeutic and medical procedures more effectively. Since its ramifications extend into all the biological and social sciences, it cannot be the exclusive property of psychiatry, psychology or any other single discipline. Psychiatry and psychology, by their very nature, will assuredly occupy a position of scientific leadership in exploring and controlling this useful phenomenon but we do not believe that a single specialty will assign itself the task of supervising all others. Wherever psychotherapy has been demonstrated to be important in the treatment, hypnotherapy has a potential contribution to make.

As more universities start teaching all aspects of hypnosis, more physicians will use it, not as an "extraordinary activity," but as just another conventional medical tool, without fanfare and without a special kind of gratification different from the usual gratification resulting from the normal practice of modern medicine (100).

REFERENCES

1. ABRAMSON, H. A.: Pseudoallergic schizophrenia: a new clinical entity. *Trans. Acad. Psychosom. Med.,* 30-43, 1958.
2. ALEXANDER, F.: Psychological aspects of medicine. *Psychosom. Med., 1*:7-18, 1939.
3. ALEXANDER, F.: Emotional factors in essential hypertension. *Psychosom. Med., 1*:175, 1939.
4. ALEXANDER, F.: Psychoanalytic study of a case of essential hypertension. *Psychosom. Med., 1*:140, 1939.
5. ALVAREZ, W. C.: *Nervousness, Indigestion and Pain.* New York, Paul B. Hoeber, Inc., 1943.
6. AMBROSE, G.: Multiple sclerosis and treatment by hypnotherapy. *J. Clin. & Exper. Hyp., 3*:203-209, 1955.
7. American Psychiatric Association: Regarding hypnosis: a statement of position. *A.P.A. Pamphlet,* Feb. 15, 1961.
8. AUERBACK, A. and GLIEBE, F. A.: Iatrogenic heart disease. *J.A.M.A., 129*:338, 1945.
9. BINGER, C. A. *et al.*: Personality in Arterial Hypertension. *Psychosomatic Medicine Monographs Series,* New York, 1945.
10. BORLAND, L. R. and EPSTEIN, S.: Psychological evaluation of hypnosis in dentistry. *J. Am. Dent. Assoc., 62*:54-65, 1961.
11. BUTLER, B.: The use of hypnosis in the care of the cancer patient. *Cancer, 7*:1-14, 1954.
12. CANNON, W. B. *et al.*: Glycosuria. *Am. J. Physiol., 29*:280, 1911.
13. COHEN, M. H.: The advantage of the use of hypnosis in the Ridley operation for cataract. To be published in *Psychosomatics.*
14. CONN, J. H.: Panel discussion, New York State Soc. Anesthesiologists. Dec. 11, 1959.
15. CRASILNECK, H. B. and HALL, J. A.: Physiological changes asso-

ciated with hypnosis: a review of the literature since 1948. *Int. J. Clin. & Exper. Hyp.*, 7:9-50, 1959.

16. DAVIS, D. B. and BICK, J. W.: Skin reactions observed under wartime stress. *J. Nerv. & Ment. Dis.*, 5:503, 1946.

17. DORCUS, R. M. and GOODWIN, P.: The treatment of patients with the dumping syndrome by hypnosis. *J. Clin. & Exp. Hyp.*, 3:200-202, 1955.

18. DORCUS, R. M. and KIRKNER, F. J.: The control of hiccoughs by hypnotic therapy. *J. Clin. & Exper. Hyp.*, 3:104-108, 1955.

19. DORFMAN, W.: Comprehensive medicine. *Psychosomatics*, 1:246, 1960.

20. DRAKE, F. R.: The iatrogenic factors in illness. *Am. J. M. Sc.*, 215:104, 1948.

21. DUNBAR, H. F.: *Emotions and Bodily Changes*. New York, Columbia University Press, 1938.

22. DUNBAR, H. F.: Psychic factors in cardiovascular disease. *New York State J. Med.*, 36:423, 1935.

23. DUNCAN, C. H. et al.: Life situations, emotions, and paroxysmal arrhythmias. *Psychosom. Med.*, 12:23-37, 1950.

24. Editorial: The art of medicine. *J.A.M.A.*, 175:898-899, 1961.

25. EICHORN, R. and TRACKTIR, J.: The relationship between anxiety, hypnotically induced emotions and gastric secretions. *Gastroenterology*, 29:422-431, 1955.

26. EICHORN, R. and TRACKTIR, J.: The effects of hypnotically induced emotions upon gastric secretions. *Gastroenterology*, 29:432-438, 1955.

27. ERICKSON, M. H.: The therapy of a psychosomatic headache. *J. Clin. & Exper. Hyp.*, 1:2-7, 1953.

28. FARINA, O.: Hypnosis in pedagogy. *Revista Psicol. Norm. e Patol.*, 6:303-360, 1960.

29. FENICHEL, O.: *The Psychoanalytical Theory of Neurosis*. New York, W. W. Norton & Company, 1945.

30. FERENCZI, S.: *Theory and Technique of Psychoanalysis*. New York, Boni and Liveright, 1927.

31. FOLIN, O. et al.: Glycosuria. *J. Biol. Chem.*, 17:519, 1914.

32. FRENCH, T. and ALEXANDER, F.: Psychogenic Factors in Bronchial Asthma. *Psychosomatic Medicine Monograph Series*, 1941.

33. GANTT, W. H.: Experimental Basis for Neurotic Behaviour. *Psychosomatic Medicine Monographic Series*, vols. 3 and 4, 1944.

34. GENDEL, B. R. and BENJAMIN, J. E.: Psychogenic factors in the etiology of diabetes. *New England J. Med.*, 234:556, 1948.

35. GORTON, B. E.: Physiologic aspects of hypnosis. In Schneck, J. M.: *Hypnosis in Modern Medicine*, 2nd Edition. Springfield, Thomas, 1959.

36. GRAHAM, D. T.: The pathogenesis of hives: experimental study of life situations, emotions and cutaneous vascular reactions. *Research. Nerv. & Ment. Dis. Proc.*, 29:987-1009, 1950.

37. GRANT, R. T. *et al.*: Observations on urticaria provoked by emotions, by exercise and by warming the body. *Clin. Sc.*, 2:253-272, 1936.

38. GREENHILL, M. H. and KILGORE, S. R.: Principles of methodology in teaching the psychiatric approach to medical house officers. *Psychosom. Med.*, 12:38-48, 1950.

39. GRINKER, R. R. and SPIEGEL, J. P.: *War Neuroses in North Africa, The Tunisian Campaign*. New York, Josiah Macy Jr. Foundation, 1943.

40. GROEN, J.: Psychogenesis and psychotherapy of ulcerative colitis. *Psychosom. Med.*, 9:151-173, 1947.

41. GUILD, J.: Hypnosis for tinnitus. *Canad. M. A. J.*, 78:426-427, 1958.

42. HALLIDAY, J. L.: Psychological factors in rheumatism: preliminary study. *Brit. Med. J.*, 1:213-264, 1937.

43. HALLIDAY, J. L.: Psychological aspects of rheumatoid arthritis. *Proc. Roy. Soc. Med.*, 35:455, 1942.

44. HARDING, H. C.: Hypnosis and migraine or vice versa. *Northwest Med.*, 168-172, Feb., 1961.

45. HINKLE, L. E. and WOLF, S.: Experimental study of life situations, emotions, and the occurrence of acidosis in a juvenile diabetic. *Am. J. Med. Sc.*, 217:130-135, 1949.

46. HOCH, P. H.: The problem of schizophrenia in experimental psychiatry. In Hoch, P. H. and Zubin, J.: *Experimental Psychopathology*. New York, Grune and Stratton, 205-217, 1957.

47. HOPKINS, J. G. *et al.*: Urticaria provoked by heat or psychic stimuli. *Arch. Dermatol. & Syph.*, 38:419-422, 1938.

48. IKEMI, Y. *et al.*: Psychosomatic aspects of gastrointestinal disorders. *Int. J. Clin. & Exp. Hyp.*, 7:139-150, 1959.

49. JOHNSON, A. *et al.*: Preliminary report on a psychosomatic study of rheumatoid disease. *Psychosom. Med.*, 9:295-299, 1947.

50. KAYWIN, L.: Emotional factors in urticaria. *Psychosom. Med.*, 9:131-136, 1947.

51. KLINE, M. V.: Situational cardiovascular symptomatology and hypnosis. *Brit. J. Med. Hyp.*, 1:33-36, 1950.

52. KLINE, M. V.: *Freud and Hypnosis.* New York, The Julian Press, Inc., 1958.
53. KLINE, M. V.: The value and limitation of hypnosis in psychotherapy: two clinical illustrations. *Int. J. Clin. & Exper. Hyp., 8*:263-268, 1960.
54. KLINE, M. V.: Personal Communication, March, 1961.
55. LIFSHITZ, K. and BLAIR, J. H.: Polygraphic recording of a repeated hypnotic abreaction with comments on abreactive psychotherapy. *J. Nerv. & Ment. Dis., 130*:246-252, 1960.
56. LINDEMANN, E.: Psychiatric aspects of the conservative treatment of ulcerative colitis. *Arch. Neurol. & Psychiat., 53*:322, 1945.
57. McDERMOTT, N. T. and COBB, S. A.: A psychiatric survey of 50 cases of bronchial asthma. *Psychosom. Med., 1*:203, 1939.
58. MALMO, R. B., BOAG, T. J. and RAGINSKY, B. B.: Electromyographic study of hypnotic deafness. *J. Clin. & Exper. Hyp., 2*:305-317, 1954.
59. MALMO, R. B., BOAG, T. J. and RAGINSKY, B. B.: Electromyographic study of hypnotic deafness. In Reed, C. F., Alexander, I. E. and Tompkins, S. S.: *Psychopathology, A Source Book.* Cambridge, Harvard University Press, pp. 243-257, 1958.
60. MARCHESI, C.: The hypnotic treatment of bronchial asthma. *Brit. J. Med. Hyp., 1*:14-19, 1949.
61. MEARES, A.: *Shapes of Sanity: A Study in the Therapeutic Use of Modelling in the Waking and Hypnotic State.* Springfield, Thomas, 1960.
62. MEARES, A.: *A System of Medical Hypnosis.* Philadelphia, W. B. Saunders Company, 1960.
63. MELDMAN, M. J.: Personality decompensation after hypnotic symptom suppression. *J.A.M.A., 173*:359-361, 1960.
64. MELLOR, N. H.: Hypnosis in juvenile delinquency. *G. P., 22*:83-87, 1960.
65. MENNINGER, W. C. and KEMP, J. E.: Psychogenic urticaria. *J. Allergy, 6*:467, 1935.
66. MENNINGER, W. C.: Psychosomatic medicine. *Psychosom. Med., 9*:92, 1947.
67. MENNINGER, W. C.: *Psychiatry in a Troubled World.* New York, Macmillan, 1948.
68. MENNINGER, W. C.: Psychological factors in the etiology of diabetes mellitus. *J. Nerv. & Ment. Dis., 81*:1, 1935.
69. MEYER, A. *et al.*: Correlation between emotions and carbohydrate

metabolism in two cases of diabetes mellitus. *Psychosom. Med., 7*:335-341, 1945.

70. MIRSKY, I. A.: Emotional factors in the patient with diabetes mellitus. *Bull. Menninger Clin., 12*:187, 1948.

71. MITCHELL, J. H., CURRAN, C. A. and MYERS, A.: A method of approach to psychosomatic problems in allergy. *W. Virginia J. Med., 42*:271-279, 1946.

72. MITTLEMANN, B. and WOLFF, H. G.: Emotions and gastroduodenal functions. *Psychosom. Med., 4*:5, 1942.

73. MOODY, H.: An evaluation of hypnotically induced relaxation for the reduction of peptic ulcer symptoms. *Brit. J. Med. Hyp., 5*:23, 1953.

74. MOSCHCOWITZ, E.: The biology of Graves' disease. *J. Mt. Sinai Hosp., 12*:828-832, 1945.

75. MOSS, C. S.: A forced hynoprojective fantasy used in the resolution of pseudo-epileptic seizures. *J. Clin. & Exper. Hyp., 5*: 59-66, 1957.

76. MORPHIS, O. L.: Hypnosis, an adjunct in the treatment of malignancy. *Trans. Acad. Psychosom. Med.,* New York, 1958.

77. PORTIS, S. A.: Idiopathic ulcerative colitis. *J.A.M.A., 139*:208-213, 1949.

78. SAUL, L. J. and BERNSTEIN, G., JR.: The emotional settings of some attacks of urticaria. *Psychosom. Med., 3*:349-369, 1941.

79. SCHNECK, J. M.: A note on the hostility component in pathological blushing. *Psychosomatics, 1*:330, 1960.

80. SCHNECK, J. M.: Hypnoanalytic study of a patient with extrasystoles. *J. Clin. & Exper. Hyp., 1*:11-17, 1953.

81. SCHNECK, J. M.: Psychogenic cardiovascular reaction interpreted and successfully treated with hypnosis. *Psychoanalytic Rev., 35*:14, 1948.

82. SCHROEDER, H. and RAGINSKY, B. B.: Uber die Harnsaureausscheidung durch den Darm und ihre pharmakologische Beeinflussung. *Arch. fur Exper. Path. und Pharmak., 168*:413-423, 1932.

83. SCHULTZ, J. H.: The problems of "hypnotic leucotomy." *Z. Psychotherap. med. Psychol., 4*:150-162, 1954.

84. SCHWARTZ, I.: Personal communication. January, 1960.

85. SCHWARTZ, I.: Personal communication. Dec. 10, 1960.

86. SEITZ, P. F. D.: Experiments in substitution of symptoms by hypnosis. *Psychosom. Med., 15*:405-424, 1953.

87. SHAPIRO, A. and KLINE, M. V.: The use of hypnosis in evaluating the physiological and psychological components in the functional impairment of the patient with multiple sclerosis. *J. Clin. & Exper. Hyp., 4*:69-78, 1956.

88. SHIRES, E. B., PETERS, J. H. and KROUT, R. M.: Hypnosis in neuromuscular re-education. *U. S. Armed Forces Med. J., 5*:1519-1523, 1954.

89. SIMONS, D. J. *et al.*: Experimental studies on headache; muscles of scalp and neck as sources of pain. *Research Nerv. & Ment. Dis. Proc., 23*:228-244, 1943.

90. SLOANE, R. B.: Recent trends in psychiatric management. *Canad. M. A. J., 83*:1084-1088, 1960.

91. STEVENSON, I. P. *et al.*: Life situations, emotions and extrasystoles. *Psychosom. Med., 11*:257-272, 1949.

92. STOKES, J. H. *et al.*: Effect on the skin of emotions and nerves. Etiologic background of urticaria with special reference to psycho-neurogeneous factors. *Arch. Derm. & Syph., 31*:470, 1935.

93. SULZBERGER, M. B. and WOLF, J.: *Dermatologic Therapy in General Practice.* 3rd ed., p. 196. Chicago, The Year Book Publishers, 1948.

94. RAGINSKY, B. B.: Hypnotism and its relation to anesthesia. *J. Conn. State Med. Assoc., 2*:11-20, 1938.

95. RAGINSKY, B. B.: Psychosomatic medicine: its history, development and teaching. *Am. J. Med., 5*:857-878, 1948.

96. RAGINSKY, B. B.: Mental suggestion as an aid in anesthesia. *Anesthesiology, 9*:472-480, 1948.

97. RAGINSKY, B. B.: Some psychosomatic aspects of general anesthesia. *Anesthesiology, 11*:391-408, 1950.

98. RAGINSKY, B. B.: Pre-anesthetic management of the dental patient. *J. Am. Dent. Assoc., 49*:672-683, 1954.

99. RAGINSKY, B. B.: Psychosomatic dentistry. *J. Canad. Dent. Assoc., 20*:479-489, 1954.

100. RAGINSKY, B. B.: On setting up a medical practice. *J. Canad. Assoc. Med. Stud. & Interns, 13*:31-35, 1954.

101. RAGINSKY, B. B.: A consideration of the new tranquilizing drugs and hypnosis for the dentist. *New York J. Dent., 27*:297-306, 1957.

102. RAGINSKY, B. B.: Discussion of Bergler's paper: Psychoprophylaxis of post-partum depression. 4th Ann. Meeting, Academy of Psychosom. Med., Chicago, Oct. 17, 1957.

103. RAGINSKY, B. B.: Psychosomatics, pharmacology, premedication and hypnosis in dentistry. *Ann. Dent., 17*:6-19, 1958.

104. RAGINSKY, B. B.: Temporary cardiac arrest induced under hypnosis. *Int. J. Clin. & Exper. Hyp., 7*:53-68, 1959.

105. RAGINSKY, B. B.: Hypnosis in internal medicine. In Schneck, J. M.: *Hypnosis in Modern Medicine,* 2nd Edition. Springfield, Thomas, 1959.

106. RAGINSKY, B. B.: The use of hypnosis in internal medicine. *Int. J. Clin. & Exper. Hyp., 8*:181-197, 1960.

107. RAGINSKY, B. B.: The use of plasticine in hypnoanalysis (hypnoplasty). Presented at the Third World Congress of Psychiatry, Montreal, June 4-10, 1961. To be published.

108. ROSEN, H. and LIDZ, T.: Emotional factors in the precipitation of recurrent diabetic acidosis. *Psychosom. Med., 11*:211-215, 1949.

109. ROSEN, H.: Hypnosis, applications and misapplications. *J.A.M.A., 172*:683-687, 1960.

110. RUBIN, S. and BOWMAN, K. M.: Electroencephalographic and personality correlates in peptic ulcer. *Psychosom. Med., 4*:309-318, 1942.

111. TONKIKH, A. V.: *Problems of Evolution of Physiological Function.* Translated from the Russian, Department of Commerce, U.S.A., 1961.

112. TUCKER, W. I.: Tension headaches. *Lahey Clin. Bull., 7*:47-53, 1950.

113. VAN PELT, S. J.: Hypnotherapy in medical practice. *Brit. J. Med. Hyp., 1*:8-13, 1949.

114. WATKINS, J. G.: Personal communication, March, 1961.

115. WHITE, B. V., COBB, S. and JONES, C. M.: Mucous colitis. National Research Council. *Psychosom. Med. Monographs,* Series *1*:1, 1939.

116. WINN, H.: Brief psychiatric approach for the clinician. *J.A.M.A., 172*:226-228, 1960.

117. WITTKOWER, E.: Studies on the influence of emotions on the functions of organs including observations in normals and neurotics. *J. Ment. Sc., 81*:533, 1935.

118. WOLF, S. and WOLFF, H. G.: *Human Gastric Function.* New York, Oxford University Press, 1943.

119. WOLFE, T. P.: Emotions and organic heart disease. *Am. J. Psychiat., 93*:681-691, 1936.

120. WOLFF, H. G.: Protective reaction patterns and disease. *Ann. Int. Med., 27*:944-969, 1947.

121. WRIGHT, B. A. (Ed.): *Psychology and Rehabilitation.* Washington, D. C., Am. Psychol. Assoc., 1959.

122. WRIGHT, M. E.: Hypnosis and rehabilitation. *Rehab. Lit., 21*:2-12, 1960.

3

HYPNOSIS IN ANESTHESIOLOGY
AND SURGERY

MILTON J. MARMER, M.D., M.SC.MED. (ANES.)

The use of hypnosis as a means of producing analgesia and anesthesia is no longer to be considered an experiment. Many valid reports of operations performed under hypnoanalgesia and hypnoanesthesia have appeared in the medical literature during the last five years (3-20). Virtually every body cavity has been entered and almost every organ operated on. However, as yet, this method has not gained complete acceptance.

Historically, mesmeric anesthesia preceded chemical anesthesia by twenty-one years. In fact, Crawford Long, who first used ether as an anesthetic in surgical operations in 1842, wrote, "At the time I was experimenting with ether, there were physicians, high in authority and of just distinguished character, who were advocates of mesmerism and recommended the induction of the mesmeric state as adequate to prevent pain in surgical operations. Notwithstanding, thus sanctioned, I was an unbeliever in the science and of the opinion that if the mesmeric state could be produced at all, it was only on those with strong imaginations and weak minds and was to be ascribed solely to the workings of the patient's imagination. Entertaining this opinion, I was the more particular in my experiments with etherization" (1).

The first attempts to perform surgery while the patient was in a mesmeric trance, were made in France by Dupotet and Recamier in 1821 (2). Jules Cloquet, in 1829, removed a breast while the patient was in a mesmeric sleep. At the termination of the operation, the woman, sixty-nine years of age, dressed herself, made a curtsy to the surgeon, and went home.

John Elliotson, who had established an enviable reputation as one of the most able physicians in London, had by 1837 participated in many medical sessions with patients under hypnosis, but he was finally asked to resign his post because of alleged charlatanism. According to Elliotson, the first surgical procedure carried out on a mesmerized patient in England, was the insertion of a seton in the neck, in 1838. Four years later, in 1842, a surgeon named Ward performed a mid-thigh amputation on a patient in a mesmeric state. By 1845, James Esdaile, in India, performed a remarkable series of operations on patients who had been hypnotized. The significance of his accomplishment in the use of mesmerism for surgical anesthesia is manifested by the fact that he reported on several thousand operations of which some 300 were major procedures including amputations, removal of scrotal tumors, repairs of hydroceles and removal of cataracts.

The more chemical anesthesia increased in efficiency, the less significant hypnotism became as a means of anesthesia. By 1860, mesmerism and surgery went their separate ways. At the end of the 19th century in England, there was again a revival of interest in hypnotism and it was demonstrated once more that surgical procedures could be performed with the patient in the hypnotized state.

Although, in the past fifteen years, new interest in the uses of hypnosis has become evident, anesthesiologists are as a rule, still more comfortable when they use drugs than when they employ less familiar psychological techniques. However, if physicians understood more clearly what can be expected of hypnosis, I believe that it would be used more widely and effectively as an adjunct to as well as a means of analgesia and anesthesia.

For most individuals, an operation is in the realm of the unknown and is generally associated with a good deal of fear and anxiety. As for anesthesia, this brings forth a feeling of even greater apprehension on the part of the average patient. As anesthesiologists, we are well aware of cardiac and respiratory decompensation and our efforts are primarily concerned with their prevention. Too little consideration has been given to the problem of psychological decompensation. We must be aware of the emotional state of the patient before and after the administration of an anesthetic. Psychic trauma is not recovered from as easily as from the physical effects of anesthesia. It is all too true that the fear of the unknown and loss of consciousness, perhaps recalling a terrifying experience during surgery in early childhood, makes the patient's anticipation of the forthcoming surgery and anesthesia a very harrowing one indeed. As Swerdlow has so aptly stated, "Mere skill in the use of a needle or in handling a gas machine and the ability to carry a patient through a surgical operation successfully does not necessarily make an anesthesiologist" (21). It is not only what drug is given but the way it is administered that is important. Raginsky has stated that a heavily premedicated patient presents a lesser threat to the emotionally insecure anesthetist than does the more wide awake patient (22).

Consider for a moment what happens to an individual when he enters a hospital for a surgical procedure. Hospitalization produces sudden and drastic changes in the patient's life. It is usually an unhappy experience, accompanied by anxiety. Going to a hospital may leave emotional scars which may persist long after physical well being has returned. The hospital is a strange environment where one is exposed to all the stresses which accompany the lack of privacy. The feeling of helplessness and abandonment produces even greater anxiety and apprehension. Operations in early childhood may produce as traumatic effects of these procedures later phobic symptoms and feelings of having been drugged, gassed or suffocated (23). Sleeplessness, restlessness and agitation are among the disturbances in emotional adjustment which have been described after surgery and anesthesia (24).

With children, one hospitalization can undermine a child's whole feeling of security. There is not only the problem of separation from parents which makes the child anxious and unhappy, but the added experience of adjustment to new and strange surroundings. There are strange faces, strange food, a strange bed and a strange routine. The child is subjected to many indignities over which he has no control, such as being undressed and having his clothes removed, having rectal temperatures taken, being fed like a baby and attending to his elimination needs without any privacy.

There is little doubt that psychological factors play an important role in the total surgical response. Relaxation by means of hypnotic suggestion will lower the tension state. It will relieve the oppressing and pounding effect of the emotions on the bodily functions. It will also influence the patient's attitudes and increase his motivation to recover more rapidly. By recognizing the patient's needs and helping him to relax, the patient's morale can be improved and the doctor can motivate him to accept the anesthesiological and surgical-medical regime.

Hypnosis is a valuable addition to the anesthesiologist's armamentarium. To be sure, hypnoanalgesia and hypnoanesthesia will never replace chemical anesthesia. Not all patients can be hypnotized as certainly as they can be anesthetized. Nevertheless hypnosis is a method which is very useful to the practicing anesthesiologist. The indications for the use of hypnosis in anesthesiology are:

1. To overcome fear, apprehension and anxiety in order to reduce the tension associated with the anticipated anesthesia and surgery.

2. For sedation, either in conjunction with or as a substitute for drug medication.

3. To increase patient cooperation and bring about peace of mind.

4. To produce analgesia and anesthesia, thereby reducing the total amount of chemical anesthetic agents used or replacing chemical agents altogether.

5. To make for a more pleasant and more comfortable reaction from anesthesia and surgery.

6. To permit the use of posthypnotic suggestions to aid in the postoperative recovery of the patient by reducing the incidence of postoperative nausea and vomiting and by permitting deep breathing and necessary coughing, thereby helping to reduce postoperative pulmonary complications. Also, to raise the pain threshold and reduce the need for postoperative narcotics, as well as to encourage earlier fluid intake and easier urinary output.

7. To produce operative amnesia.

8. To help establish better postoperative morale and motivate the patient toward getting well.

There is positive evidence that the stress state in man carries with it an increase in suggestibility (25). Yet, the opportunities for the use of hypnosis alone as a total anesthetic for major surgical procedures, have been relatively rare. Pain is not a pure or specific sensation because there are many kinds of pain. It is a result of an integration and abstraction of peripheral stimuli by the central nervous system (26). There is a tremendous variability in the reaction of any given individual to a given painful stimulus. In general there are three methods of relieving pain, namely, by modifying the perception of stimuli at the pain receptor site; by modifying the central perception of pain; and by changing the individual's reaction to pain. Beecher (27) has concluded that analgesic agents exert their principle effect on the reaction component rather than on the original sensation. There is a real difference between awareness of pain and suffering from it. It is possible to feel the pain and yet not be distressed by it. Individuals who can reduce the intensity of their perceptions can tolerate pain well (28). Pain associated with a variety of conditions can be attenuated or eliminated by hypnotic procedures. Hypnotically induced analgesia leaves the individual insensitive to pain by making him indifferent to it. Hypnosis raises the pain threshold and reduces the reaction to painful stimuli. Galvanic skin response to noxious stimuli is diminished and sometimes disappears as a result of hypnoanalgesia and hypnoanesthesia (29).

Ideal anesthesia combines the use of hypnotic techniques with reduced doses of chemical anesthetic agents. All anesthetics are protoplasmic poisons and although there may be minor surgical procedures, there are no minor anesthetic procedures. The smaller the chemical anesthetic and drug dose, the less the depression of the cardiovascular, pulmonary, renal and hepatic systems.

The preoperative use of hypnosis is an excellent method by which to allay fear and prevent psychic trauma. It is a valuable substitute for or adjunct to other means of sedation and can be a pleasant experience involving no tension whatever. Many patients will get their first good night's sleep and the first moment of calm after such an experience.

There is evidence that hypnosis can influence drug effects.

Alcohol, chloral hydrate, morphine and barbital were found to have stronger effects when used in conjunction with hypnosis (27).

For minor procedures or for surgical procedures performed in Emergency Rooms, hypnosis alone has been used to good advantage. Goldie reported on the use of hypnosis in the Casualty Department, where hypnotic techniques were used as an adjunct to or substitute for conventional anesthesia (30). The patients requiring orthopedic treatment and those needing suturing gave the best results with hypnosis. Among the operations performed were the suturing of lacerations, the reduction of fractures and dislocations, removal of foreign bodies, and incision and drainage of abscesses. Hypnosis has been especially useful under these circumstances when the patient has just eaten a heavy meal and requires emergency minor surgery.

Major surgical procedures performed under hypnoanesthesia in recent years have been operations which have not required profound surgical relaxation. Rose reported the use of hypnoanesthesia for abdominal hysterectomy (19). Kroger has done a thyroidectomy (31), and I have been able to repeat this procedure. Mason (11) reported a bilateral mammaplasty during which procedures the patient never showed any sign of pain or distress. At one point she complained of thirst and was given a drink of water while the operation continued. Tonsillectomies on adults were reported performed under hypnosis (17). Crasilneck and coworkers have recommended the use of hypnosis as a method of anesthesia in special surgical procedures where the administration of chemical anesthetics might be undesirable such as repair of the facial nerve, craniotomy for epilepsy and for chemopallidectomy (5, 6). They have also described the successful use of hypnosis in the management of patients with burns. The prolonged care of the burned patient makes for psychological withdrawal and lack of cooperation toward the treatment necessary to overcome the effects of thermal injury.

Hypnosis was successful in effecting prompt relief from pain in a fatally burned patient. In other cases it was used to good advantage in the maintenance of an adequate food intake, active exercise of painful parts, the improvement of the patient's mental attitude and the production of analgesia for the necessary frequent change of surgical dressings. The vicious cycle associated with extensive burns is not only the marked protein deficiency and toxemia from the loss of skin surface, but the excessive loss of appetite, coupled with the increased caloric needs. Starvation leads to a delay in epithelization, leaving open weeping surfaces which loses necessary amino acids and water soluble vitamins. Each general anesthetic given for repeated debridement and attempted skin grafting often leads to further loss of nutriment by the necessary preoperative withholding of food as well as possible postoperative nausea and vomiting. The patient's tolerance to pain diminishes and the subsequent administration of narcotics only serves to augment the anorexia and render the patient more immobile, thereby leading to contractures. Hypnosis has been successfully employed as a method of anesthesia for the debridement of wounds, changes of dressings and for skin grafting. Posthypnotic suggestion in these cases has served well as an analgesic agent to allay postoperative pain and allow for earlier exercise of affected parts. One of the most beneficial results of this method has been in the quantitative increase in food intake and in the correction of inanition. The importance of nutrition in determining the speed of wound healing in these cases is an established fact.

Recently, Kelsey and Baron have reported on the maintenance of posture by hypnotic suggestion in a patient undergoing plastic surgery (9). One of the problems in plastic surgery is the maintenance in apposition of two widely separated areas during the process of transfer of tissue from one area to another. In certain patients, under hypnosis, it is possible to retain them in a fixed position until the suggestion to free them is given. In the case reported, the patient was brought to the Operating Room without premedication and although the authors hoped to perform the operation under hypnoanesthesia, the patient showed evidence of discomfort at the time of incision (despite lack of response to pin prick). Local anesthesia was injected into the skin and the procedure carried out under hypnosis. The upper end of the pedicle was freed from the abdomen and inserted into the left wrist. After the dressing was applied, the patient was given the suggestion to "lock his wrist." He maintained this position for three weeks until it was released at the next operation. At this procedure, one end of the pedicle was inserted into the right foot. The left forearm was then placed in the required position on the dorsum of the right foot and the patient was commanded to "lock it." It was stressed that there would be no postoperative discomfort and that sleep would be normal. During the first three nights, the patient required small doses of sedatives to help him sleep in the sitting position. This position was maintained for twenty-eight days at which time the third procedure was performed, completing the skin graft to the foot by giving the suggestion to "unlock" the wrist. This is a remarkable achievement and opens new vistas in the possible applications of hypnosis in plastic and orthopedic surgery.

In orthopedics, hypnosis has been used to help fearful patients take their first weight bearing steps following operations for fractures. Under hypnosis, many orthopedic patients have demonstrated greater range of motion of extremities than in the waking state (32).

Ruiz and Fernandez (33) described a cataract extraction performed under hypnosis in a patient who had previously required abandonment of the procedure because of sensitivity to all local anesthetic drugs.

In urological practice, hypnotic suggestion has been used with success to facilitate cystoscopic examination and urethral instrumentation. Transurethral prostatectomy can also be performed under hypnosis in selected patients (34).

In proctology, therapeutic suggestion can facilitate the performance of proctoscopy and sigmoidoscopy. Leslie (35) has reported on the benefits to be derived from the use of hypnosis in office practice. Acute abscesses may be drained under similar circumstances. Under the influence of hypnosis and by means of deep relaxation, the anal sphincters may relax and analgesia result. Patients with intense pruritic ani without visible changes in the perianal tissues, may obtain marked relief when they are deeply relaxed and their anxiety dissipated by hypnotic suggestion. Hypnosis has also been of great benefit in aiding the patient's emotional adjustment to colostomy and in teaching him muscular control after the operation (36).

Doberneck *et al.* (8) have reported on the use of hypnosis as an adjunct to surgery. They have used hypnosis in an attempt to overcome the discomfort associated with endoscopic procedures and minor surgical procedures. They have also used it to ease postoperative pain and discomfort of nasogastric tubes, urinary catheters and the administration of necessary intravenous fluids.

The dumping syndrome is a complex problem due to the pressure of undigested food in the jejunum. This syndrome follows gastric resection in a reported incidence which varies from 2 to 45 per cent. In many instances it can be very incapacitating. The symptoms are epigastric distress, sweating, palpitation, diarrhoea, nausea, anorexia, syncope, weakness and food dyscrasias. There is no doubt that the syndrome has an organic basis but there is also a concomitant important psychological overlay as well. The latter factors may be the initiating or exaggerating mechanisms in many patients. With this consideration in mind, Leonard, Papermaster and Wangensteen (37) at the University of Minnesota have used hypnotic suggestion in patients suffering from symptoms which characterize the dumping syndrome. They chose for study, patients with persistent, incapacitating postprandial symptoms of long standing. Hypnotic suggestion was carried out first on an individual basis and then by group therapy. After the first treatment, all patients were improved and symptoms were much less in evidence. Progressive rehabilitation followed with something akin to complete relief after three to five treatments. In all, they reported success with 16 patients resulting in complete or nearly complete relief in each case. They also have employed hypnotic suggestion with complete success in the management of a patient with persistent "phantom limb" pain.

One of the best indications for hypnoanesthesia is in the field of obstetrics and gynecology. When successful this method assures the fact that the delivery will be as easy as possible on the baby, by minimizing the risk of narcosis or unconsciousness. The action of hypnotic suggestion is satisfactory in maintaining analgesia during labor and delivery. Hypnosis has also been reported as successful in the treatment of hyperemesis gravidarum (38). Kroger and DeLee have described the use of hypnoanesthesia for cesarean section and hysterectomy (3). The patient was fully conscious throughout the procedure and watched the delivery of the baby. These authors stress the need for rehearsal of the procedure. There is a difference of opinion as to the need for this aspect of the conditioning process. This operation lends itself well to the performance under hypnoanesthesia because nature has provided a nine months period of abdominal stretching with resultant muscular relaxation.

Hypnosis has been used to good advantage in dental surgery. The primary problems of the dental patient involve the fear, tension and anxiety associated with dental procedures and their effect on pain. Hypnosis has been employed successfully as an analgesic tool in operative dentistry, in exodontic, prosthetic endodontic and periodontic surgery (39). Hypnodontia has a great potential in dentistry (40). Most workers recommend its use as an adjunct to dental analgesia, for example in the insertion of a needle for the administration of a local anesthetic (41). By means of suggestion, the patient experiences no pain or discomfort while the anesthetic drug is being injected. Salivation may be controlled and there is less postoperative discomfort. When analgesia of the mouth can be induced successfully it can be maintained for long periods and the procedure becomes a comparatively pleasant one. Also, it can be quickly reinduced at subsequent visits. Claims are made that dental surgery under hypnoanesthesia may be performed in the presence of a relatively bloodless field. Although this clinical observation has been made, this phenomenon lacks experimental substantiation. The results of a recent study indicate that hypnosis and simple hypnotic suggestion are not correlated with any alterations of bleeding or clotting in normal subjects (42).

A great deal has recently been written on the use of hypnosis in the treatment of pain syndromes. Intractible pain can be successfully controlled during the hypnotic session (43). The problem is not only that of inducing analgesia at the time of the session, but that there be relief from the pain as a result of the posthypnotic suggestion. The more pronounced the organic component, the less effective is the posthypnotic control. On the other hand, pain which is primarily emotionally determined, will be more readily alleviated by hypnotic suggestion. Byron Butler (44) has documented his experiences with the use of hypnosis in the care of the cancer patient. He has recommended the use of recordings to "stand in" for the therapist when he is absent. Hypnotic techniques reduce pain and anxiety with results proportional to the depth of the hypnotic level. Butler has summarized his experiences as follows: "With an expenditure of considerable time, energy and ingenuity, a very sick suffering patient may live his last months of life with a minimum of drugs and a sense of hopefulness and cheerfulness and relative freedom from pain. His mind becomes more acute rather than dulled as with drugs. The rest of his body functions as well as it can without being further inhibited by drug action. He is a rational thinking human until death rather than a vegetating invalid as may happen after a prefrontal lobotomy. He has been supported in the last days of his life by the compassion of his physician rather than let down with drug addiction and destructive surgery. In summary, we have the mind of the patient struggling for survival aided by the mental support of the hypnologist, both fighting a losing battle for in the end cancer and death will win." Cangello has reported similar success with terminal cancer patients (45).

In general, with the use of hypnosis in the treatment of pain, Wolberg (46) has cautioned that, "The trance state revives the subject's feelings about the omniscience of authority and persons with immature personality may satisfy, in the trance state, in fantasy, the dependency need and may thus comply with the suggestions of the hypnotist even to the giving up of the functional pain both in the trance and posthypnotically. When the dependency is sufficiently great, even organic pain may be yielded. In hysterical disorders however, where pain binds great anxiety and serves a protective function, response to hypnotic commands will expose the patient to too great anxiety and he will either resist suggestions, follow commands incompletely, transfer pain to a different locus or if his dependency needs are so impelling as a force him to follow suggestions, the resulting liberated anxiety may provoke dangerous or even psychotic reactions. The key to the use of hypnosis in pain is to understand the dynamic function of the pain for the individual."

What are the practical applications of hypnosis in anesthesiology and how do you decide on which patient you will attempt hypnosis and for which one you will use only chemical anesthesia? The decision for the use of hypnosis is generally made for you by the patient. The patient determines practically everything in hypnosis, unless you are power driven or seeking ego gratification. If, during the preanesthetic interview, the patient is in good physical condition and appears to be calm and relaxed and not frightened of the anticipated procedure, there is no point in undoing it. It is not necessary for an anesthesiologist to prove that he can hypnotize and these patients can be premedicated and anesthetized in the usual way. However, given the same patient, if he is terrified, frightened, extremely anxious and apprehensive about the forthcoming procedure, a good deal of time should be spent with him to try to calm him down. Whether the proposed surgical procedure is a minor or a major one, the effect of anxiety on the patient is the same—tachycardia, hypertension, hyperventillation, sweating, etc. With such an individual hypnosis should be attempted if only to get him to relax and to gain his acceptance of the drugs you want him to have. The mere writing of an order for a barbiturate for sleep does not necessarily insure the fact that the patient will sleep. He may be so agitated that he will fight off whatever sedation could result. This is not to imply that it is incorrect to give premedication to a patient who is visibly upset. On the contrary, I recommend that if you suggest to the patient through hypnosis that he will be more calm and relaxed and you also use premedication drugs, they will be synergistic and the desired good night's rest and sleep will result. In these instances, minimal doses will be effective and in this way, the patient can come to the Operating Room without being overnarcotized. He will arrive in surgery in the optimal physiological and psychological state.

When using hypnosis with these patients you may begin with any induction technique with which you feel most comfortable. I prefer Relaxation Techniques and either elaborate them or shorten them. Although every individual handles anxiety and stress in his own way, the correct psychological approach on the part of the anesthesiologist will go far toward obtunding the psychic trauma and establishing confidence. With this purpose in mind, I have been using with most patients, what I call an Exercise in Relaxation. This is a trial attempt at hypnosis without usually mentioning the term per se, because of the misconception or misinterpretation which often accompanies it. If, during the Relaxing Exercise the patient follows suggestions and a hypnoidal level is reached more suggestion is given in the hope of reaching an even deeper hypnotic level. If this is possible, I take this opportunity to hypnotize the patient in order to take advantage of giving valuable posthypnotic suggestions. Even when it is evident that the hypnoidal level cannot be achieved, this method will help the patient attain some mental and physical relaxation and alleviate much of the anxiety and tension. This technique may be attempted on all patients, but it is most useful in patients who are poor operative risks such as those with cardiorespiratory disease or those scheduled to undergo cardiac surgery. For the patient who is allergic to the commonly used anesthetic drugs, the use of hypnosis for sedation is a boon. In order to make up for lack of time which exists in the preoperative period, a trial attempt at hypnosis can be made and repeated once or twice again if necessary at fifteen or twenty minute intervals. In this way, several patients can be seen and be taken care of without loss of time to the anesthesiologist on his afternoon or evening rounds. It also affords an opportunity of deepening the hypnotic level within a shorter period of time.

It is desirable for each individual to devise his own technique because it must sound natural. If it goes well, and if after induction of relaxation you can induce arm catalepsy for example, it shows that you are well on the way to the induction of hypnosis. Less drugs and less chemical anesthesia will then be needed. The anesthesiologist can be more calm and relaxed about the patient and the patient will be more calm and relaxed about the doctors and the procedure. With such a patient you may be able to suggest many things referable to his postoperative recovery. Therefore, you should continue with hypnosis as far as the patient permits you to go. If you can get the patient to accept the anesthetic procedure with equanimity, you have accomplished a great deal.

Most individuals are suggestible and therefore hypnotizable to some degree. However, less than 10 per cent reach a level of hypnosis deep enough to permit a surgical procedure to be performed without the use of any chemical agents. As previously stated, for minor operative procedures such as incision and drainage, removal of superficial foreign bodies, dental extractions, dilatation and curretage, etc. hypnosis may be very adequate. Also in traumatic injuries such as repair of lacerations or closed reduction of simple fractures, hypnosis alone may accomplish it. However, if the injury is more extensive a good deal more time is required than may be available at the spur of the moment. Superficial debridement may be accomplished with hypnosis, but if the situation involves the open reduction of a fracture, or an abdominal exploration if needed, as with a ruptured spleen, it is extremely doubtful that hypnosis alone would suffice.

In order to use hypnosis as the sole and total means of anesthesia, or at least to use it as the major portion of the anesthetic procedure, generally more time is needed than the night before surgery. It is for this reason that hypnosis can be used successfully with patients who are to undergo cardiac surgery. I like to use hypnosis in these cases because these patients represent the poorest risks. It is common knowledge that a patient with a bad heart is a poor surgical risk. Even more so if that heart is going to be operated on. I try to use hypnosis in these cases because three to five days are usually available preoperatively. If it can be successful, it will be of great benefit to the patient. Anesthesia for patients undergoing cardiac surgery requires the use of the least toxic medication and the lightest plane of anesthesia. In general, all that is needed for anesthesia in cardiac surgery is a combination of analgesia, amnesia and muscular relaxation to provide the surgeon with a quiet operative field to work in. It is well known that deep anesthesia may significantly impair myocardial function. The heart itself is relatively insensitive to painful surgical intervention and little analgesia is required for operations on the heart. The use of hypnosis offers a means of inducing a light plane of anesthesia in the cardiac patient without first exposing him to the hazards of deep anesthesia. Hypnosis is indicated in these patients because it is a method which is extremely effective in overcoming the fear, anxiety and apprehension which accompany the anticipated surgery and anesthesia.

Most of these patients can be hypnotized to some degree, but total and complete anesthesia requires a person capable of reaching a somnambulistic level of hypnosis. During surgery, an intravenous infusion is started in every patient to allow for the administration of fluids, blood or any drug should it be needed to maintain a smooth, safe course of anesthesia. No unnecessary risk is ever taken with any patient. Oxygen is always administered. No patient is exposed to possible noxious reflex action. For example on laryngoscopy, the vocal chords and trachea are sprayed with topical anesthesia to prevent possible laryngeal spasm or vagal arrest during intubation. Endotracheal intubation may not always be as easy in a hypnotized patient as it would be in a totally curarized one. Patients often move. However, this should not interfere with the procedure and the patient generally has no memory of this. After intubation, 100 per cent oxygen only is administered. Patients tolerate the endotracheal tube without difficulty. From time to time small amounts of .2 per cent succinylcholine solution may be added to the intravenous infusion in order to facilitate the surgery by providing a quieter operative field. The maximum total dosage of succinylcholine used in these cases varies between 25 and 50 mgm. Under hypnoanalgesia, minimal amounts of chemical anesthetic agents are needed and under hypnoanesthesia no chemical anesthetic agents are needed for these cases. When the operation is completed the patients are awakened gradually by dehypnotization after appropriate posthypnotic suggestions have been given regarding postoperative comfort and relaxation and the ability to breathe deeply and to cough easily when requested to do so. Response to posthypnotic suggestion has been very satisfactory.

The following case will illustrate the use of hypnosis in cardiac surgery (15):

> A thirty-nine year old woman was hospitalized for mitral commissurotomy. During the previous year she had had several

episodes of cerebral embolization from each of which she recovered. She was interviewed two days prior to surgery and found to be an excellent hypnotic subject. She was able to reach a deep trance level at first induction. She was seen again the next day and hypnosis was reinduced with emphasis on producing anesthesia of the chest wall. She responded very well. The morning of Surgery she was taken to the Operating Room, asleep in response to posthypnotic suggestion. She was given no premedication. She was rehypnotized in the Operating Room in response to a prearranged signal. An intravenous infusion of 5 per cent dextrose in water was begun and 100 mgm. of thiamylal sodium was injected intravenously. Endotracheal intubation was performed with comparative ease after the vocal chords were sprayed with 5 per cent hexylcaine topical solution. Throughout the procedure 100 per cent oxygen was given. To insure that the patient would remain quiet during the first valve fracture 30 mgm. of succinylcholine was given intravenously. The patient was able to open her eyes on command after each attempt at valvular fracture which was performed three times. At the termination of the operation two hours later she was given appropriate posthypnotic suggestions with regard to comfort, relaxation and the ability to breathe deeply and cough adequately. She was then asked to remove the endotracheal tube herself, which she did. She was then taken to the Recovery Room and asked to awaken and she responded immediately. This patient made an uneventful recovery, requiring no narcotic drugs postoperatively.

A surprising finding is the ease with which children respond to hypnosis. It is an excellent method for inducing anesthesia or achieving basal anesthesia in children. These youngsters will be happier, will react better, and have much greater comfort postoperatively. On recovery, these children are quieter, more comfortable and more cooperative than those who undergo anesthesia induced by means of chemical agents alone. Hypnosis may be performed successfully in younger children on occasion, but youngsters between the ages of six and fourteen are usually most amenable to suggestion. In this age group the children make good subjects because of their vivid imaginations and their ability to create a fantasy. If one uses situations with which the child is familiar, better imagery can be produced. If it is possible to have a preliminary rehearsal of the hypnotic induction the afternoon or evening before surgery, it will serve the anesthesiologist well. However, no child should ever be forced into such a situation if he is unwilling. Children admitted in the early morning for surgery, can only be seen in the Operating Room. If light premedication is given so that consciousness is not too clouded the response to suggestion is still possible.

A simple technique of indirect suggestion has proved to be an invaluable aid in inducing anesthesia for tonsillectomy in over 200 cases. It has made induction of anesthesia smoother and has aided in eliminating psychic trauma. At the termination of the surgical procedure posthypnotic suggestions of well being and postoperative comfort are given. These suggestions are usually carried out with a great degree of accuracy. It should always be remembered that suggestions of sleep and drowsiness be removed, and the suggestion to awaken directly or indirectly must be given. Admittedly, hypnosis is not successful in all instances, but where it has been successful, it has proved to be the kindest method of inducing anesthesia in children.

Occasionally, hypnosis can be used alone as a method of anesthesia. For example, a special indication would be the use of hypnosis in the maintenance of anesthesia for the control of post-tonsillectomy hemmorrhage. Recently, I was able to hypnotize a six year old boy suffering from post-tonsillectomy hemmorrhage. He received a transfusion and under hypnosis the surgery for the control of hemmorrhage was performed. The child recovered without any psychic trauma.

Children also respond well to the use of hypnoanalgesia for cardiac surgery. The following case (15) is illustrative:

A ten year old girl was admitted to the hospital for surgical repair of an interatrial septal defect. She was seen two days prior to operation and was able to enter a partial hypnotic trance by means of an image projection technique. The morning of surgery she was given as premedication pentobarbital sodium 50 mgm. and diphenhydramine hydrochloride elixir 4.5 cc. at 6:30 A.M. She was brought to the Operating Room at 7:45 A.M. in a calm relaxed state. At 8:00 A.M. after being placed on the operating table she was rehypnotized in response to a given signal. A catheter was securely placed into the right antecubital vein and 75 mgm. thiamylal sodium injected intravenously. Prior to intubation alphaprodine 10 mgm. and succinylcholine 10 mgm. were also injected intravenously. Endotracheal intubation was performed without difficulty and 100 per cent oxygen administered throughout the procedure. The incision was made at 8:30 A.M. After a right sided thoracotomy was performed, the child was put on cardiac by-pass (pump oxygenator) at 11:27 A.M. The heart was opened at 11:30 A.M. and the interatrial defect was closed with silk sutures within four minutes. During the cardiotomy the child opened and closed her eyes on command. She was taken off the pump oxygenator at 12:00 Noon and the operation was completed at 2:00 P.M. At the end of the procedure suitable posthypnotic suggestions were given and extubation was performed. The child was then awakened and was happy to know that the procedure was completed. She made an uneventful recovery and required minimal amounts of narcotic drugs postoperatively.

One of the greatest assets to be found in utilizing hypnosis in anesthesiology and surgery is in the use of posthypnotic suggestion. Posthypnotic suggestion, which may be successful even in the light states of hypnosis, can be employed to obtund nausea, vomiting and hiccoughing after operations. It may be effective in lessening the patient's response to pain, thereby reducing the need for heavy doses of narcotics. After a chest operation patients can be enabled to breathe deeply and cough up sputum more easily. Patients can be encouraged to earlier intake of fluids and to a greater ease of voiding postoperatively. Patients under hypnosis also are aware of any undue pressures in nonanesthetized areas and will always complain if an arm for example is overstretched, thereby helping avoid such accidents as brachial neuralgias and ulnar neuritis after surgery.

I do not agree with the use of drugs to enhance the opportunity for hypnotizing the patient. If the patient will let me use the drugs, he probably does not need the hypnosis. However, if you use drugs such as intravenous barbiturates to induce anesthesia, then I recommend the use of an hypnotic induction at the same

PROPERTY OF WASHINGTON
SCHOOL OF PSYCHIATRY
LIBRARY

time. Inject more slowly so that the patient can hear you for a longer period of time. Why not take advantage of the situation and tell the patient that he will begin to feel drowsier and drowsier, sleepier and sleepier? The drug will put him to sleep. At the same time he can be told that he will feel fine when he awakens and that he will be well relaxed in the Recovery Room if he goes there. If you think he will be capable of eating lunch, tell the patient he will eat his lunch and retain it. Never suggest that he will NOT vomit. Suppose the patient hears *only* the word vomit, what will happen then? Suggestions to the patient should be given in a positive semantically oriented way at the time of induction of anesthesia. Whether you use intravenous, inhalation or regional anesthesia, use words at the same time!

From all this it would seem that hypnosis is an ideal method of anesthesia for most operations. Why then is it not more widely used? The answer is that although the technical aspects of inducing hypnosis are easy to learn, successful induction and maintenance of hypnoanesthesia and hypnoanalgesia largely depends upon the interaction of many factors in the personalities of the patient and the doctor. These are little understood and many of them are not understood at all. Few of us could guarantee to produce surgical hypnoanesthesia in one in a hundred unselected surgical cases. We have no quick and certain means of determining who the promising subject will be. So then, the primary disadvantage of hypnosis in anesthesia is that not every patient can be hypnotized. For patients who are hostile to the idea or for those who will not listen, nothing can be done.

A very valid disadvantage is the time consumed. It may not always be available to a busy, practicing anesthesiologist. With the average patient one has to spend possibly fifteen to thirty minutes in order to accomplish the basic induction of hypnosis. Even the most favorable case will require an additional four or five hours work before one could feel justified to operate under hypnoanesthesia. There are also technical limitations. The muscular relaxation induced by means of hypnosis can in no way be compared to the profound deep muscular relaxation which can be produced by chemical muscle relaxants in order to meet the demands of the surgeon during a prolonged intraabdominal procedure.

As a precaution, patients who at the time of surgery are undergoing intensive psychotherapy or psychoanalysis, should not be hypnotized for anesthesia without the express permission of the psychiatrist.

Nevertheless, these disadvantages are outweighed by many advantages to be derived. Hypnotic techniques, when used by competent, ethical and skillful anesthesiologists and surgeons in the best interests of their patients and within the limitations of their specialties, will not be involved in complications due to hypnosis. Ideal anesthesia will be achieved by combining hypnotic techniques with safer, smaller doses of chemical anesthetic agents. Hypnosis is an additional useful method to be added to anesthesiological and surgical practice and should be included in the training programs in anesthesiology and surgery.

REFERENCES

1. LONG, C. W.: Account of first use of sulfuric ether by inhalation as an anesthetic in surgical operations. *South M. & S. J. n.s.,* *5*:705-713, 1849.
2. ROSEN, G.: Mesmerism and surgery. *J. Hist. Med., 1*:527-550, 1946.
3. KROGER, W. S. and DeLEE, S. T.: Use of hypnoanesthesia for cesarean section and hysterectomy. *J.A.M.A., 163*:442-443, Feb. 9, 1957.
4. BETCHER, A. M.: Hypno-induction techniques in pediatric anesthesia. *Anesthesiology, 19*:279-281, 1958.
5. CRASILNECK, H. B., McCRANIE, E. J. and JENKINS, M. T.: Special indications for hypnosis as a method of anesthesia. *J.A.M.A., 162*:1606-1608, Dec. 29, 1956.
6. CRASILNECK, H. B. and JENKINS, M. T.: Further studies in the use of hypnosis as a method of anesthesia. *J. Clin. & Exper. Hyp., 6*:152-158, 1958.
7. CRASILNECK, H. B., STIRMAN, J. A., WILSON, B. J., McCRANIE, E. J. and FOGELMAN, M. J.: Use of hypnosis in the management of patients with burns. *J.A.M.A., 158*:103-106, May 14, 1955.
8. DOBERNECK, R. C., GRIFFEN, W. O., PAPERMASTER, A. A., BONELLO, F. and WANGENSTEEN, O. H.: Hypnosis as an adjunct to surgical therapy. *Surgery, 46*:299-304, 1959.

9. KELSEY, A. and BARON, J. H.: Maintenance of posture by hypnotic suggestion in patient undergoing plastic surgery. *Brit. M. J.,* *1*:756-757, 1958.

10. TINTEROW, M. M.: The use of hypnotic anesthesia for major surgical procedure. *Am. Surg., 26*:732-737, 1960.

11. MASON, A. A.: Surgery under hypnosis. *Anesthesia, 10*:295-299, 1955.

12. MARMER, M. J.: The role of hypnosis in anesthesiology. *J.A.M.A., 162*:441-443, Sept. 29, 1956.

13. MARMER, M. J.: Hypnoanalgesia: the use of hypnosis in conjunction with chemical anesthesia. *Anesth. & Analg. Curr. Res., 36*:27-32, 1957.

14. MARMER, M. J.: Hypnosis as an adjunct to anesthesia in children. *A.M.A. J. Dis. Child., 97*:314-317, 1959.

15. MARMER, M. J.: Hypnoanalgesia and hypnoanesthesia for cardiac surgery. *J.A.M.A., 171*:512-517, Oct. 3, 1959.

16. MARMER, M. J.: *Hypnosis in Anesthesiology.* Thomas, Springfield, 1959.

17. MIHALYKA, E. E. and WHANGER, A. D.: Tonsillectomies under hypnosis. *Am. J. Clin. Hyp., 2*:87-88, 1959.

18. RAGINSKY, B. B.: The use of hypnosis in anesthesiology. *Personality, 1*:340-348, 1951.

19. ROSE, A. G.: The use of hypnosis as anesthetic, analgesic and amnesic agent in gynecology. *Brit. J. Med. Hyp., 5*:17-21, 1953.

20. WALLACE, G.: Hypnosis in anesthesiology. *J. Clin. & Exper. Hyp., 7*:129-137, 1959.

21. SWERDLOW, M. and LIPWORTH, M.: The psychological approach in anesthesia. *Anesthesia, 6*:96-99, 1951.

22. RAGINSKY, B. B.: Mental suggestion as an aid in anesthesia. *Anesthesiology, 9*:472-480, 1948.

23. MILLER, M. L.: Traumatic effect of surgical operation in childhood on integrative functions of ego. *Psychoanal. Quart., 20*: 77-92, 1951.

24. LINDEMANN, E.: Observations on psychiatric sequelae to surgical operations in women. *Am. J. Psychiat., 98*:132-139, 1941.

25. BEECHER, H. K.: The measurement of pain. *Pharmacol. Reviews, 9*:59-209, 1957.

26. GERARD, R. W.: Physiology of pain. *Ann. New York Acad. Sc., 86*:6-12, 1960.

27. BEECHER, H. K.: *Measurement of Subjective Responses.* New York, Oxford Univ. Press, 1959.

28. PETRIE, A.: Some psychological aspects of pain and the relief of suffering. *Ann. New York Acad. Sc., 86*:13-27, 1960.
29. WEST, L. J., NEILL, K. C. and HARDY, J. D.: Effects of hypnotic suggestion on pain perception and galvanic skin response. *A.M.A. Arch. Neurol. & Psych., 68*:549-560, 1952.
30. GOLDIE, L.: Hypnosis in the casualty department. *Brit. M. J., 2*: 1340-1342, Dec. 8, 1956.
31. KROGER, W.: Film: *Thyroidectomy Under Hypnoanesthesia,* 1959.
32. CHERRY, A. V.: Reported in *Scope,* April 27, 1960.
33. GOMEZ-RUIZ, O. R. and FERNANDEZ, A.: Hypnosis as an anesthetic in ophthalmology. *Am. J. Ophthalmol., 50*:163, 1960.
34. BODNER, H., HOWARD, A. H., KAPLAN, J. H. and ROSS, S. C.: Hypnosis in office practice, especially in the practice of urology. *Postgrad. Med., 28*:515-518, 1960.
35. LESLIE, L. D.: Hypnosis and its uses in proctology. *Dis. Colon & Rectum, 3*:262-267, 1960.
36. EVERETT, H. E. C.: Reported in *Scope,* April 27, 1960.
37. LEONARD, A. S., PAPERMASTER, A. A. and WANGENSTEEN, O. H.: Treatment of postgastrectomy dumping syndrome by hypnotic suggestion. *J.A.M.A., 165*:1957-1959, Dec. 14, 1957.
38. GIORIANDO, S. W. and MASCOIA, R. F.: The treatment of hyperemesis gravidarum with hypnotherapy. *Am. J. Obst. & Gynec., 73*:444-447, 1957.
39. JACOBY, J. D.: A statistical report on the practical use of hypnosis in dentistry. *J. Clin. & Exper. Hyp., 3*:117-119, 1955.
40. ROSEN, H.: Hypnosis, mental hygiene and the dental hypnotist. *J. Clin. & Exper. Hyp., 5*:101-131, 1957.
41. STOLZENBERG, J.: Psychological preparation of the patient for dental anesthesia. *Dental Items of Interest, 72*:817-820, 1950.
42. CRASILNECK, H. B. and FOGELMAN, M. J.: The effect of hypnosis in blood coagulation. *J. Clin. & Exper. Hyp., 5*:132-137, 1957.
43. ROSEN, H.: The hypnotic and hypnotherapeutic control of severe pain. *Am. J. Psychiat., 107*:917-925, 1951.
44. BUTLER, B.: The use of hypnosis in the care of the cancer patient. *Cancer, 7*:1-14, 1954.
45. CANGELLO, C.: Hypnosis for Terminal Carcinoma. Paper presented at 11th Annual Meeting S.C.E.H., San Francisco, 1959.
46. WOLBERG, L. R.: Hypnotic phenomena. *Problems of Consciousness,* 3rd Conference, 76-106, New York, Josiah Macy Jr. Found., 1952.

4

HYPNOSIS IN DERMATOLOGY

MICHAEL J. SCOTT, B.S., M.D.

INTRODUCTION

Embryologically both epidermal and neural tissues are of ectodermal origin. This common ancestry partially explains the intimate interrelationship existing between these two systems. Each may influence the other and, reciprocally, be affected by the other. Purely mental stimuli may produce somatic reactions. For example an embarrassing thought may cause blushing (vasodilation); fright may result in pallor (vasoconstriction); or mental stress produce hyperhidrosis (overactivity of the sweat gland). Cutaneous disfigurement or symptoms such as psoriasis, scarring, pruritus, or acne may produce depression, self consciousness, anxiety, etc. Therefore the presence of a dermatitis may effect the individual's emotions; conversely, emotional status may be reflected in the skin. Awareness of this basic relationship between emotions and cutaneous reactions is an important criterion for comprehensive dermatologic therapy.

Most dermatologists recognize this essential relationship but often feel handicapped by their uncertainty of how to treat the emotional factor. Each must decide whether to ignore the psychopathology, endeavor to treat it himself or refer the patient to a psychiatrist. Although there is no easy solution to these problems, psychiatrists A. H. Gottesman and Karl Menninger (8) believe the combined medical and psychological therapy by the dermatologist is probably the most frequently indicated.

If the object of treatment is not to reorganize the patient's personality, but rather to restore the individual to the degree of adjustment that he had been able to make before the onset of his skin symptoms, psychotherapy by the dermatologist or general practitioner will not need to be highly technical or greatly prolonged and will (and does) often yield excellent results.

Gottesman and Menninger (8) stress the fact that the dermatologist who would thus supplement his therapeutic program should do so scientifically, and competence in the proper handling of the emotional factors can come only from an understanding of fundamental principles of psychopathology and psychotherapy.

PSYCHOSOMATIC FACTORS IN SKIN DISORDERS

Skin disorders often result from synergistic summation of several factors, rather than one specific agent. The manifestation of disease is the product of many interacting forces: hereditary and environmental, internal and external, physical and chemical, social and psychological, etc. This multitude of etiologic forces in part explains the number of apparently divergent therapeutic approaches effective for many skin diseases. No single explanation can be postulated for the development of psychosomatic cutaneous disorders. Their diverse etiologic factors and widely varying manifestations are far too intricate.

A few pragmatic dermatologists are inclined to go no further than the assumption of a single cause for a particular dermatitis. They are content with locating a specific bacterium, fungus, allergen, etc. This sole-cause attitude of mind has perhaps an admirable cutting edge in exposing the etiology of a relatively unknown group of ailments; but it must give place ultimately to a viewpoint which recognizes multiple causation and interrelations equally fundamental as, if not more fundamental, than the single isolated cause. The psyche rarely appears in dermatoses as a sole cause and for that reason has met with more difficulty in acceptance than have fungi, bacteria, sensitization and so forth.

In my opinion psychological stimuli may (1) cause certain skin diseases; (2) precipitate others; (3) aggravate or prolong the duration of many; (4) occur concomitantly as part of a disease rather than be the cause or result of it; (5) also be produced by cutaneous disorders. Combinations of the above also occur. It is important to remember that the patient may have an emotional condition totally unrelated to the skin condition.

The psyche rarely appears in dermatoses as a sole cause but mental states and conflicts can be converted into skin disorders just as they can be converted into hysteria or phobias. The skin acts not only as a protective and defensive agent for the body, but also occasionally for the mind. The availability and erogenicity of the skin renders it vulnerable to patients with exhibitionistic, masochistic, paranoid, obsessional, compulsive, or abnormal sexual tendencies.

It has long been recognized that emotional tension may influence the course of many cutaneous diseases such as psoriasis, seborrhea, and atopic dermatitis. Both functional and somatic pruritus can be influenced by psychic distress. In neurodermatitis some believe emotions influence the skin by lowering the threshold for itching, which in turn leads to excessive rubbing and scratching. Conversely, the patient subject to an annoying, chronic, pruritic dermatitis possesses a much lower reaction threshold in stressful situations than the average individual. Skin diseases producing disfigurement or intolerable itching may understandably produce psychic or emotional sequelae. Hyperthyroidism may result in melanoderma and psychic hyperirritability.

Whatever happens in the mind is reflected in the body, and any alteration in the latter has repercussions in the former. There is a constant interrelationship between the two. It is therefore erroneous to think of any purely psychic or purely somatic disturbance. Psychic change will inevitably produce some effect on the body and somatic changes necessarily produce some psychically.

Psychic stress may elicit physiologic alterations in the skin which in turn cause or permit further skin disorders. For example, psychic tension may produce hyperhidrosis which in turn produces maceration favoring the growth of pathogenic fungi and an eventual dermatomycosis. Pruritus and discomfort from the latter may increase the emotional stress.

However, in any of these situations with an obvious emotional component, psychotherapy is beneficial. Skillfully applied, it always helps as a supportive process even if the basic disease is organic.

Examples of dermatoses with important psychic components either in etiology or aggravation are:

Phobias (Dermatopathophobias)
   Acarophobia
   Bromhidrosiphobia
   Bacteriophobia
   Cancerophobia
   Syphilophobia
   Misophobia (producing excess washing of hands)
Malingering
   Dermatitis factitia
Compulsions (many mucocutaneous changes may be produced
    including)
   Dermatotillomania
   Dermatothlasia
   Neurotic Excoriations
   Onychotillomania
   Onychophagia
   Trichotillomania
   Trichokryptomania
Paranoid tendencies
   Delusions
     Delusions of Syphilis
     Delusions of Parasites
     Delusions of Aging
Paresthesias
   Glossodynia and dermatodynia
   Pruritus
     Localized and generalized
     Primary or secondary intensification of pruritus on an
      organic basis
   Anesthesias
Neurologic
   Hyper- and hypohidrosis
   Cholinergic urticaria
   Erythema fugax
Miscellaneous
   Atopic dermatitis
   Alopecia areata
   Acne vulgaris

Dermatitis herpetiformis
Eczema (all varieties)
Lupus erythematosis
Lichen planus
Neurodermatitis
   Localized
   Generalized
Psoriasis
Rosacea
Seborrheic dermatitis
Infectious or pyogenic diseases in which psychologic elements may
    occasionally precipitate, aggravate, or clear basic conditions:
Viral
   Verruca
      Verruca planae juvenilis
      Verruca vulgaris
      Verruca accuminata
   Herpes simplex and progenitalis
   Aphthous stomatitis
Pyogenic
   Sycosis vulgaris
   Furunculosis
Others
   Venereal diseases (psychic disturbances may predispose to
     exposure).

Some may consider the above list too inclusive; others, on the
conservative side.

PSYCHOTHERAPY IN DERMATOLOGY

In general there are two types of psychotherapy; covering and
uncovering, and they may be employed in combination. Covering
therapy is designed not to disclose the subconscious material but
rather to strengthen the defense against it; reassurance, encourage-
ment, persuasion and suggestion belong in this category. Uncovering therapy aims in bringing to consciousness the subconscious
conflict with the purpose of effecting a permanent structural
change in the personality. In dermatology, hypnotherapy can be
utilized effectively in covering or uncovering forms of psychotherapy.

Blinded by achievements on the impersonal scientific side some physicians may have forgotten that the patient may be a contributor to his dermatitis and not simply its vehicle and that in any event he has something, often a great deal, to do with its outcome. Dermatologists cannot hope to do prolonged psychiatric therapy, but in many psychogenic dermatoses the underlying emotional disturbances are not difficult to discover and treat with the aid of hypnosis. Frequently some conflict exists between the environment and the emotional needs of the patient.

Psychotherapy is an indispensable adjunct in the treatment of many dermatoses and every dermatologist should offer this procedure in proportion to his ability. Considerable achievements can be attained in medicine using the naked hand and the unaided eye. No therapist can avoid the placebo effect. The psychosomatic effect is active even when specific medication is prescribed. The physician projects his opinions and hopes into the therapy he prescribes. Patients react to this psychic factor, sometimes as much as to the active ingredients in his prescription. Physicians who are impressed with tranquilizers are likely to have the best result with them; the therapeutic nihilists, less success.

We, as physicians, should not treat patients solely for their organic problems; nor should we consider the patient cured merely because the organic problem has been solved. It is our duty to endeavor to eliminate any related neurotic symptom which may be present. The patient must be treated in his totality. He cannot be subdivided into organic and psychic components for separate therapy. All agree it is inexcusable to neglect the physical disorder and offer only psychotherapy, but it is similarly detrimental to concentrate solely on physical conditions and neglect the emotional aspects. To do so frequently entrenches the psychoneurosis more deeply.

The danger always exists however that an unexplained skin lesion may be all too easily and erroneously diagnosed as a neurotic manifestation. Thus it is important that we understand the disorders under study from both the dermatologic and psychiatric viewpoints.

The potentialities of hypnosis in dermatology are limited by the insight, proficiency, and resourcefulness of the physician. The effectiveness depends upon the qualifications of both patient and dermatologist. Through hypnosis, properly administered, certain cutaneous disorders can be eliminated and many others improved. Improvement obtained during the hypnotic trance will persist post-hypnotically not only in psychosomatic dermatoses but in many organic conditions as well. The effectiveness of the post-hypnotic suggestion depends upon the depth of the trance, the nature of the suggestion, the technique employed, and the personal reaction of the subject. A suggestion may therefore remain in effect only a few moments or persist a lifetime. The effectiveness of the suggestion can be increased by repetition during one session or reenforced by additional sessions.

My results with hypnotherapy have been generally very satisfactory in patients with the following disorders: Neurodermatitis, psychosomatic pruritis vulvae and ani, nummular eczema, and neurotic excoriations. It has also proved beneficial in very carefully selected cases of resistant seborrhea, rosacea, alopecia areata, psoriasis, hyperhidrosis, chronic urticaria, lichen planus, recurrent herpes simplex and progenitalis and verrucae. In many cases it is, at any rate, as effective as anything else we have to offer therapeutically. Cutaneous surgery of every type including dermabrasion can be performed successfully under hypnosis and intractable local pain may be successfully suppressed. Paresthesia or pain from burns, trigeminal neuralgia, herpes zoster, etc., can be controlled by hypnotic suggestion as can pruritis of somatic disorders.

It is generally advantageous to employ the hypnotic procedure in conjunction with other dermatologic therapy and not to the latter's exclusion. Combined dermatologic and hypnotherapy is frequently the treatment of choice. Hypnotherapy enables the physician to obtain better rapport with the patient and helps alleviate emotional tension, depression, insomnia and other symptoms so often associated with dermatoses. In organic diseases hypnosis alleviates itching, burning, pain or tenderness, not by influencing the primary etiologic cause but often by minimizing extraneous factors (anxiety, etc.) that focus the patient's attention on the symptom. By this technique the sensations appear to be suppressed and discomfort and suffering are alleviated.

Physicians will find hypnosis not a panacea, but a valuable therapeutic adjunct in conventional dermatologic care in judiciously selected cases. Haphazard use can render no better results than the same quality application with any other modality. In unalterable cutaneous defects or diseases hypnotherapy is effective in enabling the patient, as a personality, to adjust psychologically to the emotional distress precipitated by his condition.

In assessing the value of any form of therapy, hypnosis included, it is important to know the usual course, fluctuations, and degree of spontaneous remissions expected in untreated patients. Otherwise you are apt to erroneously credit any benefit or amelioration to therapy alone.

CLASSIFICATION

In my own practice I find it convenient to classify hypnotherapy as follows: 1) Direct Suggestion, 2) Symptom Substitution, 3) Hypnoanalysis.

1. *Direct Suggestion:* Among the more common conditions for which I have employed direct suggestion during hypnosis for symptomatic relief are: a) Cutaneous itching, burning, or pain. b) Anxiety and tension associated with the dermatitis as a causative, accompanying, or contributing factor. c) Insomnia, mental depression, self consciousness, etc., precipitated by or aggravating the dermatitis. d) Controlling abnormal eating or drinking habits.

It is important that treatment be directed toward the whole patient and not the symptom alone. Emphasis in many cases is primarily aimed toward training in physical and mental relaxation. It is amazing what even one hypnotic session can accomplish with a satisfactory patient. This is especially true if the physician is familiar with the patient's personality and his needs for the particular symptom.

Some believe the effectiveness of hypnotic symptom removal in mono-symptomatic patients depends upon the significance of the symptom to the patient. When the initiating conflict no longer exists and the symptom is maintained only by conditioning or habit, the patients are excellent candidates for direct suggestive therapy. Annoying symptoms having little defensive value respond with surprising rapidity to direct suggestion.

Direct symptom removal has been frowned upon by some since it only removes the symptom, ignoring the underlying causes. Admittedly, however, a large portion of all medical therapy is directed toward symptom removal. The objection that direct hypnotic suggestion treats only symptoms and not original motivations or basic organic and mental causes should not deter one from using it. Even if we consider only symptom removal no apologies are necessary.

Must an individual be compelled to endure an unsightly dermatitis or intolerable pruritus because it is merely an indication of a deeply rooted personality conflict? Unless checked a vicious cycle may occur; the dermatitis can increase his anxiety and intensify the initial emotional conflict.

Patients deemed poor subjects for insight therapy are often effectively treated by use of direct suggestion only. It is also preferable in patients who refuse investigation of the psychodynamics of their disease but nevertheless have strong motivation for symptom removal. As with other modalities, the sooner the symptoms are treated, the easier it will be to obtain beneficial results.

Symptom removal by a gradual reduction process extended over several treatments may yield more effective and potentially safer results than an attempt at total removal during one session. Frequently it is advisable to gradually decrease the severity, intensity and frequency of an active symptom. In such a manner a previously intolerable pruritus may be decreased in intensity and frequency to a tolerable and comfortable level without depriving the patient of a symptom entirely. In a relatively very small percentage of patients complete freedom from their symptoms can be a bitter freedom. Cutaneous symptoms that persist for emotional rather than organic reasons occasionally may be either depressive equivalents or serve to control depression. Gradual symptom removal in such cases, without abrupt cessation, enables the physician to detect early indications of adverse reactions from possible total removal of the supporting emotional crutch. This procedure is especially advisable in compensated psychoses to avoid a possible decompensation.

Scratching is one means of relieving emotional tension. Functional pruritus, excoriations, or other symptoms may often advantageously be displaced from one region of the body to another less disabling, disfiguring and otherwise more satisfactory area. For instance, cosmetically repulsive neurotic excoriations of the face may be transferred to a less noticeable region without depriving the patient completely of his compulsion to excoriate his skin.

Pain and pruritus may be either organically or psychogenically based, and both components may be present to varying degree. The ability to produce anesthesia by direct hypnotic suggestion has gained considerable notoriety. Pain is not actually abolished but the emotional reaction to pain is altered. It is often preferable to avoid suggesting that patients will not feel pain or itching. Instead instruct the patient that "regardless of the sensation you feel, you will note it will not bother you in any way." With pruritus, I frequently say, "You may still feel itchy but you will no longer have any desire to scratch." Preventing scratching alleviates much of the lichenification and secondary infection associated with pruritic dermatoses and aids considerably in obtaining a cure. Wording of the direct suggestion is important and it is preferable to employ permissive statements.

2. *Symptom Substitution:* Another method of reconditioning or reeducating dermatologic patients through hypnosis is replacing one habit pattern with another more constructive pattern. The new pattern must be logical enough in the patient's mind to destroy the earlier pattern.

In selecting cases it is possible for the physician to substitute or replace one symptom with another of his own choice. The effectiveness of this procedure is partially determined by how closely the substituted symptom equates symbolically with the original symptom. The subconscious, without treatment, frequently substitutes one symptom by another spontaneously.

In symptom substitution some undesirable mental or physical outlet is replaced by a more acceptable one. Scratching, for example, can be replaced by a desire to pursue other physical activities. But know the patient. The fact that you find satisfaction and enjoyment from some particular activity does not guarantee it will be equally intriguing for your patient.

Athletic activities, painting, sculpturing, reading, verbal aggressiveness, etc., are possible replacements for scratching. Pruritus localized to an ankle may be suggested as a substitute for a generalized pruritus. Preferably the substituting symptom should have the same neurotic significance as the one it replaces; e.g., exhibitionistic or masochistic symptoms should be replaced with similar symptoms but of a more acceptable and desirable nature. Remember that whatever the undesirable skin symptom may be, it may fulfill a psychological need for the patient.

3. *Hypnoanalysis:* This is a recent improvement in hypnotherapy. In this procedure, hypnosis is combined with an analytic method of psychotherapy. In dermatologic practice, I find hypnoanalysis most useful in patients with chronic psychosomatic dermatoses.

Each of us is a maze of conflicting desires and impulses which unconsciously influence our actions. Repressed fear, hate, love, anxiety, anger, embarrassing experiences, frustration, etc., may consciously be forgotten but forever remain in the subconscious where they are capable of producing conflicts which may manifest themselves in functional disturbances.

Stored up nervous energy and conflicts finding no satisfactory outlet may produce neurotic reactions and habits. The skin can be affected in these situations and scratching is one means of relieving such tensions. Hypnosis, being a direct freeway to the subconscious, can be utilized to discover these traumatic causes.

Hypnosis also acts as a catalyst in crystallizing an opinion of the patient's reactions to his conflicts and emotions. Without hypnosis frequently months or years of psychoanalysis are required to arrive at the same conclusion. Obscure underlying conflicts, repressed anxieties, attitudes and impulses which have existed as suppressed underlying causes of neurotic behavior may come to the surface in one or two sessions. It is regrettable that in many cases hypnosis is attempted only as a last resort.

It is effective in penetrating the barrier separating man's consciousness from his underlying emotional conflicts and tensions. The patient's conscious awareness of suppressed emotionally traumatic incidents and thoughts can disintegrate a neurosis. Hypnosis can circumvent the patient's biases and prejudices which in the conscious state causes so much resistance and argumentation.

Psychoanalysis and hypnoanalysis have a common purpose, that of changing the patient's undesirable reactions by modification of his attitudes and goals. Sometimes in order to accomplish this the original precipitating traumatic event must be uncovered. However, it should be stressed that the recall of repressed traumatic thoughts and experiences does not always result in cure or amelioration of symptoms. Also it is not what is recalled that is of primary importance but instead how it can be utilized to benefit the patient.

Free discussion of pertinent experiences may give striking relief from pent-up tension. This is especially true if the patient "abreacts" or emotionally relives these recalled events with full emotional intensity of the original occurrence. The more marked the emotional release, the more successful the abreaction. Irrespective of cause, tension accompanies many chronic psychosomatic cutaneous disorders and abreactive techniques often result in amelioration or complete disappearance of the disorder.

In some instances it is a relatively simple procedure to enable the patient to recall the suppressed psychological basis for his symptoms; at other times considerable patience and skill on the part of the therapist are required.

Specialized techniques including age and memory regression, revivification, automatic writing and drawing, catharsis, dream suggestion, artificial conflicts, time distortion, as well as a variety of others may be utilized in conjunction with these three aforementioned methods in dermatologic patients.

HISTORICAL REVIEW

Reports regarding hypnotherapy in dermatology are sparse and to date little adequately controlled research has been attempted. Case reports are based primarily on personal convictions of private practitioners.

Heilig and Hoff produced herpes simplex in proven herpes virus carriers by hypnotically suggesting unpleasant, emotionally stimulating situations. Ullman (28) produced herpes simplex in a soldier twenty-four hours after hypnotic suggestion. Estrin (6) very briefly reported the use of hypnosis as a supportive symptomatic treatment for helping itching and pain in five dermatologic cases. Four of the cases had only one hypnotic treatment and the other, ten treatments. All were treated by direct symptom removal alone. One patient with a severe sunburn improved and with posthypnotic suggestion the pain could be relieved. One patient with pruritic lichen planus obtained two days' relief after one treatment. Other cases included generalized eczema, dermatophytosis plus eczematoid dermatitis, and dermatophytosis plus dermatitis medicamentosa.

Suggestion, with or without hypnosis, has been utilized for centuries in the treatment of warts. McDowell (17) reported the removal of juvenile warts by hypnotic suggestion. This patient previously failed to respond to topical therapy and roentgen irradiation. Obermayer (18) and Greenson reported a similar case with extensive juvenile verrucae on the scalp, face and neck of two years duration which previously was refractory to psychotherapy, bismuth injections, keratolytic ointments, podophyllin, solid carbon dioxide, ultra violet and roentgen irradiation. Symptoms cleared with three hypnotic sessions. Histologic examination confirmed the clinical diagnosis. Hypnotherapy was rendered once weekly for three weeks. During the first session the patient was instructed (before bedtime each night) to imagine for a few minutes that her face was covered with cold compresses and would then begin to tingle and itch. In the second session with deep relaxation the patient was told her face would feel cold and the warts would begin to tingle and fall off. In the third session the patient reported that the warts had become scaly. On awakening she was informed that no further treatments were necessary because the warts would shortly disappear. Two weeks later her skin was free of all lesions and examination after six months showed no recurrence.

Kline (13) reported the successful treatment of a chronic neurodermatitis of the hands in a 26-year-old female by using a hypnotic sensory-imagery technique. The patient reported that the condition existed from the time she was five years of age. There had been intermittant periods of remission of very short duration. The patient was depressed and defensive. She stated that she was not interested in psychotherapy but only wanted the condition on her hands cured. Treatment was undertaken on the patient's terms. A light hypnosis was rapidly induced. While under hypnosis the patient was told that her hands would begin to grow larger and larger until they were very large and then they would become very warm until they would become hot. Then they would become very cold until they would become almost freezing and then they would become very large again. In conjunction with these directions the patient was asked to visualize the hands becoming large, cold, warm and then large again. She reported that she did not feel any changes in her hands during hypnosis and could not visualize the changes. Post-hypnotic suggestions were given for these sensations to manifest themselves daily between treatment sessions. The patient was treated once weekly for six weeks. She reported that the sensations and visualizations became clearer as therapy progressed. After six weeks the patient's hand cleared completely. Utilizing the same technique, Kline later reported improvement in a forty-five year old female with chronic psoriasis. The psoriatic lesions had previously persisted for twenty years duration and had been recalcitrant to roentgen irradiation and various topical therapies.

Bonjour (2) reported the effectiveness of hypnosis in erythroderma, hyperhidrosis, and urticaria.

Hypnotic suggestion has achieved spectacular results in anxiety-tensions of children. Nail biting is primarily an anxiety reaction and Bouffe used hypnosis in onychophagia with success.

Mason (15) demonstrated improvement in both the mental and physical state of a patient with ichthyosiform erythrodermia following hypnotherapy. The patient was 16-year-old boy with congenital dermatitis. Skin grafting had previously been performed but yielded nothing but severe contractures. The hypnotic suggestion was given that the left arm would clear. After five days the horny layer softened, became friable and fell off. The skin was slightly erythematous but normal in texture and color. The erythema faded and at the end of ten days the arm was clear from shoulder to wrist. With further hypnotherapy improvement was reported as:

Region	Before Treatment	After Treatment
hands	completely covered	palms clear; fingers not greatly improved
arms	80% covered	95% cleared
back	lightly covered	90% cleared
buttocks	heavily covered	60% cleared
thighs	completely and heavily covered	70% cleared
legs and feet	completely and heavily covered	50% cleared

There was no vast change in the condition over the following year. Schneck (20) also obtained comparative over-all improvement in a patient with ichthyosis.

Encouraged by Mason's achievement, Gordon and Cohen (30) used hypnotherapy on patients selected primarily for their chronicity, and mainly from the eczema group in which psychological factors might be presumed to be operative. Some simple assessment of these factors had been attempted previously in some patients, and a few had attended the psychiatric department without, however, obtaining any appreciable benefit. The method of hypnosis adopted was simple relaxation and suggestion. Understanding and cooperation being essential, the patients were given some introductory explanation. A hypnotic trance was obtained in practicaly all patients; the depth and the ease with which it was obtained differed widely. The degree of hypnosis did not necessarily parallel the cure of the symptoms.

In non-pruritic cases their results were of interest, but not indicative that hypnosis was of any paramount value as a therapeutic measure. The reverse, however, was claimed in the much larger class of skin conditions where irritation was a prominent feature. The results there appeared to be extremely promising. Three cases were quoted in some detail. They were either cured or improved more than 80 per cent by hypnosis. These illustrate some points which appear to be important on general dermatological grounds. The value of hypnosis appeared to be fourfold: (1) It controls pruritus, sometimes even after the first suc-

ANALYSIS OF CASES TREATED

	Treated	Cured	Improved
Atopic Eczema (including generalized eczema)	15	3	4
Discoid Eczema	7	2	2
Varicose and Contact Dermatitis	5	3	1
Pruritus, generalized and nodular	3	3	0
Pruritus, anal, vulval and scrotal	5	0	3
Neurodermatitis	12	6	4
Psoriasis	7	0	2
Pompholyx	5	2	3
Urticaria	1	1	0
Alopecia Areata, severe	4	0	0
Rosacea	1	1	0
Total	65	20 [sic!]	19

Patients still under treatment and improving steadily	20
Patients tending to relapse	3
Failures	3

Average previous duration of symptoms........9 years
Average length of hypnotic treatment........3 months

cessful hypnotic session. If this relief can be obtained following previous failure of internal drugs or external applications, the patient obtains great confidence and cure is likely. (2) Rapport with the patient is greatly facilitated. (3) Insight is obtained by the patient into the part he plays in the production of his own disease. (4) It has an important reeducative value. Many patients learn auto-suggestion and are able thereby to control their own pruritus.

In a subsequent article, Gordon investigated the effect of hypnosis in 144 dermatological patients. The suggestion was given patients during hypnosis that the skin condition and irritation would be resolve and the skin return to its normal state. The antipuritic effect of hypnosis was often marked. Psychotherapy was later added to hypnosis. Dr. Gordon found the psychic factor was important in degrees varying from 100 per cent down to 50 per cent in a wide range of common skin disorders. One boy of twelve, who had had eczema and asthma from the age of two, was completely cured of both in about six sessions. He was still clear two and one-half years later. The series included many patients with atopic eczema and some of them had been extremely resistant to treatment. In another patient with dermatitis herpetiformis of ten years duration, the condition had been controlled by arsenic, but this had to be withdrawn because of severe and obscure retinal lesions. These improved when the arsenic therapy was stopped but the dermatitis relapsed. Both skin and eye lesions cleared rapidly under hypnosis and psychotherapy and remained so two years later.

Cheek (4) listed the following skin diseases as meriting consideration for hypnotherapy:

1. Acne vulgaris
2. Herpes Simplex
3. Herpes Zoster
4. Dermatomyositis
5. Lupus erythematosus
6. Scleroderma
7. Psoriasis
8. Eczema
9. Neurodermatitis
10. Dermatitis venatata
11. All thermal burns
12. Any acute debilitating inflammation of the skin threatening life
13. All forms of warts
14. Hyperhidrosis

Cheek also stressed knowing what the skin condition means to the patient. He recommends investigations with ideomotor response to the following questions:

1. Is the disease like that of any friend or relative with whom you may have identified yourself?
2. Are you using the disease in any way as a form of punishment to yourself or someone you know?
3. Do you feel you can recover from this disease?
4. If not, does your inner mind know why you are pessimistic?
5. Are you willing now to use hypnosis to remove symptoms and permit healing to occur?

Sinclair-Gieben and Chalmers (25) described a controlled trial in the treatment of warts by hypnosis. In a pilot study the warts of six patients disappeared within three months when treated by medium hypnosis. One remaining patient, who was mentally defective, failed to respond. Fourteen patients were then treated by well-established methods of inducing hypnosis. Once a state of hypnosis was induced it was suggested that the warts on one side of the body would disappear, and that on awakening the patient would perform some specified action as described. Only patients with bilateral and multiple common warts of at least six months' duration were admitted to the trial, and only one side of the body was treated. This was always the side with the larger or more numerous warts. Ten patients reached an adequate depth of hypnosis and four did not. The time taken for cure on the the treated side was between five weeks and three months. In the four patients whose hypnosis was only slight no benefit was obtained. If the original seven patients are included, sixteen of twenty-one consecutive patients could be hypnotized to an adequate depth. The matched controls showed that the cure of warts can be effected by hypnosis. Improvement was always on the treated side, but the hypnosis must reach a certain depth. Those who lost their warts all showed posthypnotic suggestion in that after awakening they performed actions suggested to them. In those who received no benefit, such suggestion had failed.

The genuineness of blister formation being induced by direct hypnotic suggestion has been doubted by many. The general method is to touch a specific cutaneous area with a bland instrument (glass rod, fountain pen, etc.) and simultaneously give vivid suggestions that the site is being burned. The area is then protected by an occlusive dressing for a predetermined period and then examined for bulla formation. Bullae identical to those produced by thermal burns reportedly have been so produced. An individual with a sensitive vasomotor system is stated to be essential for success. I have never attempted this procedure. Pattie (19) states that in the past fifty-five years only ten articles have been recorded accurately enough to substantiate that this phenomenon occurs. He concluded it is an established fact although the mechanism is not clear.

The psychosomatic concept pertains to the interaction of emotions and bodily functions in the production of symptoms. Certain cutaneous diseases should be objectively observed and treated as dynamic, constantly fluctuating adaptations to the stresses and strains to which the patient is exposed both externally and internally.

There is a definite trend in dermatology toward the psychosomatic approach in treatment when indicated. The introduction of psychiatric thinking into dermatologic disorders enables a physician to attain therapeutic results far beyond those expected from organic therapy alone. Theoretically some use of psychotherapy could be made in any skin condition which has an emotional component. This holds true whether the emotional disturbance is a factor in the production of the illness or is merely the result of organic distress. Whether psychotherapy is utilized merely for supportive therapy, symptom removal, symptom substitution, or toward uncovering subconscious motivations and conflicts as contributory or etiologic factors in disorders of the skin, hypnosis is invaluable in enabling the physician to secure rapid and effective results.

Hypnotherapy is an effective multifunctional technique permitting directness and acceleration in psychotherapy. Best results with hypnotherapy can be anticipated in cases where the cause is primarily emotional and less where organic components predominate.

In private practice, patients with primarily somatic disease seldom are therapeutic problems in comparison to those with primarily psychosomatic or functional complaints. In the latter group, difficulty is frequently encountered in securing satisfactory response to conventional medical therapy alone. In such instances combined dermatologic and hypnotherapy is frequently the treatment of choice. It is generally advantageous to employ the hypnotic procedure in conjunction with other dermatologic therapy, not to its exclusion.

Physicians will find hypnosis not a panacea, but a valuable adjunct to conventional dermatologic therapy in judiciously selected cases. Orientation in psychodynamics is a basic prerequisite for successful hypnotherapy.

REFERENCES

1. ARNOLD, H. L.: Stress dermatoses. *A.M.A. Arch. Dermat. & Syph.*, *67*:566, 1953.

2. BONJOUR, J.: Influence of the mind on the skin. *Brit. J. Dermat. & Syph., 41*:324, 1929.

3. BRANDT, R.: A tentative classification of psychological factors in the etiology of skin diseases. *J. Dermat., 14*:81, 1950.

4. CHEEK, D. B.: Possible uses of hypnosis in dermatology. *Med. Times,* Jan., 1961.

5. ERICKSON, M. H.: Hypnosis in medicine. *Med. Clin. North America, 28*:639-652, 1944.

6. ESTRIN, J.: Hypnosis as a supportive symptomatic treatment in skin diseases. *Urol. & Cutan. Rev., 45*:337-338, 1941.

7. GORDON, H.: Hypnosis in dermatology. *Brit. Med. J., 1*:1214, 1955.

8. GOTTESMAN, A. H. and MENNINGER, K.: The dermatologist and the psychiatrist. *Arch. Dermat. & Syph., 59*:367, 1949.

9. GREENSON, R. R. and OBERMAYER, M. E.: Treatment by suggestion of verrucae planae of the face. *Psychosomat. Med., 11*:163-164, 1949.

10. HORAN, J. S.: Management of neurodermatitis by hypnotic suggestion. *Brit. J. Med. Hyp., 2*:2, 1950.

11. HORAN, M.: The psychogenic aspect of dermatology. *Practitioner, 127*:675-685, 1931.

12. KARTAMISHEW, A. I.: Hypnosis in psoriasis. *Dermat. Wchnschr., 102*:260, 1936.

13. KLINE, M. V.: Psoriasis and hypnotherapy. *J. Clin. & Exper. Hyp., 2*:318, 1954.

14. LeCRON, L. M.: *Techniques of Hypnotherapy.* New York, Julian Press, 1961.

15. MASON, A. A.: A case of congenital ichthyosiform erythrodermia of Brocq treated by hypnosis. *Brit. Med. J.,* Aug. 23, 1952.

16. MENNINGER, K.: Observations of a psychiatrist in a dermatology clinic. *Bull. Menninger Clin., 1*:141, 1947.

17. McDOWELL, M.: Hypnosis in dermatology. In Schneck, J. M.: *Hypnosis in Modern Medicine,* First Edition. Springfield, Thomas, 1953.

18. OBERMAYER, M. E.: *Psychocutaneous Medicine.* Springfield, Thomas, 1955.

19. PATTIE, F. A.: The production of blisters by hypnotic suggestion; a review. *J. Abn. & Social Psychol., 36*:62-72, 1947.

20. SCHNECK, J. M.: Ichthyosis (simplex) treated with hypnosis. *Dis. Nerv. Syst., 15*:211-214, 1954.

21. Scott, M. J.: *Hypnosis in Skin and Allergic Diseases.* Springfield, Thomas, 1960.
22. Scott, M. J.: Hypnosis in dermatologic therapy. In LeCron, L. M.: *Techniques of Hypnotherapy.* 1961.
23. Seitz, P. F. D.: Experiments in substitution of symptoms. *Psychosom. Med., 15:*405-424, 1953.
24. Selye, H. and Frontier, C.: Adaptive reactions to stress. *Psychosom. Med., 12:*149-157, 1950.
25. Sinclair-Gieben, A. H. and Chalmers, D.: Treatment of warts by hypnosis. *Lancet,* Oct. 3, 1959.
26. Sneddon, I. B.: Mind and skin. *Brit. Med. J., 1:*472-475, 1949.
27. Stokes, J. H.: Effect on the skin of emotional and nervous states. *Arch. Dermat. & Syph., 22:*803, 1930.
28. Ullman, M.: Herpes simplex and second degree burns induced under hypnosis. *Am. J. Psych., 103:*830, 1946.
29. Wisch, J. M.: Hypnosis in psoriasis. *Dermat. Wchnschr., 100:*234, 1935.
30. Gordon, H. and Cohen, K.: The value of hypnosis in the treatment of skin diseases. *Excerpta Medica, 6* (Sec. 13) :361, 1952.

5

HYPNOSIS IN OBSTETRICS AND GYNECOLOGY

RALPH V. AUGUST, M.D.

Chapters on the use of hypnosis in many areas of medical practice are here presented by a variety of authors, each a specialist in his own field. This testifies to hypnosis being an interdisciplinary science. It also frees this writer of the need for discussing historical background and theoretical explanations for the mechanism of hypnosis. Instead, first hand knowledge based on personal experience will dominate this chapter.

Medical specialization still requires attendance at the meetings of various specialty groups, each of which bears on my own work. Each society tends to emphasize its own particular viewpoint, sometimes nearing the exclusion of all other thinking. I find it necessary for maintenance of proper perspective to think in terms of hypnotherapy at obstetrics-gynecology conventions and to do an about face at meetings for the study of hypnosis. This presentation in *Hypnosis in Modern Medicine* will be oriented to obstetric and gynecologic management.

My thesis shall be termed, "An obstetrician-gynecologist reviews the employment of hypnosis for the purpose of improving his therapeutic results." The implications are threefold. Firstly, the doctor must be capable in his chosen field of obstetrics-gynecology. Secondly, hypnosis must serve as an adjunct to other therapy. It must never be an end unto itself. Thirdly, this is one area of medical practice where pragmatism is paramount. As an addendum, the author will give evidence of the additional service provided his patient when her doctor also employs hypnosis, a service often impossible to duplicate with all other therapeutic modalities.

The obstetric patient differs in many respects from her gynecologic counterpart.

DIFFERENCES BETWEEN OBSTETRIC AND GYNECOLOGIC PATIENTS

| | Patient | |
Area of Comparison	Obstetric	Gynecologic
1. A desirable product obtainable	almost always	never
2. Duration of "disease"	self limited, usually nine months	endless, often progressively worse
3. Usual general physical condition	good	ailing
4. Systemic organic involvement	always	not necessarily
5. Somatic and psychic involvement	usually somatopsychic	more often psychosomatic
6. Age	usually 17-40	not limited to these ages, often older
7. Marital status, husband involvement	usually associated (always initiated by male)	not necessarily so (rarely initiated but often aggravated by either presence or absence of male)
8. Hospitalization required, (in our society) sooner or later	always	less often
9. Surgical therapy required	always	sometimes, current therapy tends to be less frequently surgical, more often medical and psychologic
10. Incapacitating for varying periods	less often	more often
11. Favorable, possibly happy and desirable situation	should be, and usually is	almost invariably not
12. Availability to employment of hypnotherapy	in groups or as an individual	individual

HYPNOSIS IN OBSTETRICS

The medical management of pregnancy must be structured
differently from that of every other area of practice. As a rule, the
obstetrician is confronted with a healthy, young, adult female seek-

ing care for a "disease" of limited duration. He must simultaneously care for two individuals of differing physiologic capacity, and do so through one portal. Although he consistently views obstetric care as insurance for maternal and fetal health, his patient often considers maintenance of her comfort to be his most important responsibility. A third party may sometimes require management because of his vested interest as the expectant father.

No regularly recurring somatic alteration of the norm is encountered more frequently than pregnancy. None will be so frequently colored by psychic symptomatology. The devoted obstetrician must simultaneously be a psychotherapist as well as an organotherapist. Hypnosis can rarely be life saving, but will be often beneficial to the child bearing female.

This area of practice may be outlined as follows:

I needs, II therapy, and III results.

Needs

These may be subdivided as they occur during the temporal divisions of the gravida's life.

First Trimester: Nausea with or without vomiting may begin at or about the time of the first missed menstrual period. It may continue throughout pregnancy. This may become severe enough to cause considerable weight loss and even require hospitalization, or it may be mild and fleeting. About 50 per cent of pregnancies are so complicated, usually beginning about the sixth or eighth week, and often terminating spontaneously at about the sixteenth week. It is believed that hyperemesis and ptyalism result from subconscious rejection of pregnancy (18, 19).

These symptoms are amenable to hypnotherapy. Drug therapy also will often be effective. Writing a prescription or dispensing sample medications (of which we have a goodly number and variety) is much simpler for the busy obstetrician. I do so. After medications fail to control symptoms I resort to hypnosis. In my practice, this routine has always succeeded, although the duration of time involved may of itself have been responsible for some cures.

Ptyalism is infrequently encountered. However, when present, it is most distressing. The onset and duration are similar to those of nausea and vomiting. Therapy required is usually much more intensive. Tranquilizers, barbiturates, and belladonna derivatives are often helpful, rarely adequate. Hypnotherapy has, in my experience, provided satisfactory control in every case.

Such evidence of emotional instability as sleeplessness, restlessness, weariness, and anorexia are frequently encountered. These will usually respond to tranquilizing, ataractic, analgesic, anorectic, and sedative drugs. When needed, hypnosis becomes a valuable adjunct to therapy.

Frequency of urination and/or constipation are often attendant on pregnancy. These symptoms are associated with pelvic vascular engorgement and pressure of the uterine mass. They frequently appear early in the first trimester, may persist throughout pregnancy, and are often accentuated during the last month or two, especially after lightening. Medication other than sedatives is of little value. The tranquility derived from hypnotherapy is most satisfying. It effectively leads to the gravida's acceptance of these physiologic concomitants.

Cramps or vaginal bleeding as portents of abortion may be encountered. These are amenable, in part at least, to hypnotherapy, and will be discussed later.

Second Trimester: Tiredness and backache are frequent complaints at this time. The gravida two, in particular, will bring these symptoms to her physician's attention. "Why did she feel so good during her first pregnancy, and why do these symptoms bother her now?"

She forgets that the child already borne is now a full time responsibility. She may also fail to realize that frequent lifting and carrying her youngster, particularly if he be large and not yet ambulatory, would be sufficient for creating a backache in men far stronger than she.

Employment of autohypnosis permits these patients to ignore, overlook, or to compensate for these symptoms. Explanation followed by resultant sensible adjustment of work schedules lessens the burden and may alone be sufficient for tranquilizing the "tired mother."

More serious second trimester problems are vaginal bleeding and lower abdominal cramps. Either of these may signal an impending abortion. These symptoms may first appear during the early part of the first trimester or at any time prior to the onset of labor. Cramps may result from a variety of causes such as tiredness, constipation, or any one of many intercurrent diseases. They may be nothing more than Braxton-Hicks contractions. Yet, they must be viewed with concern. Vaginal bleeding is always serious. Although cervical erosions and malignancy must be ruled out, the obstetrician needs to consider first and foremost the danger of abortion, the possibility of placental (abruptio/previa) separation. Such a problem, particularly when repeatedly encountered in the same patient (the chronic aborter), demands every measure of available therapy. Bed rest and medication are always indicated. Hospitalization may be needed. Hypnotherapy has been of immense help in my practice. The tranquilizing effect of hypnosis may turn the tide. It certainly eases the burden for the patient and to some degree for her husband. It may even tranquilize the obstetrician once he is no longer saddled with his patient's excited family.

Third Trimester: Backache becomes a more common complaint as the physiologic tumor increases in size. The nausea and vomiting which resulted from subconscious rejection early in pregnancy may now be replaced by physiologic and anatomic problems. The stresses and strains on the bones and joints are readily understandable, so they are noticed and promptly brought to the physician's attention. Displacement of the gastrointestinal organs and pressure on the bladder may induce heartburn, constipation, and frequency of urination. All of these are necessary, although not desirable, concomitants of terminal pregnancy.

These symptoms are logically present. Most obstetric patients can understand these logistics, ergo most will evidence the complaints. Explanation and "talking it out" at the hynoidal level will, for a good number, lead to acceptance and an improved outlook. Hypnotherapy will do so for many more.

Vaginal bleeding and/or cramps are now, as they are at any other period of pregnancy, the most serious complaints. Again, as previously stated, the obstetrician must employ every measure at his command. Awareness of placenta praevia, abruptio placenta, and premature labor alerts him to proper therapy. Bed rest, medication, hypnotherapy, and possible surgical intervention permit him to individualize management and to mobilize all resources in the direction of a favorable termination.

Labor and Delivery: At this time, all other symptoms fade into insignificance. Only pain is the all pervading problem. The perception of uterine contractions, and, most of all, the anticipation of a journey through "the valley of the shadow of death," these are the problems of labor and delivery!

So often, gravid patients engage an obstetrician, not for prenatal or postnatal care, not for attention to the newborn, rarely even for maintenance of their own physical well being, but for relief of anticipated discomfort. Most patients take for granted that their obstetrician is a capable technician and an intelligent doctor. Their choice will often be determined by the promise, overt or implied, of most adequate comfort at the time of delivery.

Although some (25, 29) feel that hypnosis in obstetric care is most valuable prior to and subsequent to delivery, I disagree. From my experience, most patients need support during labor and delivery. This can be psychologic, chemical, or both. When the former meets her needs, the latter may be markedly diminished or entirely eliminated. A combination may be termed "balanced" analgesia-anesthesia. Training for hypnotherapy and its employment during pregnancy paves the way for its utilization during labor and delivery. Lack of such preparation, however, is no bar.

There are both maternal and fetal indications for reduction or elimination of chemo-analgesia and chemo-anesthesia. The poor risk mother, the one with cardiac or pulmonary disease, the patient with multiple allergies, the one who has recently ingested food, and the emotionally disturbed patient are all prime candidates for hypnoanodynia. Fetal prematurity and fetal embarrassment are even stronger indications for substituting hypnotherapy for chemotherapy. The newborn's entire life may depend on a few minutes of maternal therapy.

Postpartum Period: This interlude is required for restoration of mind and body to the nonpregnant, so called normal, state. Certain problems may be encountered. Afterpains, hemorrhoidal and episiotomy discomfort, gaseous distress, and lactation problems are most frequent. The patient trained to employ hypnotherapy is impressed by their absence. Her sisters in adjoining beds may complain. She feels very well. In fact, her alertness, vigor, and general well being are most remarkable. I wish that this were just as universally true of patients employing terminal, delivery hypnoanesthesia without prior training. I have not found it to be so.

The trained (conditioned) patient enjoys her hospital stay. Posthypnotic suggestions have adequately prepared her. Whether she wishes to nurse her baby at the breast or on the bottle, appropriate suggestions will aid in promoting or suppressing lactation. Early, pleasurable ambulation is always suggested. Many a patient is so enthusiastic that rising from the delivery table, walking to the wheelchair, and riding to her room is permitted. Requests to eat and drink as desired are always granted immediately following delivery. Most patients will readily partake of toast and coffee. Thus normal physiology and rapid restoration to the norm are permitted.

Therapy and Hypnosis

Modality: Hypnosis may be employed as an ataractic. It is the tranquilizer par excellence. By diversion of attention and focus on desirable channels it induces the most amazing and satisfying euphoria, yet does so without danger of overdosage or drug addiction. Only physician understanding and patient cooperation are required.

Hypnoanalgesia may be induced in a similar manner at any time during pregnancy, labor, delivery, and the postpartum period. Moderate intensity of hypnosis and, more conveniently, posthypnotic suggestions will raise the level for pain tolerance. As previously mentioned, posthypnotic suggestions will relieve most conditioned patients of postpartum discomforts. This requires that one be particularly circumspect less organic problems be masked. In the good hypnotic subject, the anus, episiotomy, leg veins, and breasts should be regularly checked for the purpose of promptly diagnosing any pathology.

Labor may be induced by means of hypnotic suggestion (23). It may also be speeded or slowed in a similar fashion. I have done all three with good hypnotic subjects. This, however, is more of academic than of practical importance. A good subject is required. The indications for such procedures are few except in the presence of terminal labor, fetal distress, or placental bleeding.

Hypnosis for anesthesia is of greater value for obstetric delivery than for any other surgical procedure. Here and only here is general anesthesia, massive enough for an adult of 150 pounds and upward, employed with almost total disregard for a seven pounder receiving the same dose. Hypnosis can be intensified from an ataractic or analgesic dose to one of anesthetic proportions. It can be freely fortified with chemicals, and terminated at will. There have been no contraindications or untoward sequellae to its use in the delivery room.

Hypnosis has still another use, that of inducing amnesia. Many of life's experiences are fleeting enough that tolerance can be easily obtained. Yet, painful memories may be relived ad infinitum. A patient may experience only several terminal painful contractions, but the reliving and retelling of these may, over a period of time, magnify them to no end. This can be and should be controlled with amnesia through the medium of hypnosis. Similarly, time distortion may be employed to sublimate unfavorable situations in favor of pleasant ones (8). Such management may be extremely helpful to her obstetrician in that it will enhance his reputation every time she recalls these pleasant memories, at bridge club, the hair dresser's, and various other places where obstetrician's reputations are made. More seriously, she will not only be spared painful memories but will be more likely to accept her role as a wife, a mother, and possibly as a mother again.

Method: Three differing approaches may be employed for induction of the hypnotic trance (26, 28).

The authoritarian method consists of hypnotist commands and patient performance as directed. He advises; she follows. His orders are graduated in such a manner that her actions become increasingly automatic. The ordered performance is usually motor rather than sensory. This method sacrifices intensity or depth of trance at the alter of induction speed. Repeated eye closure and counting techniques are commonly employed examples.

The authoritarian approach has been described as the paternal in contrast with the permissive or maternal. With the latter method all suggestions are presented in such a manner that the patient may feel free to accept or reject, follow or ignore each one. Careful and clever presentation leads her to follow a preplanned course of acceptance.

The third, or cooperative approach consists of accepting without restructuring the patient's presenting pattern of behavior and employing it for trance induction (13, 14).

Each of the foregoing general approaches to trance induction requires only intelligent and studied physician('s) verbalization together with the patient('s) attention and acceptance. The effectiveness of trance induction will be directly proportionate to the intensity of motivation (of both physician and patient). It will also parallel the degree of rapport.

Judicious semantics are important to good patient-physician relationships (3). They are essential to satisfactory hypnotherapy. The obstetrician must not only keep this in mind for himself, he must also constantly impress this on the ever changing hospital personnel who will be aiding in the care of his patients. A simple procedure such as the drawing of blood at the initial complete examination will illustrate the significance of proper verbalization.

I never say, "I'm going to stick you," or "I'll be injecting you with this needle," or "I have to jab you and it won't hurt you very much."

I do say, "I'll be pressing this (needle and syringe) against your arm. You may feel a little pressure, that's all. I need a sample of blood for a blood count, Rh determination, blood type, and serology test. You can be pleased that all four tests will be done on the same sample so that we need to do this only once."

A variety of devices may be employed for aiding trance induction. The Chevreul pendulum, hypnodisc, Stokvis color contrast card, metronome (26), brain wave synchronizer (20), plus others have been used. The patient may be requested to fix her gaze on a ceiling spot, a fountain pen, a cigarette lighter, or her own thumb nail. Eye fixation is the usual key to commanding attention with each of these devices. Proper verbalization must accompany.

"Autogenic training," "Psychoprophylactic preparation for

painless childbirth" (6, 7), and "Natural childbirth" (11, 12) are methods similar to or identical with hypnotherapy. Similarly, Christian Science healing makes use of suggestion to a degree sometimes difficult to differentiate from hypnosis.

Employment of Hypnosis: The trance itself. The depth of trance obtainable may be extremely variable. This does not matter. The adequacy is all important. Intensity sufficient for the patient's needs is desirable. No more is needed.

Conditioning: Hypnosis may be employed without prior conditioning. Rapport is probably more intense between the gravid patient and her obstetrician than it is in any other therapeutic situation. This patient is usually highly motivated. The maternal instinct will compensate for many lesser problems. She rarely has anything to hide, for the obstetrician has already examined her completely.

Conditioning may be initiated during the first month of pregnancy for the patient with hyperemesis. I have done so a day prior to delivery and at various times in between these extremes. Usually, several to a half dozen sessions of group conditioning suffice. A lesser number of individual sessions will do as well (3).

Patients may be conditioned in groups or singly. Fundamentally, hypnosis results from a special type of interpersonal relationship. The presence of only patient and physician is advisable because this permits of a closer and more intimate relationship. Concentration is facilitated for her. A greater variability of techniques is possible for the physician. The speed of hypnosis can be adjusted to the patient's needs and capacity for performance. Individual problems can be more conveniently discussed. Special situations such as blindness and deafness can be more readily managed.

Group conditioning has its own special advantages. There is economy of time involved in teaching. Group motivation and learning from others are a great help to many. Somnambulists set fine examples for the others. There is a certain degree of uniformity among obstetric patients. All are within a fairly well defined age group. All have similar problems and probably identical motivation. Yet the groups are ever changing as some patients deliver and new ones are added. Repetition of teaching and omission of some desirable ideas, for one or another individual, are bound to occur with group conditioning. Some patients learn poorly or not at all. It has been difficult to single out one member of a group and confront her with the desirability of employing chemoanesthesia rather than hypnoanesthesia for delivery.

Balanced Analgesia-anesthesia: Hypnosis may be employed as an ataractic, analgesic, anesthetic, amnesic, in any combination, or as all four. The patient's needs may be met without any particular attention, with hypnosis alone, with chemoanalgesia and/or anesthesia, or with any combination. Elimination of large or dangerous amounts of chemical analgesics and anesthetics should be every obstetrician's goal. Small amounts well within the bounds of safety should cause no concern. If these be administered alone or in combination with hypnosis, or if hypnosis alone be used, and if this meets the patient's psychologic and physiologic needs, it is good therapy. Patients will vary in their needs. The same patient will make different demands at different times. It behooves her obstetrician to meet the situational requirement of the particular moment.

The Obstetric Situation: This consists of certain constants and variables. The pregnant female and the unborn child are always center stage. The attending physician and, almost as invariably in our society, the hospital together with its personnel are in this picture. The expectant father is an integral factor and almost always present during labor and delivery. Other relatives such as expectant grandmothers often manifest their presence.

The laboring female may be a grandmultipara having her umpteenth delivery or, a primigravida. She may require but a single contraction prior to fetal expulsion, or may labor many hours before terminating with cesarean section. She may enter the hospital for induction of labor by appointment or be rushed in by ambulance because of massive hemorrhage. She may be physically and/or emotionally in excellent health, very ill, or at any stage between the two extremes.

The expected infant may be intensely desired, as it would be after long and costly therapy for infertility. It may be undesirable for any one of a host of reasons. It may be a potentially ill child as with an expected Rh problem. It may be dead in utero or, worse yet, born mained or as a monstrosity. It may be large or small, at term, premature, or postmature.

The obstetrician may be tired or comfortable, hurried and harried, or relaxed. He may have serious problems of his own, or not a care. He may like the patient, be most intimately friendly as a result of caring for her through many illnesses over a number of years, or he may be treating her only because she contributes to his income.

Obstetric delivery in a hospital is certainly different from that in the home. I wish to speak only of the former. The mechanical facilities available, and, to a greater degree, the nursing personnel will affect the management of labor and delivery. This is doubly true when hypnotherapy is employed. Psychosomatically oriented nurses and aides facilitate employment of hypnosis. Careless conversation, inconsiderate care, and even noisy and disturbed patients in adjoining beds may prevent maintenance of a satisfactory trance. Any factors which tend to create disturbance or increase apprehension are objectionable.

The presence of a resident staff capable of administering adequate chemoanesthesia is invaluable to good obstetric care. It lessens the obstetrician's responsibility, also decreases the need for adequate hypnoanesthesia. Similarly, the absence of such ancillary personnel, in our hospitals as in many others, increases the desirability of hypnoanesthesia besides placing a greater burden on the obstetrician.

The expectant father can be tolerated, considered as an additional person requiring tender loving care, or employed as an aide for providing his wife with psychologic support. Some hospitals not only permit but encourage the husband's presence throughout labor and delivery. At the other extreme, he may be excluded completely. Ours permit his presence only during labor. Hypnotic rapport may be transferred from the obstetrician to the husband or to any properly coached hospital personnel. This lessens the need for the physician's presence. The conditions regulating my work do not lend themselves to a lightening of responsibility in this manner. Therefore, I employ analgesics such as Demerol whenever desirable during labor. I try to be present terminally and for as much more time as other responsibilities permit.

Patient care during labor and delivery must at all times serve the one primary purpose, that of terminating with a normal healthy mother and a normal healthy baby. Hypnosis must serve this purpose. If only the hazard of chemo-analgesia and anesthesia is limited or eliminated through reduction of quantities of chemicals administered, then hypnosis has served well.

The obstetrician is in a much better position for employing hypnosis than any other physician, even better than that of the psychiatrist. He has done a complete physical and a fairly adequate laboratory examination. He has become her confidante and general health adviser. Rapport comes easily to the gravid female. She is in a subservient position which readily permits the obstetrician to assume the father figure. Hypnosis is goal directed and limited, as therapy is always terminated after a preordained duration of time.

Results

I have personally employed hypnoanesthesia for over 1300 deliveries. Recently, 1000 consecutive obstetric deliveries were documented (3). These included management of cesarean section, forceps deliveries, episiotomy, both first and second degree lacerations, transverse arrest, prolapsed fetal parts, placenta praevia, abruptio placenta, retained placenta with manual removal, and ruptured uterus. Other conditions encountered in this series were hypertensive heart disease, toxemia with albuminuria, acute gastroenteritis, pneumonia, high temperature elevations of unknown etiology, heart disease with decompensation, diabetes, syphilis, Hodgkin's disease, pulmonary sarcoidosis, terminal carcinomatosis, and an acute appendicitis with appendectomy.

The following table shows the various anesthetic modalities employed.

Type Used		Number of Patients
Hypnoanesthesia		850
With prior conditioning	387	
Without prior conditioning	463	
With or without prior conditioning, requiring chemo-anesthesia	36	
Conditioned and requiring chemotherapy	14	
Nonconditioned and requiring chemotherapy	22	
Kind of chemo-anesthesia used		
Local—Novocain 1 per cent	17	
Trilene	8	
Multiple	6	
Pudendal block	2	
Saddle block	2	
Ether	1	
Other than hypnoanesthesia		150
Pudendal block	34	
Trilene	34	
Multiple	32	
Ether	14	
Local	13	
Saddle block	7	
Cyclopropane	2	
Psychoprophylactic education	8	
Precipitate	6	
Total		1000

It will be noted that hypnoanesthesia was attempted in 85 per cent, and that only 46 per cent of these patients had been previously conditioned. Of the 850 patients, with and without prior conditioning, 95 per cent required no chemoanesthesia of any kind.

Others (1, 5, 9, 17, 22) have described satisfactory employment of hypnosis for obstetric delivery. The average obstetrician may not have the time, the need, or the desire to complement his care with hypnotherapy, particularly not this frequently. Yet, each one will find many opportunities for improving his patient care in this manner, when he so wishes.

GYNECOLOGY

Definitive therapy in this specialty has been, until recent years, more often surgical. Ever since the discovery of and widespread use of antibiotics, therapy has tended to be medical, psychologic, or both. The interaction of psyche and soma with the resultant complex of symptoms is probably more frequently encountered in the specialty of gynecology than in any other area of medical practice. Hypnosis may serve as prime or adjunctive therapy only when psychologic or psychiatric problems are involved.

Gynecologic disease is rarely pediatric. Beginnings usually parallel the onset of menstruation. The frequency of such illness increases with the years, often reaching a peak at the menopause. Such complaints may, in any one person, become cumulative.

Menstrual problems may be classified as those associated with too little, absence of, irregularity of, excessive, or painful menstruation.

The menarche in white females living in the temperate zone usually occurs at about thirteen years of age. A later onset may be either a hereditary characteristic or evidence of organic disease. Whereas the etiology of such a problem would most rarely be psychogenic, subsequent irregularity, and especially amenorrhea in the nonpregnant female, may often result from psychogenic factors. Although asymptomatic infrequency of menstruation should lead to no concern, it often does. The patient may question her "normalcy." She may be desirous of regulating sexual contacts for the purpose of controlling the size of her family. Psychologic investigation followed by proper lines of therapy will either induce more regular menstruation or reduce the need for this. Symptom removal is not indicated. Understanding, initially by the therapist and subsequently by the patient herself, will remove this problem. Hypnosis may serve as a short cut to understanding and to therapy. Use of age regression, recall, and posthypnotic suggestion permit economy of physician's time and patient's expense.

The etiology of menometrorrhagia must be sought prior to therapy. When unknown, it may be first treated medically, then surgically with a dilatation and curettage. If this proves to be unsuccessful, some patients will respond to psychotherapy. Others will require hysterectomy. Hypnotherapy may here also serve most efficiently to hasten improvement. The order of employing the therapeutic modalities listed will save the therapist embarrassment and the patient untoward results. Menometrorrhagia which is etiologically functional should always be treated only with psychologic means.

Dysmenorrhea, premenstrual tension, and associated headaches and backaches are common complaints. Mittleschmerz is less frequently encountered. The etiology of all these is usually functional, often representing resentment of the feminine role (27). As a result, psychotherapy should be most efficacious. Yet, most patients so afflicted will shun this type of therapy because it is time consuming, expensive, or because they prefer to abstain from care which brands them as "mental patients." Hypnotherapy may be more acceptable because the foregoing objectionable factors are reduced or eliminated. Hypnoanalysis can be most effective. The therapist must, however, avoid direct symptom removal for such an approach might lead the patient to seek other outlets for manifestation of unresolved conflicts, which would subsequently worsen her general health. Even when successful, direct symptom removal is limited by the patient. I find the latter objection to be more valid. The former has not been encountered in my practice.

D. W. was a pretty, eighteen year old, white college student. She worked in a supermarket on weekends. Dysmenorrhea began shortly after the menarche at age twelve. It continued with such severity that neither work, nor study, nor even play was possible for two days out of every twenty-eight. She was able only to take analgesics and to remain in bed.

Her history obtained at the hypnotic level was much more revealing. She became twelve years old on February 12, 1953. Two days later, she was guest of honor at a birthday party. The menarche appeared. This together with the irritation attendant on wearing a perineal pad for the first time was doubly embarrassing because none of the other little girls had as yet begun to menstruate. Her mother said it was just "her sick time." So she feigned a headache and went to bed. This procedure continued each month, at first with varying intensity of headache, subsequently with increasing severity and multiplicity of noxious symptoms.

Wonderingly, I asked why her twelfth birthday party had been postponed two days. She thought for a minute then answered that her birthday (that year) fell on a Thursday. The children of her age group were free of school attendance on Saturday, two days later. After our visit had terminated, and the patient left, I called our local newspaper office to verify that February 12, 1953, fell on a Thursday. It did. Yet the patient was unable to verify this or any other such birthday in a similar manner at the waking level.

Suffice it to say that discovering the origin of her initial complaints and understanding the effects of habit formation permitted marked improvement and negated the necessity for continued inconvenient confinements to bed.

Diminution followed by cessation of the menses signals the initiation of another of life's phases (10). The human female often thinks of this transitional period as the termination of the desirable portion of her life rather than as another beginning. She is concerned over her decreasing physical attractiveness, the possibilities of losing libidinous activity, and the need for facing an empty future devoid of responsibilities. The single girl and the widow, both feel themselves relegated to an inferior position in the presence of younger and presumably more attractive women. The mother has now accomplished that for which she was created. The most important task, giving birth to children, has been completed. Although the responsibilities, skill, care, and intelligence attendant on motherhood and marriage may require far more than the begetting of children, she may accept this truism only at the conscious level. Subconsciously she fears most of all that she will now be no longer needed, a most depressing thought. Is it any wonder that involutional melancholia and other psychoses commonly occur at this time of life?

Vasomotor symptoms (hot flashes) and a whole host of anxiety reactions characterize "the change of life." Hormonal agents, sedatives, tranquilizers, and psychic stimulants are often useful. These may prove adequate. Intensive psychotherapy may be needed. Hypnotherapy, providing an opportunity for patient self understanding, evaluation, and acceptance, will help many. Psychologic rather than medical or surgical therapy is most frequently indicated because climacteric symptoms are to a large degree psychic in origin.

Symptomatology resulting from sexual interaction is far more frequently encountered in the female than in the male. Either the presence or the absence of psychologic and physical contact with the opposite sex may become the most significant of etiologic factors. Societal status, marriage or lack of it, economics, and pregnancy are also controlling factors. Frigidity or sterility are resultant complaints which bring these patients to the gynecologist. Pseudocyesis may confront either the obstetrician or gynecologist.

The etiology of frigidity is rarely organic. The young lady with external development defects such as total absence of the vagina may present herself for treatment after failure to consummate marriage. The girl with inadequate breast development will seek therapy much earlier. The one with gonadal insufficiency or total failure of heterosexual differentiation may never seek therapy. She may not know of what she is missing. However, the total number of people with such developmental or organic problems are few.

Frigidity may follow male ineptness or lack of consideration. It may result from female lack of orientation and understanding. Most frigidity problems are functional in origin (4, 19).

FRIGIDITY

Etiology	Frequency	Totality		Associated Noxious Symptoms
		Relative	Absolute	
organic	extremely rare	rarely	usually	rare
functional	common	usually	rarely	common

Cultural bias teaches the little girl to fear and to avoid homo- and, most of all, heterosexual contact. She is taught to shun the former and to reserve the latter for some future time. Sexual activity is often equated with the bad, abhorent, distasteful, and unclean. Maternal prohibitions will so often create filial inhibitions.

This is not so for the lad. He learns of sexual practices through his peer group. Freedom of discussion leads first to bravado of expression, subsequently to greater lattitude of understanding. Besides, he feels no concern over becoming pregnant. Shame and responsibility become of less concern for him than they do for her.

Some women can be sexually aroused yet fail to experience an orgasm. Others will be libidinously satiated in a variety of ways such as with "petting," "necking," fondling, kissing, and with loving speech and acts of kindness. The likelihood of a child's propinquity fulfilling love needs is far greater with a mother than it is with a father. There is a great variance in the need for love and in the readiness for orgiastic response from one time to the next. Some women, apparently, have no such need at any time. A multitude of psychologic problems in addition to culturally ingrained bias may prevent one from so doing. The mother who is fearful for her child's health may refuse sexual relationships altogether or, at best, respond without orgasm. Her husband will not be inhibited to the same degree. Does the female's response represent a higher form of love? Should the gynecologist interfere?

Obviously, single or infrequent episodes of frigidity will cause no concern. Therapy is needed when such a pattern has been established to the degree that either or both wife and husband are no longer happy. Attention becomes ever so much more desirable when the usual concomitants of dysmenorrhea, pelvic pain, backache, severe headaches, and dyspareunia make their appearance. Each of these is in its own way a manifestation of the primary problem, unhappiness linked with misunderstanding and with failure to accept the feminine role. Psychotherapy or hypnoanalysis are needed. Mere symptom removal should not be practiced for it will no more suffice than will surgery or the administration of medications. Even the unearthing of traumatic material must be carefully managed. It must be fed back to the patient only after she is psychically ready for understanding and acceptance. A complete history and physical examination may be followed by explanation and suggestion indicating the advisability of hypnotherapy. The hypnotic trance is induced for more intensive investigation followed by retraining with the permissive approach. If necessary, authoritarian guidance is also employed. Results have been good.

C. H. was a twenty-one year old laboratory technician. Her husband was of the same age. Her only pregnancy had terminated favorably with a child now fourteen months old. There had been no coitus for eight weeks following her delivery. She had been blessed with an apparently normal libido prior to her delivery, but was now cursed with frigidity. No contraceptives had ever been used. Physical examination revealed an attractive, healthy, young, adult, white female of average weight and height. She had a partially relaxed entroitus, a vagina of better than average size, and absence of any sensitive areas. There was good tone in the levator ani and constrictor vaginae muscles.

She readily and avidly accepted the hypnotic trance, despite this being her initial experience, because she had been referred for hypnotherapy. Misinformation and misunderstanding were discovered to be her problems. She was advised of the normalcy and propriety of marital sexual relationships attuned to her husband's desires. Anatomic and physiologic details about her genitals were explained. Sensations obtainable were pictured verbally. An authoritarian manner was employed to suggest that she *enjoy* intercourse. She was seen again one week later. Intercourse with pleasure had been enjoyed five times in the previous seven days. She had culminated with a climax each time.

Sterility or infertility always involves two people. It may be primary, or secondary following any number of prior pregnancies. It normally tags on the skirts of the climacteric. A number of interacting variables, both functional and organic, may prevent pregnancy. Therapy must begin with a thorough investigation of both partners. All organic problems must be sought and treated when possible. Only subsequently is investigation and therapy of functional factors indicated. When such is needed, hypnosis becomes a valuable adjunct. It is a rapid method for learning psychological background, for removing problems which might interfere with consummation of coitus by the male and satisfactory cooperation by the female, for altering the vaginal flora, and for reducing female tensions and tubal spasm. Hypnotherapy may also aid in the production of regular ovulatory cycles and in more nearly normal vaginal hydrogen ion concentration, although we do now have some excellent hormonal preparations which will produce similarly satisfactory results with far less physician effort (2).

Hypnoanalytic investigation may uncover the imprudence of

pregnancy. Subconsciously, she may have a deep seated antipathy for pregnancy, and may be submitting to therapy in order to satisfy family or social demands. She may be doing so as a last ditch effort to sustain a marriage on the verge of dissolution. Then, we serve her best by failing to aid in her conscious desires. Thus, psychologic investigation by a capable physician cognizant of her problems and entrusted with her care can favorably alter the course of her entire adult life.

Pseudocyesis, although rare, can be a most formidable problem. It has been seen at all ages of the childbearing period and into the climacteric. Etiologically, it probably results from either an intense desire for or fear of pregnancy (15). Most of the women presenting this picture have never previously been pregnant. Yet they are acquainted with the signs and symptoms expected of them. Amenorrhea, nausea and vomiting, pica, breast changes, abdominal enlargment, striae, quickening, and weight gain may be present. These changes may be progressive, consonant with normal alterations expected in pregnancy. Early diagnosis may be difficult, but failure to palpate a progressively enlarging uterus and absence of radiologic evidence of a fetal skeleton are conclusive. Such a patient has deeply seated emotional problems. Divulging the diagnosis to her must be carefully managed. Psychiatric care is often needed.

Special problems such as leukorrhea and obesity are commonly seen in the gynecologist's office.

Leukorrhea

The etiology of leukorrhea, with or without pruritis, is most frequently organic, rarely functional. Satisfactory evaluation which has ruled out organic causation must be followed by psycho- or hypnotherapy. Here again, mere symptom removal is contraindicated. Conflicts and other subconscious material must first be discovered then properly managed. Functional leukorrhea will respond only to functional therapy.

Obesity

Being excessively overweight is almost always an organic manifestation of functional disease. Although it might require consideration as being the curse of prosperity, this is not invariably true.

I have seen economically impoverished people become obese on bread and potatoes. Obesity is certainly not limited to adult females, yet they are simultaneously most susceptible and most desirous of cure.

Why does an apparently intelligent, otherwise healthy, adult female overeat to the degree of requiring medical attention to help her lose weight? Still more strange, why do so many present themselves with the statement, "I want you to *make* me lose weight"?

With the exception of poor familial eating habits, obesity is the next to the last chapter following functional disease which employs overeating as a compensatory or covering mechanism. The last is loss of attractiveness, disfigurement, organic disease, and an earlier demise. These are a high price to pay for failure to understand and to correct emotional problems.

Ataractics, anorectics, sedatives, and diuretics, as well as dietary control all have their place in the process of weight reduction. Understanding and acceptance leading to emotional stability is the *sine qua non*. Psychotherapy may be needed, particularly for treatment of deep seated emotional conflicts. The cost in time and dollars may be considerable, even prohibitive. Hypnotherapy may be most satisfactory, and will usually consume less time and dollars.

I have not as yet succumbed to the temptation of group hypnotherapy for this problem. Others (16, 21) are apparently well satisfied with such an approach for economic reasons. I have found individual hypnoanalysis to be most effective. This, combined with medication and dietary regulation, have been productive of satisfactory results in most cases.

Office Procedures

Tubal insufflation, cervical cautery or biopsy, catheterization, or even a proper pelvic exam may be most disconcerting and well nigh unto impossible with some patients. Induction of a light to medium trance will facilitate these procedures.

Gynecologic Surgery

Hypnosis may be employed to prepare the patient for surgery, for surgical anesthesia, and for providing postoperative comfort. Suggestions prior to surgery may prepare the way for all three or for only pre- and postoperative tranquility.

The initial trance state should be terminated with suggestions leading to postoperative comfort. A patient so treated will not only become a better surgical risk, but also will recover more certainly, more promptly, and with less distress.

A. M., a pretty twenty-five year old mother of four, had been hospitalized for vaginal hemorrhage. The history and physical examination revealed an incomplete abortion indicating the need for uterine curettage. The fact that this was an extramarital pregnancy, and that her husband had been sterilized several years previously, probably contributed to a pronounced degree of emotional distress. Induction of a deep trance permitted her the enjoyment of a peaceful night preoperatively, and postoperative asymptomatic recovery. In addition, the anesthesiologist was delayed, so I proceeded with surgery in his absence. No chemoanesthesia was required.

Gynecologic surgery rarely requires hypnoanesthesia. However, the patient needing an emergency D&C because of severe and continuing hemorrhage may be a poor anesthetic risk, particularly if she had recently ingested a full meal. This has been encountered a number of times, with a D&C easily performed while employing only hypnoanesthesia on each occasion. From my experience, the emergency patient can readily understand the need for acceptance of suggestions leading to a satisfactory trance. The physician need only to be certain of himself. Convincing the patient easily follows.

Pronounced emotional distress, recent ingestion of food, multiple allergies contraindicating use of the usual chemical anesthetic agents, fear of chemoanesthesia and/or spinal anesthesia, and advanced cardiac or pulmonary disease may serve as indications for hypnoanesthesia. Unfortunately, no form of chemical anesthesia will provide continuing postoperative comfort as will posthypnotic suggestions.

Carcinoma

Terminal and incurable carcinomatosis provides an unlimited and little explored field for employment of hypnotherapy. Understanding, acceptance, and analgesia are boons which no other therapeutic modality can grant.

D. M. expired of generalized carcinomatosis in her 38th **year.**

She had found time for mothering six children, varying in age from two to nineteen, plus active participation to the very last in church and community affairs. A total mastectomy had been performed on 5-1-56. She was apparently in good health when last seen for postpartum care on 5-12-58. Ten months later, back pain led to hospitalization and radiologic examination which revealed metastatic malignant involvement of the lungs, liver, thoracic and lumbar spine, rib cage, pelvis, and both femurs. She was discharged on 4-13-59, apparently well enough to resume her normal activities plus taking a thousand mile automobile trip to Florida for a month's vacation the following winter. She was rehospitalized on 11-3-60, and remained so until her death on 12-25-60, four and a half years after the initial diagnosis of carcinoma and one and a half years after evidence of generalized metastatic lesions.

Chemical analgesics, radiotherapy, and hypnotherapy provided her with an unusual degree of comfort. Autohypnosis daily with an analgesic capsule only once or twice a week were employed during the last year of her illness. Although bedridden for the last few months she continued quite comfortably with a complacency and acceptance rarely seen except in the well conditioned hypnotic subject.

SUMMARY

The what and the when of hypnosis in obstetrics and gynecology have been presented. Space has limited discussion of methodologies. The good obstetrician-gynecologist must be concerned with many disciplines. There are times when medicine, surgery, psychiatry, and hypnosis are indicated.

Hypnosis for investigation and for therapy has an unique and most important niche in the obstetrician-gynecologist's armamentarium. It can result in amelioration and in cure when nothing else will. Therefore it behooves him to be sufficiently conversant to make proper referrals when indicated, or better yet, to be adequately skilled for employment of hypnosis to serve his patients properly.

REFERENCES

1. ABRAMSON, M. and HERON, W. T.: An objective evaluation of hypnosis in obstetrics. *Am. J. Obst. & Gynec.*, *59*:1069-1074, 1950.

2. AUGUST, R. V.: Hypnosis: An additional tool in the study of infertility. *Fertil. & Steril.*, *11*:118-123, 1960.

3. AUGUST, R. V.: *Hypnosis in Obstetrics*. New York, McGraw-Hill, 1961.

4. AUGUST, R. V.: Libido altered with the aid of hypnosis: a case report. *Am. J. Clin. Hyp.*, *2*:88, 1959.

5. BALL, T. L.: The psychoprophylactic preparation of pregnant women for childbirth in the Union of Soviet Socialist Republics. *Ann. New York Acad. Sc.*, *22*:578-580, 1960.

6. BONSTEIN, I.: *Psychoprophylactic Preparation for Painless Childbirth*. New York, Grune & Stratton, 1958.

7. CHERTOK, L.: *Psychosomatic Methods in Painless Childbirth*. London, Pergamon Press, 1959.

8. COOPER, L. F. and ERICKSON, M. H.: *Time Distortion in Hypnosis*. Baltimore, The Williams and Wilkins Co., 1954.

9. DELEE, S. T.: Hypnotism in pregnancy and labour. *J.A.M.A.*, *155*:750-754, 1955.

10. DEUTSCH, H.: *The Psychology of Women*. 2 Vols., New York, Grune & Stratton, 1945.

11. DICK-READ, G.: *Natural Childbirth*. London, William Heinemann, 1933.

12. DICK-READ, G.: *Childbirth Without Fear*. New York, Harper & Brothers, 1953.

13. ERICKSON, M. H.: Naturalistic techniques of hypnosis. *Am. J. Clin. Hyp.*, *1*:3-8, 1958.

14. ERICKSON, M. H.: Further clinical techniques of hypnosis: utilization techniques. *Am. J. Clin. Hyp.*, *2*:3-21, 1959.

15. FRIED, P. H., RAKOFF, A. E., SCHOPBACH, R. R. and KAPLAN, A. J.: Pseudocyesis: A psychosomatic study in gynecology. *J.A.M.A.*, *145*:1329-1335, 1951.

16. GLOVER, F. S.: Use of hypnosis for weight reduction in a group of nurses. *Am. J. Clin. Hyp.*, *3*:250-251, 1961.

17. HOFFMAN, G. L., JR. and KOPENHAVER, D. B.: Medical hypnosis and its use in obstetrics. *Am. J. Med. Sc.*, *241*:788-810, 1961.

18. KROGER, W. S. and DELEE, S. T.: Hypnoanesthesia for cesarean section and hysterectomy. *J.A.M.A.*, *163*:442-444, 1957.

19. KROGER, W. S. and FREED, S. C.: *Psychosomatic Gynecology.* Glencoe, Ill., Free Press, 1956.
20. KROGER, W. S. and SCHNEIDER, S. A.: An electronic aid for hypnotic induction: A preliminary report. *Int. J. Clin. & Exper. Hyp.,* 7:93-98, 1959.
21. MANN, H.: Group hypnosis in the treatment of obesity. *Am. J. Clin. Hyp.,* 1:114-116, 1959.
22. MOYA, F. and JAMES, L. S.: Medical hypnosis for obstetrics. *J.A.M.A.,* 174:2026-2032, 1960.
23. RICE, F. G.: The hypnotic induction of labor: six cases. *Am. J. Clin. Hyp., 4*:119-122, 1961.
24. SCHULTZ, J. H. and LUTHE, W.: *Autogenic Training.* New York, Grune & Stratton, 1959.
25. TAYLOR, H.: (Panelist) Hypnosis in Obstetrics, Annual meeting Soc. Clin. & Exp. Hyp., Cleveland, Ohio, 1961.
26. WEITZENHOFER, A. M.: *General Techniques of Hypnosis.* New York, Grune & Stratton, 1957.
27. WILLSON, J. R., BEECHAM, C. T., FORMAN, I. and CARRINGTON, E. R.: *Obstetrics and Gynecology.* St. Louis, C. V. Mosby, 1958.
28. WOLBERG, L. R.: *Medical Hypnosis,* Vol. I. New York, Grune & Stratton, 1948.
29. ZUSPAN, F. P.: (Panelist) Hypnosis in Obstetrics, Annual meeting Soc. Clin. & Exp. Hyp., Cleveland, Ohio, 1961.

6

HYPNOSIS IN PSYCHIATRY

JEROME M. SCHNECK, A.B., M.D.

Psychiatric hypnotherapy denotes the use of hypnotic settings and methods for the application of psychotherapeutic techniques and principles. Hypnosis is used, in this sense, for the purpose of facilitating psychotherapy. The frequency with which these settings are employed vary considerably, but therapy may be designated hypnotherapy specifically if the hypnotic features play a significant role in the total treatment process. The hypnotic methods vary too, in keeping with the needs and aptitudes of patient and therapist for good utilization of the measures themselves.

In a broad sense psychiatric hypnotherapy should apply to the use of hypnosis for any aspect of psychiatric practice. For example, Bowers and Berkowitz (1) have reported on its incorporation into electroconvulsive therapy. It helped to mitigate some disturbing after-effects associated with electroconvulsive procedures, and apparently permanent amnesia related to ECT was dispelled through utilization of hypnosis. But the current status of psychiatric hypnotherapy identifies it as largely a form of psychotherapy. Hypnotic methods are adjuncts in such therapy, and they are frequently of fundamental importance. The core of effective hypnotherapy, however, is good psychotherapy. And an important feature of psychiatric hypnotherapy is its adaptability to flexible employment in that it is not bound to any one theoretical orientation. Hypnotic methods may be joined with psychotherapy of any theoretical persuasion should the therapist wish to adapt its use to his purposes. Basically of course, the needs of patients are of fundamental concern and the hypnotic methods and settings are aimed at assisting patients in gaining relief from distress, with greater self-understanding to be achieved whenever possible. Hypnotherapy called hypnoanalysis consists of the fusion of hypnotic methods and theory with psychoanalytic method and theory. Again, hypnoanalysis itself need not be confined to any one orientation in the broader realm of psychoanalytic practice. Analysis of resistance and transference can constitute part of hypnoanalytic practice as it does in equivalent psychoanalytic experience not involving the use of hypnosis (Schneck, 2).

THE USE OF PSYCHIATRIC HYPNOTHERAPY

Hypnotherapy should be confined by the practicing psychiatrist to problems for which he would not hesitate to employ his skills were hypnotic methods themselves to play no role in treatment (3). Such methods are not to be employed for problems beyond the confines of the psychiatrist's basic aptitudes. If experience has been limited largely to the neuroses, hypnotherapy should not serve as an experimental venture in dealing with psychotic problems. General psychotherapeutic experience with the latter would obviously be an essential. To move beyond the range of one's legitimate experience may seem clearly to be proscribed, yet it is attempted too often when therapists have not overcome the feeling of magical potency so long associated with hypnotic techniques. If a therapist practices hypnotherapy within the sphere of his basic competence there need be no concern about risks and dangers any more than would apply under similar circumstances to other areas of medical practice. With acquisition of hypnotherapeutic skills superimposed on fundamental psychiatric training, there is no need to stress dangers in any special way. Indeed the potential risks do not exceed those encountered in numerous medical, surgical, and psychiatric procedures. It is sufficient to mention the necessary safeguards of therapeutic abilities and good knowledge of psychodynamics. To stress hazards beyond this impedes progress in the proper development of psychiatric hypnotherapy.

Hypnotic techniques have been used effectively as adjuncts in treatment for a variety of psychiatric problems including anxiety reactions, conversion reactions and anxiety hysteria with special reference to phobic difficulties, obsessive-compulsive reactions, character disorders, neurotic depressive reactions, and certain facets of schizophrenic problems. Hypnotherapy has been used for many psychophysiologic reactions and specific problems in interpersonal relations including family difficulties. Some of the psychophysiologic disturbances include gastrointestinal upsets, cardiac arrhythmias, migraine, neurodermatitis and psoriasis, and psychogenic dyspnea. Benefits have emerged with psychological complications of multiple sclerosis. The gamut of psychiatric disabilities need not be listed because at one time or other, if one were to study the history of hypnosis over the past century, virtually all psychological problems have fallen within the range of hypnotherapeutic efforts. The hysterical disorders have probably come in for greatest attention with claims of success. Occasionally some therapists may find them difficult to ameliorate. Obsessive-compulsive difficulties are usually acknowledged to be more refractory than the hysterical problems, yet at times some therapists report especially favorable results.

The character neuroses probably can be assisted more than is usually reported, but those of great severity tend to be refractory. Psychopathic personalities present special difficulties in psychotherapy, and hypnotherapy is no exception, but isolated claims are favorable although they are perhaps based on few cases. Mild depressive reactions are undoubtedly ameliorated with relatively greater ease than severe depressions. The latter are so frequently refractory. With them many therapists are reluctant to employ hypnotherapy without hospital supervision. The great risk, of course, is the suicidal potential. Less experience with the psychoses has been reported than with the neuroses (46). Schizophrenic patients may experience help of a type that varies with the patient (44, 45). One such example is a feeling of protective support associated for some patients with a good interpersonal relationship intensified by child-parent identifications within the hypnotic setting. Yet care is required with paranoid patients who may focus on the fantasy of insidious control as part of hypnotic mechanisms. They tend to elaborate pathologically the implications of the hypnotic relationship. If hypnotherapy is used for paranoid problems or for psychotic reactions in general, a hospital setting is often desirable unless the psychiatrist possesses special experience not only with hypnotherapy, but in dealing with seriously disturbed patients as part of his daily practice.

Alcoholics are felt often to be readily hypnotizable. Those with mild problems are seen more consistently than patients with severe difficulties. The latter call for psychiatrists especially efficient in the treatment of alcoholism as well as experienced in the use of hypnotic methods. Alcoholism is difficult to treat, yet as is true of all the disorders, one encounters occasional claims of special success. Hypnotherapy has long been used for amnesic reactions, especially those associated with more pervasive hysterical disorders. Many amnesias can be cleared under hypnosis but it is most desirable to attempt longer term assistance for the fundamental personality difficulties. This view would apply also to the many symptoms that have at some time been approached hypnotherapeutically. Yet relatively short term therapy has frequently been of great help in assisting with pervasive, fundamental personality problems beyond specific symptom complaints.

The hypnotic setting with its varying intrapsychic and interpersonal significance for individual patients has often been in itself a helpful measure to expedite relief from anxiety in patients with anxiety states and with conditions in which overt anxiety has been a prominent feature. The setting has been helpful for patients in permitting them to work through on ideational and affective levels the problems with which they were contending. This facilitation of change varies in degree and time with many patients without any direct relationship necessarily to the specific classification of disability. Within hypnotic settings there is a trend toward greater ability to work effectively on consciously available issues, preconscious material that comes to the surface better at such times, and unconscious material of significance which becomes consciously available more readily within the hypnotic interpersonal contact. The latter permits helpful exploration of determinants in symptom formation with resolution of conflicts, although at times symptoms may be relieved without such exploration by virtue of the psychological forces favorably influencing such change within the doctor-patient relationship.

An undetermined number of such symptomatic cures are permanent, and they have been known to be accompanied by more extensive and meaningful personality improvement apparently as a result of concurrent psychological reorganization set in motion by the more circumscribed symptom alteration. In the same way, a favorable change in the dynamic core of one symptom may evoke a series of changes resulting in amelioration of other symptoms apparently bound to the same dynamic issues. This contrasts with the opposite trend of symptom substitution that occurs when any one symptom, as a surface aspect of a problem, is suppressed rather than resolved. This suppression and symptom replacement by a counterpart occurs, as should readily be admitted, in all therapeutic encounters whether or not hypnotic methods are employed (Schneck, 48).

When the hypnotic setting and methods enhance abilities of patients to work effectively therapeutically, the past and present may be explored in many ways. Events may be restudied and reconstructed, attitudes and interpersonal relations re-evaluated, patterns of personality functioning elucidated, and goals redefined. The rapidity with which significant data are unearthed can at times be controlled effectively to conform to the needs of patients. Insights may be elicited indirectly with some methods and the timing with which they become consciously available to patients may be manipulated satisfactorily through the use of specific suggestions or with induced amnesias in the case of patients capable of achieving such amnesias. Hypnosis may be a strong stimulus to effective thinking through and working through of psychological problems on all levels, and achievement of insight is often more rapid. Productivity in general may be enhanced. The use of hypnosis appears often to diminish total treatment time although claims on this score are unfortunately exaggerated. Yet there is always the possibility that with proper management some reduction may well occur in many instances. More important is the betterment of the treatment situation as a whole and the assistance supplied patients in achieving therapeutic goals. This enhancement is too often obscured by stress on brevity, although rapid amelioration of problems is of legitimate concern.

Effective hypnotherapy does not call for compulsive reliance on hypnotic technique. Hypnosis may be introduced into sessions whenever indicated for special purposes in the judgment of the therapist. His clinical experience is the base for determining when hypnosis should or should not be employed, and he guides the coordination of hypnotic and non-hypnotic interview content. The degree of his activity or passivity is determined by his intentions. In hypnoanalysis, for example, he may choose a passive role more frequently than in other types of hypnotherapy, yet there are opportunities for considerable flexibility in his manner of operating. Behind the choice lies the interplay of the patient's and therapist's personalities and the latter's theoretical focus.

The manner and extent to which efforts are made in treatment to have patients gain insight into the nature of their problems varies considerably. This relates also to the ability of hypnotherapeutic and analytic methods to elucidate the nature of psychological dynamisms in the course of treatment. Until recently the usual emphasis has been the role of hypnosis in coping with the mechanism of repression. Probably this emphasis was based on attempts to use hypnotherapy primarily to uncover buried memories. There has been ample demonstration more recently that a variety of significant dynamisms have been brought into sharp focus in hypnotic settings with several techniques. They include projection, isolation, condensation, symbolization, identification, introjection, and rationalization (Schneck, 4). Clarification of their operation is most likely to occur in either short-term psychoanalytically oriented hypnotherapy or long-term hypnoanalysis.

SELECTION OF PATIENTS FOR HYPNOTHERAPY

The decision by a relatively inexperienced psychiatrist to employ hypnotherapy must be based on several considerations. His clinical judgment regarding his own aptitudes for dealing with the basic problem presented by his patient during initial consultation is fundamental. His previous work with similar problems for which hypnotherapy had been employed, his professional reading, instruction in hypnosis, and opportunities for supervision, are to be considered also in the decision to use hypnosis. The more experienced hypnotherapist has less of a problem in deciding whom to accept, and has more concern with dissuading patients from seeking hypnotherapy when it appears to be contraindicated. Few experienced psychiatrists would wish to limit their practices to hypnotherapy exclusively.

Hypnotherapy may be considered for patients requesting it when the problem seems suitable for its use and when the requests are based apparently on a realistic view of possibilities for successful outcome. Expectations are often unrealistic, however, and disappointment is likely to be the outcome in such instances. An example is the notion of cure in one or two sessions for deep-seated personality problems of long standing, perhaps with a history of one or more therapeutic failures in previous psychiatric treatment. Such examples are certainly not unusual. Some requests may appear to be accompanied by reasonable expressions of awareness regarding the desirability of mutual cooperation in therapy, the need for patience as concerns time required for treatment, and related issues. Yet at the same time patients may harbor unconscious fantasies about hypnosis, some of which may impede treatment if they are not dealt with successfully. The existence of unconscious fantasies about hypnosis is not remarkable. The importance of the fantasies has to do with what they reveal about the general personality functioning of the patient and their significance for therapeutic management.

In requests for hypnotherapy patients experience fantasies of omnipotence and masochistic submission, the satisfaction of dependency needs and sexual strivings both heterosexual and homosexual, as well as symbolic death and rebirth equivalents. The fantasies may be even more complex with a variety of combinations. Many patients requesting hypnotherapy do not necessarily desire it and a number of hidden determinants are present in the deceptive search for hypnotherapy and hypnoanalysis (Schneck, 5). It is important for therapists to recognize them because of their significance in the initiation and conduct of treatment. Patients may desire psychotherapy, but with ambivalent feelings, and the search for hypnosis may be a way of establishing initial contact.

During a phase of intensified resistance with one therapist, inquiry about hypnosis may be an indication of the wish to change psychiatrists. Requests may reflect the wish to change doctors during a period of negative transference, and as in the previous example the expressed wish for hypnotherapy specifically may actually be deceiving. Also, the alleged wish may cover the more fundamental search for a new therapist when the patient feels no gains have been achieved in previous treatment or when the speed of recovery has not been sufficiently satisfying for the patient. Deceptive requests for hypnotherapy are at times a way of acceding to pressure by others who favor such treatment, whereas actually the patient is voicing, through making this contact, an essential agreement to psychotherapy in general. Whether or not hypnotherapy is decided upon and initiated should depend on the therapist's evaluation of the patient's suitability for it. At times it may be advised against. On occasion, hypnotherapy may be indicated regardless of the original deception. The latter, in addition to being discerned by the therapist, may be evaluated with the patient during the course of treatment to the extent deemed appropriate. If requests by patients are not judged adequately, significant problems of resistance, transference, and counter-transference may arise.

Whether patients request hypnotherapy or the psychiatrist decides during the course of treatment that its use may be of potential advantage, there are forces which are involved intrinsically in the relationship that unfolds. For the psychiatrist there is his confidence in his abilities, the significance of hypnotic relationships for him, his true, casual acceptance of hypnotic procedure as a legitimate scientific tool in medical treatment, and the absence of highly charged emotional associations fostering troublesome countertransference reactions and interfering with smooth technical functioning. For the patient there are the positive and negative influence of his level of intelligence that would permit an understanding of what is expected of him in the hypnotic setting, the impression made on him by what he has seen or heard in connection with hypnosis specifically and psychiatric treatment in general, his reactions to the psychiatrist as a person and therapist, and the aforementioned unconscious implications of hypnosis as they apply to him. When hypnotherapy is suggested by the doctor rather than the patient, the latter's conceptions and misconceptions may be elicited soon after initial contact as an outgrowth of a discussion regarding the patient's views about a variety of possible treatment procedures. If hypnotherapy is considered after treatment has been conducted on a non-hypnotic level, it may be approached usually in a more direct fashion. The more that is known specifically about a patient or inferred indirectly, the better the psychiatrist is able to evaluate the manner in which he proceeds with induction and the application of hypnotherapeutic principles.

INDUCTION AND TERMINATION OF HYPNOSIS

Induction and termination are discussed in a separate chapter. Brief reference will be made here to certain aspects of both in order to highlight the writer's views and preferences and special points of interest.

Each therapist follows his inclinations in accordance with his training, experience, and personality needs. He must modify his methods to suit the requirements of different patients also. His tone, use of words, timing, application of direct and indirect suggestions, and general manner among other elements are adjusted to serve the requirements in each instance. The degree to which an authoritative approach is employed and the manner in which non-authoritative techniques are used vary among therapists and in relation to patients.

There are numerous modifications of methods for inducing the trance (47). Many fall under two general but not mutually exclusive categories. They are the ocular or visual fixation and the hand levitation methods. For several years, although employing both, the writer favored the former simply because it suited better the needs and abilities of most patients and was less time consuming for routine office practice. In recent years he has favored his modification of the latter, in the form of a two stage hand levitation method. Most patients use it as well as, or more easily than ocular fixation and it often is even more rapid although it should be emphasized that within convenient limits for office use, time is not an urgent issue. After a few sessions, hypnotic induction generally presents no problem and is quite rapid. The first stage involves focus of attention by the patient on his hand which is lifted voluntarily and slowly an inch or two or three from his lap. This is helpful in overcoming delays, sometimes quite marked, if voluntary activity is discouraged. Then suggestions simply convert the voluntary movement into an involuntary action by centering attention on automatic bending of the elbow and contraction of arm muscles. Variations of the remainder of the induction parallel routine maneuvers of the hand levitation technique are described by Erickson (6).

Although it is often stated that relatively normal people respond to induction better than those with psychological disturbances, no special problem exists in psychiatric practice consisting largely of neurotic patients. Most experienced hypnotherapists readily achieve inductions exceeding 90 per cent on initial encounter and often the figure is much higher. There is a difference, however, in the frequency with which patients experience complete posthypnotic amnesias in therapeutic settings as contrasted with demonstration or experimental settings. Approximately 25 per cent of subjects in the latter groups tend readily to develop such amnesias. Ten per cent or less of psychiatric patients demonstrate complete amnesias early in their work with hypnotherapy. Differences in the dynamics of the settings, interpersonal relationships, and associated impulse tendencies and defenses undoubtedly account for this difference. Treatment settings that are not of the routine office practice variety permit generally the development of types of trance behavior more likely to involve complete posthypnotic amnesias too. Indirect or modified techniques need not include mention of the word "hypnosis" at all, but these are generally reserved for special situations (2, 7).

Many patients reveal their personality problems significantly during induction and these can serve as important guides in treatment. They may manifest evidences of compliance, dependency, aggression, negativism, skepticism, masochism, sexual excitement, and varying degrees and aspects of impulse control. Their fantasies at such times are very revealing. Many psychosomatic reactions are evident or reported and they involve organ systems including the respiratory, cardiovascular, gastrointestinal, and musculoskeletal. Tachycardia and altered breathing rates are quite common. Frequently these are somatic expressions of anxiety in relation to the conscious and unconscious significance of hypnosis as a new experience. Occasionally miniature, transitory, conversion phenomena are observable in initial inductions (10). Thus induction can serve virtually as a concentrated setting for the expression of psychosomatic, hysterical, obsessive-compulsive, and other reaction patterns.

At times one encounters stress on the importance of differentiating between the stage of induction and the fully developed hypnotic state, especially in terms of the proper timing of therapeutic work and related concerns. It is important to realize, however, that one must not divide stages too decisively in that the personality interactions and intrapsychic activities in all phases of hypnotic sessions, including induction and termination, are intimately entwined and from a view of therapeutic significance and movement must not be divorced from one another. One example of this view would be the definite relatedness of the fantasy activity within the hypnotic setting (no less aside from it) being pertinent in its connections with and transitions into the fantasies of the post-induction period and the termination phase as well.

Compared to other portions of hypnotic contacts, termination of hypnosis has received relatively little attention. Troublesome aspects when mentioned are generally exaggerated, and among psychologically qualified practitioners difficulties appear to be quite infrequent. Yet Williams was able to collect accounts of difficulties in dehypnotization from several sources and the issue of potential problems deserves its share of serious attention (8). Sometimes the dynamics of the problems involved are subject to investigation and understanding. When Rosen discussed such cases he felt the problems were similar to those of patients who refuse to leave the office at the end of ordinary therapy sessions (9). Overlapping dynamisms highlighted such behavior as a form of acting out.

Under the heading of "depth reversal during termination of the hypnotic state" I pointed out, in connection with dehypnotization, that termination is not necessarily undirectional in the sense of gradual change from so-called deeper levels to lighter levels of hypnosis with final emergence from it. Not only does the process vary in rapidity, but the movement may be reversed with immediate deepening as termination is started, followed by lightening again. The reversal may occur several times from start to finish, with biphasic and multiphasic responses. Depth may lessen at first, increase, decrease again, and so on. Three examples of issues encountered on investigation of patients' reactions are: 1) the wish of the patient to continue in hypnosis with its gratifications and those of the hypnotic interpersonal relationships, 2) the interest of the patient in attending to unfinished business pertaining to therapeutic material on which he had been concentrating, and 3) the relinquishing of defenses by the patient who had been guarding himself against the threat of unconscious conflict during the hypnosis. Thus, as is true of the trance state, reactions during induction and termination, as reflected in depth reversal, are not simple ratio responses to specific instructions. They reflect behavior based on dynamic, complex processes in the intricate fabric of personality functioning.

TRANSFERENCE, COUNTERTRANSFERENCE, RESISTANCE AND DEPENDENCE

Fundamental transference and countertransference issues and problems encountered in psychotherapy are to be found also within hypnotherapeutic relationships. The hypnotic relationship, however, often involves an intensification of certain aspects of transference. The intensified themes are connected with fantasies of hypnosis referred to earlier. Sexual feelings and control wishes and requirements are especially highlighted. It can be observed often that the introduction of hypnosis into treatment effects in some patients a crystallization of the transference in ways that are directly or indirectly evident within the range of total hypnotic behavior and with impressive clarity. The hypnotic transference may be heterosexual or homosexual. Recognition by the patient of its sexual implications may occur even though there had been no conscious awareness of such sexual leanings in psychotherapy preceding the introduction of hypnotic methods. Also, hitherto unconscious homosexual feelings may come to conscious awareness spontaneously with the inclusion of hypnotic procedures. For some patients the induction methods themselves, with their implicit closer psychological ties, foster an identification of hypnosis with heterosexual or homosexual involvements. Therapists should be sensitive to all signs of transference reactions and to countertransference. With such sensitivity and awareness therapists are in an improved position to gauge all phases of treatment procedure with subtle elements of timing, management of anxiety, interpretation, and the caution inherent in dealing with fine points of interpersonal transactions.

Transference reactions may become evident directly in feelings consciously experienced by patients and verbalized by them within the hypnosis. They may come to the fore in hypnotic thoughts, fantasies, and dreams. They may express themselves in facial appearance and body movements. They may be reflected in a variety of reported spontaneous sensory experiences. Such happenings are usually ignored in non-analytic contacts, but they are intrinsically important, can be explored, and can be clarified in hypnoanalytic work. Attention to alterations in the state of the ego as indicated here can play a significant role in hypnotherapy.

Hypnotic transference issues and reactions can be analyzed within the hypnotic setting. And the varieties of manifestations of resistances in the course of treatment are amenable to analysis also. Gradually these points are becoming more widely recognized although the resistance to accepting them is apparently part of the emotional resistances on a professional level to hypnotherapeutic activity in general. Heretofore much stress has been placed on the use of hypnosis to bypass resistances and avoid transference concerns. Should this be the goal of a therapist it must be seen as his choice. It is not a necessity. On the contrary the analysis of transference and resistance plays an integral role in the intensive work of hypnoanalysis. Evidences of transference and resistance appear during induction and termination of hypnosis as well as in the midst of the general hypnotic setting. The time for focusing on such evidence for purposes of exploration and specific analysis is a matter of clinical judgment.

In addition to questions raised about the management of resistance and transference is that of dependence in relation to the hypnotic contact. It has long been claimed that the patient experiences excessive dependence on the therapist by virtue of the hypnosis. It is said that the dependence is rather lasting and difficult to resolve, and if an attempt is made to break it the risk is presented of relapse from any apparent gains achieved. The writer's impression is that the opposite emerges from clinical experience. Dependence seems less than in non-hypnotic contacts. Dependency problems are amenable to analysis as are other issues. Favorable changes are not intimately linked with dependency satisfactions. Relapses associated with excessive dependence are as frequent or more frequent in non-hypnotic therapeutic and analytic settings. The concern over excessive dependence in hypnotic therapy has been greatly exaggerated. Some patients with strong dependent needs will attempt to express them in the hypnotic relationships and in others too, and this becomes a matter of therapeutic management. The tendency of a therapist to encourage dependence consciously (without good control and with specific therapeutic intent), or unconsciously, is a problem of his own and a countertransference issue rather than a problem inherent in, and peculiar to hypnotherapy.

Manifestations of transference, resistance, and dependency issues are reflected in hypnotic behavioral patterns of excessive compliance, negativism, tendencies toward detachment, denial of sensori-motor experience, need to control and to be controlled, reassured, encouraged, praised and criticized. Countertransference is commonly reflected in needs and efforts of therapists to control excessively, and power fantasies in this connection are well known. Overt anxiety is common in countertransference reactions. Guze has mentioned feelings of guilt in therapists when they recognize their own sexual impulses toward subjects. He referred also to hostility developing in a particular doctor when he observed exaggerated resistance or compliance in his patient (12). Meares has dealt also with related concerns (13). Therapists may avoid the use of hypnosis or an interest in the subject owing to fear of sexual fantasies that may be stimulated toward patients. They may fear activation of aggressive impulses toward some patients in the hypnotic setting. I have pointed out that certain people unconsciously identify hypnosis with death (2). This plays a role in transference, countertransference, and resistance issues in the hypnotic interpersonal relationship for therapist and patient. The link between the hypnotic state and re-birth fantasies is significant for some patients and it influences the transference. It may be involved more frequently than is recognized and may influence the belief in remarkable possibilities for hypnosis entailing simple, authoritative suggestion (Schneck, 14).

HYPNOTHERAPEUTIC AND HYPNOANALYTIC TECHNIQUES

Technical procedures in hypnotic settings overlap those employed without the use of hypnosis. This would apply, for example, to conversational exchange and to free association. But some methods are rather peculiar to hypnosis. Regression and the use of experimental conflicts apply here. Occasional techniques such as automatic writing may be attempted with or without the use of hypnosis. However, such procedures involving intense concentration often result in the patient entering an hypnotic state even though the therapist, especially if he be inexperienced, does not recognize it.

Conversational exchange during hypnosis may be more productive at times than during non-hypnotic interviews. This may occur because of facilitation of productivity through hypnotic relaxation, freer flow of ideas with decreased anxiety, and the tendency for easier access to preconscious and unconscious material during hypnosis. Occasionally a patient may become less verbal in hypnosis as a defense against revealing thoughts and feelings brought to the fore under pressure of an intensified transference. This happens under the stress of sexual and aggressive impulses. The therapist should be aware of this possibility and the reactions are usually subject to analysis.

Free association sessions may be conducted in the hypnotic setting as without it. Again, in general there is a tendency toward greater productivity and the points mentioned regarding conversational exchange are pertinent here too.

Automatic writing is possible with varying degrees of facility among patients. Some write freely almost immediately. Others require time to accustom themselves to the procedure. The writing may be fluid and psychologically transparent. Often it is cryptic with condensations, substitutions, displacements, and subject to many other dynamisms remarkably similar to those found in dreams. Eyes of patients may be open or closed as deemed desirable. They may be aware of what the hand is writing as the writing appears. They may be partially aware or unaware. This may often be directed and controlled by the therapist in suitable patients. Automatic writing may be achieved in the form of visual imagery rather than manual effort and this procedure is often helpful. Automatic writing is helpful in eliciting factual information, retrieving lost memories, clarifying aspects of resistance and of transference reactions.

Hypnotic drawing may be used in hypnosis as voluntary or automatic activity and its purposes are similar to those just mentioned. Drawing and writing may be done on posthypnotic suggestion. Meares pointed out that hypnography should be integrated with hypnoanalysis and waking psychotherapy. His use of the term hypnography pertains to the hypnotized patient's projection of psychic material in black and white painting. In hypnosis the patient associates to his productions. He considers it useful for patients who do not talk readily in hypnosis and states that graphic expression of conflicts is therapeutically beneficial beyond verbal expression of the same conflicts (15).

Scene visualization is a form of hypnotic imagery. The term is used in connection with visualizations of essentially realistic everyday settings. They serve as the focus for projection of concerns and conflicts, some of which may be brought to light or to more clear-cut expression, through such visual representations. Scenes may appear spontaneously or on suggestion.

Hypnotic dreams may bear such close structural resemblance

to nocturnal dreams as to be essentially indistinguishable from them (16). They may be simple or complex in accordance with the manner in which the patient tends to express himself in this fashion and in keeping often with the form and content of his spontaneous nocturnal dreams. The variety of dream mechanisms employed in the latter are evident in the former and the analysis of hypnotic dreams is often therapeutically beneficial. Hypnotic dreaming may occur spontaneously or on suggestion. Hypnotic suggestions may influence subsequent nocturnal dreams. Scene visualizations and hypnotic dreams may form a continuum for any one patient. Problems may be depicted, explored and analyzed in a series of such visualizations and dreams. Scenes and dreams may emerge in some patients with greater freedom initially if suggestions tend to structure the settings and content. Some patients immediately, and other patients in time, visualize hypnotic scenes and dreams freely without such assistance. Symbolizations, condensations, displacements and substitutions, representations by the opposite and a broader array of mechanisms are readily discernible. Scenes and dreams reflect resistances and transference relations in abundance and are subject to analysis within the hypnotic setting or subsequent to the hypnosis sessions as is deemed clinically expedient. In hypnosis, forgotten dreams may be retrieved, new dreams stimulated, and previous nocturnal dreams continued in some new fashion or concluded in a new way (Schneck, 16).

Hypnotic age regression may facilitate recall of early experiences and it may help to clarify early attitudes and modes of personality functioning. In regressed states there is greater or lesser degree of contact with the environment. For example, a patient may be so involved in an earlier age period that he feels subjectively part of that period instead of engaging in simple recall. At the same time he is aware to some degree of his current environment and contact with the therapist. Yet an occasional patient is so involved in earlier happenings that distortions occur in current perceptions. He may misidentify his environment, seeing it as consistent with past events, and he may identify the therapist as someone participating in past happenings. It is at times stated or implied that a patient achieving age regression invariably is able to experience posthypnotic amnesias. I believe there is no essential correlation here. Furthermore patients easily achieving one of the modes of hypnotic functioning now outlined do not necessarily demonstrate efficiently any ability to achieve the others. Another important point is that there is no direct correlation between the ability to perform hypnotically in each of the ways described, and the ability to do well therapeutically. Capacity for special hypnotic behavior is a reflection of total personality functioning, and such functioning with its complex ingredients involves a large variety of crucial elements that influence general therapeutic activity. The notion that a "good hypnotic subject," which often implies dramatic behavior, is likely to be a good candidate for treatment is erroneous. A patient's hypnotic behavior is to be examined and explored and accepted for what it is so that it may be utilized fruitfully within the range of total therapy. Should such hypnotic behavior prove to be of little or no practical assistance it need only to be set aside and treatment continued without it.

Hypnotic chronological age regression is generally the goal of therapists and experimentalists. This is distinguishable from what is designated as hypnotic dynamic age regression. The latter is easier to observe when patients regress spontaneously so that specific age levels are not defined by the therapist. Concern with such levels and preoccupation with substantiating evidence may lead to the disregard of important, intruding elements considered to be inconsistent with a "successful" hypnotic response. In dynamic regression there is concurrent reliving of different time periods at the same moment, so that a temporal setting at one age level may merge with a spacial setting appropriate to another level. Affective and ideational experience pertinent to different age levels may fuse in curious fashion. The fusions occur because of the dynamic relatedness of the different time periods with the problems on which the patient is dwelling. These dynamic fusions can be very important within the therapeutic context, and the spacial-temporal distortion and fusion is consistent with the concept of dynamic hypnotic age regression as differentiated from chronological regression that has been stressed so much in clinical and experimental reports.

The dynamic view encompasses more completely the recognition of spontaneity and psychological fluidity and change inherent in hypnotic subjects studied in longitudinal and cross-sectional perspectives (Schneck, 16, 17). It seems often to be assumed that the ability to function well with regression techniques is virtually indicative of ability to make good progress in treatment. This is not true and probably much time is taken up needlessly with attempts to achieve regression, essentially of the chronological type just mentioned. Its potential dramatic elements have appeal to some and countertransference issues must be kept in mind on this score.

In lieu of free association, "controlled" associations may be attempted. Here, on signal, the patient is asked to respond with an idea or emotion that immediately occurs to him. The stimulus may be a word, for example, to which such associations are requested, and in investigations along certain directions the stimulus words may be selected for their inferred dynamic significance for the patient.

Some paients work effectively with induced visual and auditory hallucinations the nature of which is intended to have direct reference to the problems on hand. These experiences may be structured or unstructured depending upon the needs of investigation at the time. By studying the feelings and attitudes projected onto hallucinated figures, much can be learned in treatment. By auditory hallucinations, the writer refers basically to impressions of external stimuli impinging on the subject. In the case of such visual experiences, the subject would have his eyes open. Such experiences are encountered less frequently than aforementioned phenomena and, as a result, are encountered less in treatment settings.

Experimental conflicts may be used for patients capable of developing complete posthypnotic amnesias. Conflict situations are suggested to patients in line with anticipated reactions based on known behavioral patterns of the patient. After emerging from hypnosis, with the conflict suggestions buried by posthypnotic amnesia, the patient is observed, assuming success of the expedient, to engage in actions consistent with the suggested conflict and linked with his basic problems. Uncovering the forgotten material then demonstrates the relationship between the posthypnotic behavior and the buried conflict, with the goal of enabling the patient to gain insight into his method of coping with stress situations and the unconscious determinants in his methods of functioning (18). Relatively few patients can utilize this approach because of the amnesias generally required. But when experimental conflicts can be employed they are potentially helpful, though, as in the case of other methods, not invariably so.

There are additional hypnotic techniques available in hypnotherapy and hypnoanalysis. Some will be mentioned in passing, and the literature may be explored for details. They include the induction of dual or multiple personalities, role playing by patient and therapist, utilization of symbolic stories to parallel conflict issues, the incorporation into the hypnotic setting of various psychological test procedures (Rorschach Test, Thematic Apperception Test, Word Association Test, House-Tree-Person Test, and others) (Schneck and Kline, 19, 20), time distortion methods (21), and sensory hypnoplasty (22). Again it should be stressed that these and the aforementioned methods may be used individually and in combinations. The choice depends on demonstrated ability by patients to use them constructively. The writer favors starting with the most technically simple devices, introducing more difficult and complex operations only when necessary. Verbalization measures as in conversational exchange and free association are examples of the former, along with visual imagery procedures that many patients can manage without too much difficulty and with a little practice.

CASE REFERENCES

It is not possible to illustrate all the complexities of psychiatric hypnotherapy in one detailed account of a patient. Several brief "case references" will be given therefore, to highlight aspects of hypnosis in psychiatry, although here too only a small fraction of pertinent issues is revealed. More information can be acquired by the interested reader directly through the bibliography appended.

Case 1: Characterological Problems: It is possible in a hypnotic setting to investigate a variety of characterological problems and personal relationships. In relieving anxiety and depression in a thirty year old patient, some issues examined included his hostility toward his father, fear of figures in authority, competitive feelings toward other men, conflicts between ambition and the need to escape responsibilities, masculinity-femininity conflicts, and various elements in an unhappy marriage. There were thirty-eight sessions in treatment, not all of them involving hypnosis. Hypnotic methods employed included conversational exchange with the patient in hypnosis, free association, visual imagery with scene visualization, evaluation of spontaneous sensory and motor phenomena, recall of nocturnal dreams, completion of dreams not adequately recalled, posthypnotic suggestions promoting therapeutic progress, and hypnotic suggestions for direct alleviation of anxiety (Schneck, 4).

Case 2: Resolution of Symptoms Related to Incest Barriers: A young woman sought treatment because of her reaction of nausea and distaste whenever she came into some physical contact with her father or when she anticipated such contact in everyday settings. During treatment, much material arose in connection with her relationship to a current boyfriend. With the use of hypnotic methods stressing visual imagery in the form of scene visualizations and hypnotic dreams, she became aware of identifications between this boyfriend and her father. She gained insight into her incestuous longings and her symptoms as defensive measures. Eventually she sought intercourse with her fiancé, an experience which would have been her first, and a happening in which she was capable of participating only on resolution of the underlying oedipal conflict (Schneck, 23).

Case 3: Hypnotic and Nocturnal Dreams: A patient had a water phobia. In hypnosis she was to visualize a scene representing the first appearance of her phobia but the only thought that came to mind was the series of water dreams she had experienced. To save time she was told she would now dream again only the most significant one in this series. She described a hill and lake scene, with people diving into the water. She rowed away. Then the scene switched to a river setting, but it was no longer her dream. She was caught in a current that carried her downstream, an actual event. This reminded her of another dream that preceded this happening. Someone was drowning, someone she couldn't identify. With visual imagery technique the identification was pressed and it turned out to be her father. This stirred up considerable anxiety with which, however, she was able to cope. It clarified death wishes toward him and incest longings as in the case of the previous patient. These and related problems were worked through and the water phobia disappeared. The removal of the phobia was only part of a hypnoanalysis lasting more than 300 hours for this patient with a character neurosis (Schneck, 24).

Case 4: Spontaneous Sensory and Motor Phenomena: A young man experienced for several sessions, in hypnosis, a disturbance in equilibrium. He felt as if his entire body were swinging in a wide arc. As the hypnoanalysis continued it was discovered that these feelings were related to sexual stimulation. Prior to their onset, the patient had been exploring his psychosexual development. The patient revived memories of early childhood when he would be in bed between his parents, playing "a sandwiching game" with them. The feelings he experienced occurred then, as well as in more recent dreams connected with sexuality and the transference relationship. The patient also described the feeling of his head being turned toward the hypnoanalyst while the patient was actually lying on the couch looking at the ceiling. Analysis of this phenomenon revealed homosexual components in the transference (Schneck, 25).

Case 5: Automatic Writing: During extensive treatment, the patient employed a variety of hypnotic techniques to assist him with an impotence problem. They included free association, visual imagery with scene visualizations and hypnotic dreams, regression, psychological test procedures combined with hypnosis, and other measures. The point to be stressed here pertains to the characteristics of his automatic writing. It showed: distortion of letters; elimination of letters in words; child-like scrawls; extraneous lines; perseverative repetition of single words; perseverative movements over parts of individual letters; running together of words without appropriate spacing; use of vulgar terms not employed in speech during interviews; tendency toward fusion of letters; irregular spacing of letters; altered timing during writing; substitution of one letter for another because of similarity in form, phonetic association, and psychodynamic significance; use of one letter to represent an entire word through phonetic equivalence; word distortion through misspelling; use of the first letter of a word to represent the entire word followed by use of the same letter to represent an entirely different word. The automatic writing was specifically helpful in the clarification of ambivalent feelings toward his parents, his own sexual strivings, and certain aspects of the doctor-patient relationship (Schneck, 26).

Case 6: Recaptured Dream and Its Hypnotic Extension: A patient developed a head shaking symptom. It was determined that the symptom appeared on waking from sleep one morning. In hypnosis it was possible to have the patient redream the material of the preceding night. Then he spontaneously continued the dream in hypnosis. The original dream had terminated unfavorably with his rejection by his daughter. The hypnotic extension permitted him to reorganize spontaneously the conflict issues in the dream and to bring it to a favorable termination. This resulted in a disappearance of his symptom. The occurrence is somewhat unusual, and indicative of certain aspects of adaptabilities inherent in ego functioning within the hypnotic setting (Schneck, 27).

Case 7: Hypnotic Evaluation and Removal of an Amnesia: Hypnosis has been known for some time to be effective often for lifting amnesias. A soldier developed an amnesia for a period of unauthorized absence. It was possible under hypnosis to retrieve forgotten episodes and to study their dynamic significance. The patient was concerned on one level with the welfare of his wife and children. This was related to his absence without leave. His wife was identified unconsciously with his mother. He recaptured many events, feelings and attitudes in connection with his mother who had turned prostitute under adverse financial circumstances.

Memories and associations pertaining to this time period were repressed, as were the more recent events that became highly charged because of affective associations with his early childhood and his relationship with his mother. Not only was the amnesia symptom removed, but the patient gained significant insights into his behavior and problems that could serve him well thereafter. In the military setting it was possible to set one and a half, and two and a half hour sessions that appeared to be helpful in avoiding disruption of important explorations. This can be done in private practice, but it is usually more difficult under conventional office arrangements. Length of sessions in relation to therapeutic advantages and disadvantages probably warrants additional study (Schneck, 28).

Case 8: Homosexual Identifications of Hypnotic Experience: Early in his hypnoanalysis, a patient developed spontaneous bilateral hand anesthesia, inability to raise a leg as a result of hypnotic suggestion, a light feeling in his head on termination of hypnosis, tachycardia, and a need to deny the existence of the hypnotic state, among other reactions. It was possible, through his associations, to analyze the implications of these happenings. They served as expressions of underlying concern about homosexual leanings, loss of his penis, passivity, and loss of control. Analysis of the homosexual transference early in treatment did not interfere with continued efforts and with his hypnotizability. In the past, implications had been made that learning the significance of hypnotic relationships would preclude development of a hypnotic state. This is usually not true and the forces involved are more complex than implied in this expression of opinion (Schneck, 29).

Case 9: Precordial Pain and Hypnotic Abreaction: Dramatic hypnotic abreactions are most frequently associated with circumstances that are highly affect-laden and often associated with wartime or equivalent traumatic settings. A soldier experienced precordial pain which could be explored and removed after dramatic catharsis under hypnosis. The pain arose as a result of his identification with a friend who was killed in action, having been shot through the heart. Involved in symptom formation also was identification with the sorrow of the friend's wife, and guilt in relation to both. Effective relief was possible for the patient after general medical examinations with appropriate laboratory studies had shown no structural pathology, when he relived the wartime experiences with evaluation of pertinent concurrent and childhood happenings and emotional involvements (Schneck, 30).

Case 10: Extension of Psychoanalytic Themes: Hypnoanalysis provides opportunities to supply additional substantiation of psychoanalytic concepts and theories, to formulate new concepts and theories pertaining to personality development and functioning, and to elaborate observations noted in the growth of psychoanalysis (Schneck, 31). Some time ago, Freud discussed the psychological significance of the mythological Medusa's head (32). He did not supply a case report. One is available in that of a young man who presented during hypnoanalysis a recaptured dream from the age of seven. He was aware of the Medusa's head with snakes forcing it backwards, and in the dream the Medusa's head was actually his own. He awoke in terror. During hypnosis sessions his verbalizations at this time reflected a homosexual transference. The qualitative nature of the transference at certain points in hypnoanalysis have a bearing not only on hypnotic functioning in general, but on the timing for the emergence of specific memories of which this serves as one example. Little or no attention had evidently been focussed, incidentally, on the Medusa's head symbolism since Freud had given it his attention 40 years earlier.

Case 11: Incest Experience During Hypnoanalysis: In psychiatric practice one occasionally encounters patients who reveal actual past incest experience. Incest fantasies are, of course, not unusual. Incest experience occurring during analysis is worth noting especially (Schneck, 33). The sexual contact involved brother and sister, and the latter was in treatment. It was possible to study some of the underlying ingredients in the experience during hypnoanalytic work. She was substituting for a girlfriend who had left her brother. She also substituted for their mother, both of them having been involved in special mother-child problems. The patient experienced the incestuous relationship as an expression of her need to deny she was a woman, because she believed normal femininity would, for her, have precluded such behavior. It was in fact a denial of her femininity.

Case 12: Aspects of Hypnotic Regression and Revivification: A patient in her fifties was helped considerably in hypnoanalysis for severe gastrointestinal allergies. In hypnotic regressions, frequently spontaneous, she revivified early experiences, and when doing so she would not verbalize concurrently. It seems that in her intense reliving of the past, she maintained only a thread of contact with the present through the hypnoanalyst. Some revivifications involved the emotional impact of sexual sensations when in contact with her father, at the age of 12, emotional attachments to mother and siblings in early childhood, and traumatic episodes relating to dating experience, loss of a pet dog, and a whipping by her father. The patient claimed the hypnotic experiences seemed more "real" than the original happenings. It is known that at times in treatment an analyst-father identification was of considerable significance for her. It is conjectured that at certain times the current setting in terms of the transference influence, superimposed on, and merged with revivified happenings, resulted in a fusion accounting for this impression of greater reality in the hypnotic setting. This fusion is consistent with the concept of dynamic hypnotic age regression mentioned earlier (Schneck, 34).

Case 13: Hypnotic Treatment for Cardiospasm: A patient had been given a diagnosis of cardiospasm two years prior to hypnotherapy. He complained of eructation, regurgitation, lacrimation, dysphagia and weight loss. One year prior to hypnotherapy, passage of a mercury-weighted tube brought brief, temporary relief. Two esophageal roentgenograms revealed achalasia and dilatation. Hypnotherapy involved first some efforts to allay anxiety and reduce muscular tension. This was followed by some improvement. Then a silent numerical count conditioning technique for the patient to use in reducing spasm helped additionally. Finally spasm and relief were hypnotically induced during fantasied food ingestion, with even greater relief. The patient gained fifteen pounds. He then received forceful dilation under surgical care after weeks of daily esophageal washings. There was temporary change, with relapse, but the degree of prior hypnotherapeutic improvement remained unchanged. Attempts at more extensive personality investigation were successful in achieving understandings pertaining to various aspects of personality functioning, but no practical results were evident in any greater progress in symptom relief. Additional efforts at hypnotherapy for partial or complete relief of cardiospasm would appear to be worthwhile (Schneck, 35).

Case 14: Symbol Clarification in Hypnoanalysis: Hypnoanalysis is capable not only of confirming, but of extending psychoanalytic concepts and themes (Schneck, 36). For example, it has been known that body parts may be invested with phallic significance. It was possible to show that for a patient in hypnoanalysis, the heart could serve as a phallic symbol. The issue was clarified when the patient retrieved and emotionally relived a frightening dream with obvious display of discomfort, accompanied by groaning and complaints of pain. He was concerned about damage to his heart which he proceeded to identify with his penis on the basis of recollections from childhood when he viewed the hearts of fowl that were eviscerated by his mother in her household chores. Castration anxiety was quite pronounced in this patient's problems.

Case 15: Psychopathology of Fainting: A patient in his late twenties had a history of fainting episodes in childhood and adult life. Some points to be considered in fainting episodes are hysterical syncope, vasodepressor syncope, and carotid sinus reactions (37). Fainting in people with personality problems has been considered also a mechanism for blocking ego functions when serving a role of primitive defense against overwhelming stimuli (38). Among the several fainting episodes experienced by this patient was a crucial event at the time of an operative procedure in childhood. Hypnoanalytic reconstruction of events and associated dynamics revealed that the personality matrix for fainting consisted of passive, masochistic submission to a dominant, highly influential mother whose pressure on the patient was felt by him as stifling and pervasive. When happenings were psychologically associated with this core relationship, fainting reactions were triggered. As the patient matured, the episodes diminished. The crucial operative scene was revivified during spontaneous hypnotic regression. Here again the hypnotic setting affords opportunities for extending and clarifying psychopathological issues encountered and studied originally in non-hypnotic psychotherapy and analysis (Schneck, 39).

Case 16: Visual Imagery, Transference, and Identification: A thirty-six year old man entered hypnoanalysis because of stuttering dating back to childhood. The speech difficulty appeared in a variety of settings. Following improvement, it was observed that he had trouble with his speech when arriving for his sessions. This was investigated further with elicitation of the frequently encountered issue of increased anxiety when in contact with figures of authority (Schneck, 40). In hypnosis it was suggested that, without conscious control, imagery would appear and would represent directly or indirectly the problem of his anxiety and speech difficulty in connection with office visits. He saw himself walking down a flight of steps into a dark basement. He was frightened, felt someone was there, but did not know who it was. He saw a figure he could not identify. He was encouraged to scrutinize the person carefully. It was his father. The doctor-father identification in relation to the current setting and problem was now clear. The symbolism in the imagery, often related to investigation of the unconscious with attendant anxiety, was believed by him to be specifically connected with concern lest his masturbation be discovered. His anxiety was consistent with that he experienced during investigation of his sexual problems.

The fear of criticism was pertinent to his early contact with his father and it played a role in the current transference setting. In hypnosis he encountered a reactivation of feelings during his youth when talking with his father about masturbation during which he was accidentally discovered. In an earlier hypnosis he had revealed the severe stuttering that had set in immediately upon this discovery by his father. He had the greatest difficulty now when saying the word itself (masturbation). When he blocked in his speech, he felt people might consider him mentally unbalanced. Further hypnotic interviews dealt with recollections of being warned about insanity by his father, should his masturbation continue. The patient was startled in hypnosis when he suddenly realized that at the time of this warning there was a psychotic girl living in the building in which he had his home. Further, this girl had a stutter and he became aware of having identified himself with her. During a subsequent hypnoanalytic session he mentioned that he was puzzled by a tendency to hold his breath when he stuttered. His younger brother had engaged in breath-holding as a child and the patient felt there was a connection. With a scene visualization technique he saw himself with his own child who was now manifesting the same behavior. He was concerned and became quite attentive to the child. Then he recalled his parents' worry that breathholding might lead to the death of his brother. Correlating this material, the patient saw his own behavior reflecting a search for attention and solicitous concern by others toward him. In part his speech problem reflected his attempt to elicit unconsciously this type of response from others.

Case 17: Assurance of Illness Reversibility: It has been possible to demonstrate with examples from hypnotherapeutic efforts that some patients appear to have, as a major goal in treatment, the need to reassure themselves only about the reversibility of their illnesses. This goal seems to be part of the broader issue of retention of symptoms for secondary gain (Schneck, 41). Treatment is terminated by the patient when this goal is reached, and it may occur soon after the start of therapy, or following some delay. Some improvement, however, must occur first. Areas for such improvement are stated by the patients, but after it occurs, and at the point of termination, the presence of this improvement is usually not verbalized spontaneously. Furthermore, reasons offered for discontinuing treatment are inconsistent with information volunteered at the start of treatment. A patient in his forties sought hypnotherapy for chronic gastrointestinal distress requiring much care with eating habits in order to prevent physical discomfort. He was shy and inhibited and limited in his social contacts. He was very fault finding and felt victimized by society. He claimed that previous, prolonged psychiatric treatment had not helped him. He simply wanted symptom removal now without further personality investigation. Yet he spontaneously proceeded to speak about himself much, revealing his experiences, problems, and critical judgments. He said he had countless general medical studies that were not helpful. Various forms of medication had done him no good. During the first few hypnotic sessions he freely proclaimed he felt no better. Then he discontinued these assertions. Finally, only when eventually asked about his reactions, did he begrudgingly admit that he was experiencing some symptom relief. Shortly afterwards he terminated treatment. The reason he gave was that he had decided to seek help through general medical channels although, as mentioned above, he had said earlier that several extensive medical studies and treatment efforts suppled no relief at all.

Case 18: *Failure of Hypnotherapy:* Failures may be due to many elements a few of which include technical errors, inappropriate application of hypnotherapy, special transference problems in the hypnotic interpersonal relationship, inability of the patient to use hypnotic techniques effectively, and fundamental problems of the patient in relation to any form of treatment including hypnotherapy (Schneck, 42). A 30 year old patient was having difficulties with nausea, anorexia, and inability to gain weight. The verbal exchange in previous psychotherapy was deemed by him to be unsatisfactory without special additional applications and hypnoanalysis seemed to him to supply an extra ingredient. He said he had not been helped in his previous psychiatric encounter. Initial work with hypnosis produced varying results and he was encouraged to look beyond his surface wishes. He was superficially bright, sexually repressed, and had difficulty in revealing himself during interviews. It was learned that in previous psychotherapy he developed resistances toward deeper exploration of personality problems. Efforts were made again and appeared to be rewarding only briefly. He did not seem to be able to surmount continuing resistance barriers and terminated contact. He wanted treatment essentially without exploration and believed hypnotherapy would serve his purpose. It was of interest to him really as a means of bypassing his fundamental problems but he was apparently unable to achieve this goal at this point.

Case 19: Psychopathology of Blushing: An unmarried woman in her thirties sought treatment two and a half years after the onset of pathological blushing with accompanying anxiety. It started when taking dictation from an employer and spread to involve other encounters with men. Finally it extended to social settings and contact with women also. Hypnoanalytic settings revealed problems incorporating masochism and exhibitionism, guilt in relation to sexual expression, fear of discovery and being judged. The hypnoanalytic exploration also revealed an important addition to previously reported ingredients as outlined here. The patient found that she was equating the blushing with orgasm which it represented in parallel and was a substitute for, in certain settings. The mechanism of isolation was utilized by this patient as a major defense, and it was consistent with some obsessive features in her make-up, beyond hysterical, conversion elements. The hypnoanalytic setting proved capable of penetrating this barrier and exposing it to scrutiny and proper evaluation. The isolation barrier seems more amenable to reduction in some patients within a hypnotic setting than in settings where hypnosis is not used (Schneck, 42).

Case 20: Hypnotherapy for the Control of Anxiety: Hypnotherapy may relieve anxiety in some patients even though it has been present for many years. Results are often difficult to predict and a trial at treatment is helpful. The use of hypnosis for attaining such relief appears often to be more effective than nonhypnotic methods. Other symptoms are sometimes relieved concurrently when a common dynamic core is present. With diminution of anxiety, improvement tends to take place in interpersonal relations. The degree to which insight therapy is attempted varies with apparent capacities of patients and their expressed desires based on past conditionings and current needs. Relief from some anxiety sometimes opens the way for more deep-seated changes. It may even be a necessity before the patient will permit more extensive explorations. Relief must be balanced with assessment of motivation if deeper investigations are considered (Schneck, 43). A patient in his forties was hostile toward psychiatry and psychoanalysis, claiming lack of success in several therapeutic ventures. In accordance with his wishes, symptom relief was stressed with hypnotic relaxation techniques. Anxiety was extreme and his attitudes quite ambivalent. He seemed unable to decide at times whether to minimize the relief he was experiencing or to express gratefulness for some relief. Suggestions encouraged conscious and unconscious work on underlying problems but he was not encouraged to verbalize any understandings he might reach in order to avoid a clash with his expressed attitudes toward uncovering techniques. However, when the patient was somewhat more at ease he spontaneously acknowledged improvements in interpersonal relations. The patient's work eventually took him abroad. During his weeks of treatment care was taken not to press for thorough, rapid relief because of his precarious psychological state entailing paranoid coloring and indications of prepsychotic functioning. The hypnotic setting in a sense would assist the patient in achieving the measure of betterment that he was capable of sustaining and that he required.

CLOSING REMARKS

Psychiatric hypnotherapy implies the judicious use of a hypnotic setting and hypnotic methods within the framework of psychotherapy. The best principles of psychotherapy must be employed with careful selection of suitable patients. Selection pertains to needs and strivings of patients in keeping with what hypnotherapy can potentially offer, and the clinical judgment of the therapist is the deciding element in the decision to incorporate hypnosis into treatment. It is not so much the issue of diagnostic categories that determines the use of hypnotherapy. Rather it is the past experience of the hypnotherapist with hypnotic methods and his abilities to treat patients for the problems they present, whether or not the therapist were to introduce hypnotherapeutic devices at all. Understandings pertaining to hypnotic behavior, the hypnotic doctor-patient relationship, and related concerns are part of the broader framework of psychotherapy and keep pace with the over-all developments unfolding in modern concepts of dynamic psychiatry. Studies in scientific hypnosis are contributing not only to newer developments in psychiatric practice, but also to experimental psychological investigations, personality explorations, and theoretical issues relating to the behavioral sciences.

REFERENCES

1. Bowers, M. K. and Berkowitz, B.: Clinical observations on the effects of electroconvulsive therapy in the hypnotic state. *J. Nerv. & Ment. Dis., 118*:355, 1953.
2. Schneck, J. M.: *Studies in Scientific Hypnosis.* Baltimore, Williams and Wilkins, 1954.
3. Rosen, H.: Hypnosis—Applications and misapplications. *J.A.M.A., 172*:683, 1960.
4. Schneck, J. M.: Hypnotherapy in anxiety and depression. In Burton, A.: *Case Studies of Counseling and Psychotherapy.* New York, Prentice-Hall, 1959.
5. Schneck, J. M.: Hidden determinants in deceptive requests for hypnoanalysis. *Int. J. Clin. & Exper. Hyp., 9*:261, 1961.
6. Erickson, M. H.: Historical note on the hand levitation and other ideomotor techniques. *Am. J. Clin. Hyp., 3*:196, 1961.
7. Erickson, M. H. and Kubie, L. S.: The successful treatment of a case of acute hysterical depression by a return under hypnosis to a critical phase of childhood. *Psychoanal. Quart., 10*:583, 1941.
8. Williams, G. W.: Difficulty in dehypnotizing. *J. Clin. Exper. Hyp., 1*:3, 1953.
9. Rosen, H.: Dehypnosis and its problems. *Brit. J. Med. Hyp., 5*:18, 1954.
10. Schneck, J. M.: Comment on a miniature conversion reaction during the induction of hypnosis. *J. Gen. Psychol., 47*:235, 1952.
11. Schneck, J. M.: Depth reversal during termination of the hypnotic state. *Psychoanal. Rev., 43*:506, 1956.
12. Guze, H.: The involvement of the hypnotist in the hypnotic session. *J. Clin. Exper. Hyp., 4*:61, 1956.
13. Meares, A.: A note on motivation for hypnosis. *J. Clin. Exper. Hyp., 3*:222, 1955.

14. SCHNECK, J. M.: Hypnosis—death and hypnosis—rebirth concepts in relation to hypnosis theory. *J. Clin. Exper. Hyp., 3*:40, 1955.

15. MEARES, A.: Hypnography—a technique in hypnoanalysis. *J. Ment. Sc., 100*:965, 1954.

16. SCHNECK, J. M.: Clinical and experimental aspects of hypnotic dreams. In Kline, M. V.: *Clinical Correlations of Experimental Hypnosis.* In Press.

17. SCHNECK, J. M.: Dynamic hypnotic age regression. *Am. J. Psychiat., 113*:178, 1956.

18. McDOWELL, M.: An abrupt cessation of major neurotic symptoms following an hypnotically induced artificial conflict. *Bull. Menninger Clin., 12*:168, 1948.

19. SCHNECK, J. M.: Hypnotic scene visualization and the word association test. *J. Gen. Psychol., 46*:29, 1952.

20. SCHNECK, J. M. and KLINE, M. V.: The h-t-p and t a t in hypnodiagnostic studies. *Brit. J. Med. Hyp., 5*:3, 1953.

21. COOPER, L. F.: Time distortion in hypnosis. *Bull. Georgetown Univ. Med. Center, 1*:214, 1948.

22. RAGINSKY, B. B.: The sensory use of plasticine in hypnoanalysis (sensory hypnoplasty). *Int. J. Clin. & Exper. Hyp., 9*:233, 1961.

23. SCHNECK, J. M.: Fragments of a hypnoanalysis. *Dis. Nerv. Syst., 12*:369, 1951.

24. SCHNECK, J. M.: The hypnoanalysis of phobic reactions. In LeCron, L. M.: *Experimental Hypnosis.* New York, Macmillan, 1952.

25. SCHNECK, J. M.: The elucidation of spontaneous sensory and motor phenomena during hypnoanalysis. *Psychoanal. Rev., 39*:79, 1952.

26. SCHNECK, J. M.: Automatic writing during hypnoanalysis. *J. Gen. Psychol., 46*:233, 1952.

27. SCHNECK, J. M.: The role of a dream in treatment with hypnosis. *Psychoanal. Rev., 34*:485, 1947.

28. SCHNECK, J. M.: The hypnotic treatment of a patient with amnesia. *Psychoanal. Rev., 35*:171, 1948.

29. SCHNECK, J. M.: Some aspects of homosexuality in relation to hypnosis. *Psychoanal. Rev., 37*:351, 1950.

30. SCHNECK, J. M.: Psychogenic cardiovascular reaction interpreted and successfully treated with hypnosis. *Psychoanal. Rev., 35*:14, 1948.

31. SCHNECK, J. M.: A hypnoanalytic note on a Medusa's Head dream. *J. Nerv. & Ment. Dis., 131*:80, 1960.

32. FREUD, S.: Medusa's head. In *Collected Papers*. London, Hogarth, 1950.

33. SCHNECK, J. M.: Incest experience during hypnoanalysis. *Int. J. Clin. & Exper. Hyp.*, 8:147, 1960.

34. SCHNECK, J. M.: Special aspects of hypnotic regression and revivification. *Int. J. Clin. & Exper. Hyp.*, 8:37, 1960.

35. SCHNECK, J. M.: Hypnotherapy for achalasia of the esophagus (cardiospasm). *Am. J. Psychiat.*, 114:1042, 1958.

36. SCHNECK, J. M.: A hypnoanalytic note on the heart as a phallic symbol. *J. Nerv. & Ment. Dis.*, 126:401, 1958.

37. BARNES, R. H.: Fainting: a review of the neuropsychiatric aspects. *Am. J. Med. Sc.*, 231:109, 1956.

38. FENICHEL, O.: *The Psychoanalytic Theory of Neurosis*. New York, W. W. Norton, 1945.

39. SCHNECK, J. M.: Hypnoanalytic observations on the psychopathology of fainting. *J. Clin. & Exper. Hyp.*, 5:167, 1957.

40. SCHNECK, J. M.: Hypnoanalytic therapy with case illustrations. *Am. J. Psychoth.*, 10:536, 1956.

41. SCHNECK, J. M.: Concept of assurance of illness reversibility. *Dis. Nerv. Syst.*, 17:191, 1956.

42. SCHNECK, J. M.: A hypnoanalytic exploration of the psychopathology of blushing and erythrophobia. *Psychoanal. Rev.*, 43:111, 1956.

43. SCHNECK, J. M.: Hypnotherapy for the control of anxiety. *Dis. Nerv. Syst.*, 14:274, 1953.

44. BOWERS, M., BRECHER-MARER, S. and POLATIN, A.: Hypnosis in the study and treatment of schizophrenia—a case report. *Int. J. Clin. & Exper. Hyp.*, 9:119, 1961.

45. ELLIS, A.: Hypnotherapy with borderline schizophrenics. *J. Gen. Psychol.*, 59:245, 1958.

46. GALE, C. and HERMAN, M.: Hypnosis and the psychotic patient. *Psychiat. Quart.*, 30:417, 1956.

47. KLINE, M.: A visual imagery technique for the induction of hypnosis in certain refractory subjects. *J. Psychol.*, 35:227, 1953.

48. SCHNECK, J. M.: Symptom relief, authority substitution, and suggestibility. *Dis. Nerv. Syst.*, 20:583, 1959.

7

HYPNOTHERAPY FOR CHILDREN

GORDON AMBROSE, L.M.S.S.A.

INTRODUCTION

The treatment of adult neuroses by hypnotherapy and hypnoanalysis is still meeting with a certain amount of incredulity, suspicion and unfortunately with the release of emotions which should be under control, particularly in the psychiatrist. The unanalysed practitioner, it could be argued, has not acquired the insight necessary to understand his or her aggression against a method of treatment which is beginning to be assessed now, not so much clinically but from the research point of view. With children the use of hypnosis does not seem to produce quite so much bitterness. Is it because the psychological treatment of children can be accepted as largely empirical and based on suggestion?

It has been found over the years by the writer that childhood problems must be treated first by rational understanding of the child mind and secondly by treatment aimed at explanation and insight for the child himself. By rational understanding is meant a knowledge of the various schools of thought in child psychiatry. No physician can treat a child psychologically without a knowledge principally of the teaching of Freud. Nowadays the concept, just as in adult psychiatry, has broadened and we have acquired understanding of the psyche since 1910 which has enabled us to bring a greater knowledge to the underlying psychological dynamisms of the human intellect.

It is tempting to analyse the reasons for interest in hypnosis, which is apparently revived every fifty years or so. Has hypnosis finally come to stay? If the question is primarily asked in relation to child psychiatry some of us would answer "yes"! Those of us who have used it as well as other methods of treatment could answer in the affirmative because hypnosis, probably more so than in adults, appears still to be the method of choice in the anxiety problems of children. The nervous child seems still to be the best "vehicle" for testing this maneuver against a background of tension, fear, guilt, etc.

The child is the barometer of the parents. It is probably because the child is so suggestible to the adults in his environment that the psychiatrist sees the child in the first place. Naturally this must depend upon the interpretation of the child as well as the behaviour of the parents, and it is out of place to discuss the problem of the genesis of dis-ease. It is because the child allows suggestion to play such a great part in the conformation of his problems in early and later life that we find the key to turn the lock of treatment. If suggestion aids in the building up of neurosis, suggestion should be used in the destroying of the inadequate structure and the re-building with more adequate and better supporting bricks.

It has never been argued that hypnosis is not the weapon of suggestion par excellence. It is the suggestions given during hypnosis which enable the child to face his difficulties more adequately. But most of us understand nowadays that suggestion and hypnosis, although valuable, cannot be the whole answer to any psychiatric problem. Hypnosis has a drawback. It seems to repress more readily the emotions which wish to come to the surface. In psychiatry we want to avoid relapse. The symptom first presented is the key to the underlying conflict. We must not repress the conflict by suggestion but must release it and show the patient what it means.

At first sight this object of treatment might appear to be a deterrent when dealing with children. It might be argued that adults can intellectualise about their symptoms, but that a child will find it more difficult. This, fortunately, is not true. The child is quick to see, appreciate and understand his conflict. The use of hypnosis in these circumstances can enable the child to look around, as it were. During the hypnotic session the child evaluates

his problems. He can visualise, as on a large screen, the particular
conflict which may be revealed. It is at this point that we ask ourselves how does hypnosis accomplish this? Even if the conflict is
revealed what can the child do about it? Here again it is tempting
to compare the child with the adult. The genesis of the traumatic
situation leading to the neurosis in the adult is, the reader will
agree, older and thus more conditioned than in the child. The
neurotic pattern has had a longer innings in the adult. It will be
more structurally embedded, it will take a greater amount of suggestion to release and finally to eradicate it. What will happen
in the child?

Freud's concept that the hypnotist takes over the role of the
father cannot entirely be ignored. It does in fact offer a more
easily acceptable theory with children. If we agree that the child
develops a neurosis because of his "barometric" feelings towards
the parents, then who more easily can rid the child of his ill-
conceived rationalisations. The break-up of the patterning, providing the child can intellectualise and gains sufficient insight,
must be more readily accomplished for the conditioning is less
"chronic." Suggestibility is never entirely absent in our lives, we
simply become more difficult to influence. The idea that our
father is God in the first five years of our lives must be a most
powerful factor for good or ill in the life of the child. The objective father (psychiatrist), unemotionally attached to the child, is
a most potent and valuable ally—few children will fight him. We
cannot say this when dealing with our adult patients, for the aggressive component has become more determined and the father
must sometimes be defeated and ultimately destroyed. To the
child the idea of obedience is reassuring. The strong, loving
father is a necessity. This is what the child is searching for—he
finds this in the psychiatrist but even more so in the hypnotist.
He is willing to submit to the father and this would seemingly be
the reason why nearly 100 per cent of children can be hypnotised.

What brings the child for treatment in the first place? It has
already been suggested that parental difficulties will be projected
to the child. It is platitudinous to describe this factor and indeed
since Otto Rank's theories there have been attempts at broaden-

ing the theory of the problems of childhood behaviour. Thus Kelsey (6) has described a pre-uterine genesis of stress and anxiety being projected through the cord itself. He suggests that gastro-enteritic problems, diarrhoea and constipation can be acquired before birth, just as a cord 'round the baby's neck at birth might explain breathing problems, e.g., asthma, later on in life. In other words a "fixation" can appear before birth. Moodie (9) described engrams which followed the child into adulthood, i.e., any trau-matic episode followed by inadequate repression would result in the formation of an engram and naturally in problems associated with any memory of the original trauma. It will be appreciated by the reader how difficult it might be to illustrate the concept of pre-uterine stress by research. However, Freud's contention that phantasy is of the same value as memory allows us further con-jecture, and particularly the use of substances such as Lysergic Acid (4, 10, 11) has enabled us to test the truth or falseness of this statement. Hypnosis has helped clinically in the same way.

The author (1) took a series of cases that were apparently "cured" of their acute attacks of asthma, but were still showing isolated attacks of less severe asthma. Six children were chosen, their ages ranging between eight and fifteen, for a pilot study, and each of these children was hypnotized to a deep level of hypnosis. The assessment of a deep state was made in each case by the cri-terion that the child had to phantasise his or her psyche leaving the soma, i.e., they would imagine their minds being separated from their bodies—that their minds were going up and up some stairs which seemed to them to lead to a wonderful land of grass and snow-capped mountains; their bodies would remain in the chair, their minds were higher and higher in this make-believe heavenly world. They were then given suggestions that they should think of themselves becoming smaller and smaller and younger and younger, until they would feel about one year old— then gradually a few months old, then weeks and days. They would eventually see a cave and imagine themselves inside the cave. Only one exit was to be seen and this was a little slit which they could see rather like the end of a passage. They would feel warm and comfortable and would go towards the exit and try to get through.

As they were trying to push through they would feel unable to do so. They would have to lean sideways and have to go out head-first (it was taken for granted that they had all presented in actuality as a vertex birth). This of course was the attempt at reproducing the phantasy of their respective births.

Three of the children became obviously temporarily uneasy and it was discernible that their colour changed. Two became increasingly breathless and showed obvious fear and discomfort. After a few moments suggestions were given that they would push through and emerge into sunlight feeling a sense of relief, comfort and ease of breathing which they had never felt before. Of the six cases so treated none of them have relapsed. These patients will continue to be followed-up, but after three years no relapse has yet been recorded in any of the children so treated.

It would appear therefore that some claim must be made for birth-trauma of a psychological nature contributing to the pathology of childhood ill-health. If the baby escapes from this hazard he approaches the next one with at least a better chance of success. Oral, anal and urethral problems can be explained in part by the attitude of the mother. It is nowadays accepted that the success of breast-feeding depends largely upon the stability of the mother. We might coin a phrase and say: "The fewer the conflicts the easier the flow." If the food passes easily to the stomach it passes as easily through the bowel. If the mother causes a problem at the mouth she will repeat the pattern at the anus. How much the child will aid in this pattern is more difficult to explain. But both child and mother will symbolise food as love and the tug-of-war commences. The child, desperate in his efforts to gain love at every conceivable moment will tax the patience and understanding of his mother. Possibly the first interpretation of the child is now called for—if he is satisfied that love is being demonstrated to his satisfaction we could argue that all will be well. If the mother herself must prove that she is loved by her child, as a result of her own problems of childhood when she was uncertain of her own love from either parent, she concentrates too much on the excretory apparatus of her baby—she becomes the "Syrup of Figs, or Magnesia Mother." This is the mother who will not tolerate aggression—she is unconsciously too aggressive herself. The family history is bound to be repeated, and the child commences a pattern of illness. Whether the illness will be released as a psychiatric problem or a psychosomatic one is nowadays immaterial, and whether one child develops a skin reaction, another asthma and yet a third anxiety, it could be claimed that basically the sick child is the anxious one. It is tempting to promulgate a theory of "all for one and one for all" when confronted with a psychiatric or paediatric problem.

It will be appreciated that in a chapter of this description the history of childhood illness must necessarily be sketchy, but some explanation should be given before tackling the use, abuse and value of hypnosis. From what has been said, however, it will be seen that a sick child has been "sick" in the formative years. To reveal the first five-year problems is a difficult task with children, although even more so with adults. Psycho-analytic techniques must be used in the majority of psychiatric problems if early memories and phantasies are to be exposed, but this method is tedious and cannot be successful with every child. Hypnotherapy offers a technique which, although skilled and demanding of adequate knowledge, will nevertheless be rewarding, and it is possible to cut down the number of interviews which will be necessary to produce the desired result. In other words hypnosis can be used to hasten the means to an end.

HYPNO-ANALYSIS AND DREAM INTERPRETATION

Hypno-analytic techniques with the child vary little from those used with the adult, but the more elaborate methods are not indicated. Thus the author has seldom found it necessary to use mirror-gazing or automatic writing in a child's treatment. It will be found in practice that once the child attains the hypnotic state suggestions can be given in a direct way, but advantage must be taken of the fact that dreams, post-hypnotic suggestion and auto-hypnosis are all easy of attainment. Particularly should children be taught the benefit of the dream and its interpretation, and they should always be taught auto-hypnosis. Children are quick to value a means of combatting sickness in itself. There is acute perception in many cases that a positive attitude to sickness is the right one. Many ill children are kept that way by unconscious conflicts in either parent, although it is usually the mother's feelings of which the child is more intuitively aware, to his own detriment.

TECHNIQUE OF INDUCING DREAMS: CASE HISTORY

The technique of inducing a dream in the child is simple. The hypnotherapist, however, must be aware of what he is searching for in his patient. His own intuition is of paramount importance, hence the necessity for knowledge of psychological interpretation. If a child complains of fear that something dreadful will happen to one of his parents the analyst must be aware of the psychiatric implications of death-wishes and ambivalent feelings present in us all. If a child describes his terror of thunderstorms and fears that it will rain until a flood appears, it would not be good psychiatry to offer direct suggestions that these symptoms will disappear because "Mummy and Daddy love you; you will never again fear a thunder-storm, all your fears will vanish . . ." The child is telling the analyst: "I have done something I am ashamed of, I will be punished for this and the punishment will come from God." Some children will be able to verbalise their fears in one or two sessions and will immediately respond to enquiries directed towards religious upbringing. With other children we receive blank denial or silence. If the child, notwithstanding hypnosis, cannot put into words the fear which is repressed, then the hypnotist calls for a dream. This will be given in the form of a post-hypnotic suggestion. The dream should preferably be analysed by the patient, but occasionally the analyst will have to help the child to a fuller understanding of the underlying conflict revealed by the dream. In this respect it should always be appreciated that the dreamer is aware of the conflict unconsciously revealed. With the usual methods of psychotherapy it might be that several sessions are required in order to break up the dynamisms revealed, but with hypnotic interpretation, i.e., interpretation achieved by the child in the hypnotic state, this time factor can be controlled and months of treatment cut down to weeks.

In relationship to dream interpretation using hypnosis, it is not always necessary for a profound knowledge of symbols to be a requisite. Hypnosis is a form of dream in itself. As the patient relaxes and enters the deeper stages of hypnosis it will be realised that if he is asked to imagine himself at the age of seven or eight, pictures of past events will be released. The child may, for example, say that he remembers being on a farm and seeing the animals. He may recall anxiety-provoking memories or pleasant ones. He may speak of school or home, and gradually with a little gentle probing traumatic episodes will be revealed.

A child of fifteen complained of the fear of dark clouds. If she thought a storm or rain was imminent she would become panicky and anxious. She refused to go out of the house until she had listened to the daily weather forecast on the wireless. She insisted that when it rained it would continue until there was a flood. This behaviour started when she was nine, and gradually got worse until the entire household was controlled by her behaviour. In a deep hypnotic state she was regressed to the age of nine and said she could remember nothing. When asked if she could recall anything at an earlier age she said that at six she nearly drowned. She was then told that before her next session she would have a dream. The subsequent dream revealed that she was trying to get her spade and bucket from a ledge and was balancing precariously to do this. She suddenly lost her hold and fell into the sea. She was rescued in the nick of time. She was asked how this tied up with her fear of rain, the inference appearing to be obvious. However, she said she remembered her mother saying that she would fall into the sea one day if she didn't listen to her. Asked if her mother was in the habit of making statements like this, she said that her mother would often suggest that unpleasant things might happen if she were rude or naughty. Further enquiry, while she was still in the hypnotic state, revealed that she was a child who had always been interested in religion. She said she read books about the Bible. She had three different versions of Noah and the Flood. At this point she asked the analyst if he believed in God. "Do you think God is in this room?" The analyst gave her his interpretation of faith and the ability to grow up and find God within oneself. She was then told that a dream would reveal her real fear. Subsequently her next dream was analysed under hypnosis. It revealed guilt about a sexual misdemeanour with a boy next door. She was chastised by her mother and a great fuss was made. After eight hypnotic treatments, which revealed much guilt, anxiety and aggressive feelings towards her mother, the situation was relieved to the extent that the child could travel about and had lost her fear of floods.

INSIGHT MORE EASILY ACQUIRED IN THE HYPNOTIC STATE

Few children will be adequately treated if phobias are not investigated and explanations given. It is surprising how certain children will apparently deny the interpretation of traumata in the waking state, but in the hypnotic state they find understanding easier of attainment.

A girl of thirteen was vomiting and could not eat. Her weight loss was two stone in five months. The parents were naturally anxious and hypnotic treatment was sought as a last resort. The history was simply that five months previously she had a fat girl friend who told her the "facts of life." She started her periods at about the age of eleven and at the time her mother gave her some knowledge of sex, emphasizing that if the periods stopped a baby was to be expected. The child did not gather that a male was necessary in this process. The fat girl-friend embellished some of these facts two years later. The patient feared that if she became fat this would mean the presence of a baby. It was revealed under hypnosis that the girl had used a suppository for constipation just before the symptoms commenced. Further unconscious material was released by dreams which revealed a traumatic episode at the age of three, when the child had gone to live with an aunt and uncle. During hypnosis she saw a doll in bed with the relatives. She said she could see her uncle "doing something with her aunt." The mother could remember that ten years earlier her daughter could not sleep and would be taken into the parents' bed. She also became constipated and suppositories and enemata were given.

This was after her visit to the relatives. In the waking state she was given explanations along the following lines. The primal scene was explained and the suppositories used, it was suggested, were allied with the phallus. She was told that she phantasised a baby within her and was trying to vomit it out. She was afraid of getting fat like her friend for fear of the confirmation of a phantasy pregnancy. It is hardly surprising that the patient was quite unable to accept this interpretation, but the analyst continued to repeat it while she was under hypnosis. Within three months the girl was eating well and was putting on weight. Certain problems in the parents' marriage required discussion, but the child's symptoms abated after the fifth or sixth hypnotic session. Previous psychiatric help and hospitalization had failed in this case.

It is felt by the author that anorexia nervosa in children offers a valuable field for hypnosis, which will be found the method of choice if rapid results are to be expected.

SUPERFICIAL METHODS OF HYPNOTHERAPY: PSYCHOSOMATIC PROBLEMS

It will readily be understood that the cases illustrated were treated by hypnoanalytical means. In general practice the physician, and especially the doctor not versed in analytical techniques, might be reluctant to commence a form of treatment which demands skilled psychiatric knowledge. Can cases of anxiety and illness in children be treated by a more superficial method? Undoubtedly hypnosis can be used at a more superficial level. The use of direct hypnotic suggestion could be tolerated in asthma, for example. The asthmatic of today can so easily become the chronic bronchitic of tomorrow. It is important to control the spasm of asthma which, if allowed to continue, may proceed to status asthmaticus—a dangerous condition. Clinical research has shown that a child who is told immediately preceding the hypnotic state that: "You will be more in control of your body by your mind," will show relaxation and a greater confidence in his ability to control the symptoms.

A stethoscopic examination will reveal the presence of rales and rhonchi, but the general state of the child will surprise the onlooker. If the child is capable of acquiring a reasonable state of hypnosis much can be accomplished by simple reassurance and explanation. It must be remembered in this respect that the parents, particularly the mother, are deeply anxious and some time should be devoted to probing the state of the family unit. Asthma is a sign of aggression, or rather the inability to release this emotion. The general practitioner will be in the best position to judge the psychological unrest etc. within the family. Some attempt must be made to analyse the difficulties encountered in the environment. The relationship of the child to brothers and sisters, jealousy reactions and the mother's aggression should be explored. But during or before this time much can be accomplished with the child victim by hypnotic treatment. It may even be found that the mother must be analysed and the father given an understanding of his role in the family. But while the asthma is being controlled the rapport of the doctor to the parents can be utilised in the psychological explanation.

The enuretic child can often be successfully treated by a more superficial approach. It should be realised in this respect that bed-wetters hate the condition and are only too willing to cooperate in any treatment which is not frightening. Many enuretics subjected to osteopathic methods, for example, are only too willing to embrace a treatment which avoids "bending them up and down," as one child described it, and seek hypnosis as a haven of refuge from frightening methods of treatment.

It is not emphasized that simple directive suggestions are all that are necessary in this condition. Some attempt will have to be made to give the parents insight into the significance of the bed-wetting act. The symbolism of the act should be recognized. The wet bed does often represent the sexual desire of the child for the mother, for not only does the act get attention (in lieu of love), but the male child is using the urine as a phantasy of his desire for sexual relations with his mother. If the bed-wetter is punished and the word "dirty" etc. used to decry his habit, the nocturnal enuresis becomes a magnified guilt when nocturnal emission occurs later. The child of thirteen "wetting" his bed with the seminal discharge is an echo of himself at the age of five or six being "dirty" by wetting his bed with his urine.

It is interesting that in certain cases of phobia of ghosts, relief of the fears has been accomplished by recalling the emotions which accompanied bed-wetting during the patient's first five years—the wet sheets and the angry mother become the "ghost" of which he was afraid years before. If the phantasies of childhood can be revealed, many people who "dabble" in Christian Science, faith-healing etc. find, much to their astonishment, healthier outlets and a greater value in more adequate sublimation.

It is considered that if directive attempts are made to abolish this habit, for example by bell-ringing techniques, regimes of exercises for the bladder etc., the dynamism of the act is further repressed and the child may need treatment for guilt and fear at puberty or adolescence. Hypnosis should be reserved for re-educative procedures. The "habits" of the first five years are to be repeated as the patterns of later life. It is easier to reveal these patterns and de-condition them early in life rather than later.

EPILEPSY

Ideopathic

In the discussion of this grave illness it is not intended to pursue the subject at any length. If the reader is interested he can refer to other literature on the subject (1, 2). The author has treated cases of Grand Mal, but this problem is best dealt with by hypnoanalytical means and demands not only patience but also an understanding of the psychological dynamisms to be expected. The fit is analytically seen by some authorities as the need for the orgasm, and an epileptic child will be seen to illustrate grave inhibition of his emotions. It is not unusual to find birth traumata, as in the asthmatic child. Loss of consciousness in the birth canal itself and prolonged labour is very often said to be a concomitant of the later epileptiform seizure.

While treating Grand Mal in children with hypnotherapy it is usual to work under a cover of modern drugs used in this condition. As treatment takes effect it may be possible to cut down the medication.

Petit Mal

Hypnosis should be reserved for this condition. It is surprising how successful hypnotherapy can be and several authorities have stressed the ease of treatment and its value (5, 7).

It is usual to see children who have been subjected to much physical treatment and the parents will seek hypnotic aid as a last resort. Their attitude has very often much to do with their child's illness—although this statement is nowadays a platitude.

The hypnotherapist's difficulty is to remove the idea that Petit Mal is purely a physical illness and that only drugs will have any effect on its course. However, the child is quick to seize upon a technique which offers it a haven from its feelings of being different from other children. Whether the child is too fat, too thin or too anxious, whether it is suffering a skin complaint, asthma, stammering or has a scoliosis, the doctor must try to put the child at ease, remove his doubts and be prepared to play the role of the ideal father—the father who will temporarily take over his problems as his own and will be the barrier between the child and the outside world. This attitude will inspire confidence in the patient. When a transference situation is created the child will begin to show improvement.

The technique of treating Petit Mal cases is no different from the treatment already outlined in other conditions. The child should be encouraged to speak about his problems, discuss his dreams, air his grievances, express his aggression and deal with his fears, guilts and the like. It is preferable to work in the deep state, but depth is no bar to treatment. The number of fits will be dramatically affected as the confidence of the child is gained. As the parents become less obsessed by the condition and the child is allowed to get on with life, so a corresponding lessening of the attacks will be noted. Patients should be seen at least 12 times during the early days and asked to report back for reinforcement treatment when control has been gained over the smyptom. Autohypnosis should be taught and is easily learnt (1). It is always worth while to use the technique of rebirth in these cases, as outlined previously.

STAMMERING

It is intended to avoid the various theories about stammering. The stammerer is first and foremost suffering from an inhibition of aggressive drives. It has been mentioned that spasm will be seen at both ends and a history of constipation is not unusual in this condition.

A boy of thirteen always thought that his stammer had commenced at the age of six. Under deep hypnosis he remembered that during a trip abroad with his parents, when he was eight, he had an inability to move his bowels for nine days. The door of the lavatory he used was covered with glass and he felt that people outside could see him at stool. When he arrived back home he stammered. Further analysis of oral problems as well as his attitude towards his parents and their attitude toward him, resulted in the cure of the stammer after a year's treatment.

The patient should be trained to enter a deep state of hypnosis and it must be insisted upon at this time that he will not worry about the condition. Many of the cases seen for hypnosis will have been treated by speech therapists and this will be found of value during directive suggestions that the child will be able to put the theoretical and practical treatment of the speech therapist to better use. In all pediatric problems, suggestions should be given that the worry associated with the condition will cease. It is surprising how the child will be able to absorb and act upon this suggestion, returning to the therapist with a greatly enhanced positive attitude towards his problems.

Parents again will be found intimately associated with the fundamental factors in stammering. They become self-conscious of their child's efforts to break the habit and will often have used various methods of trying to overcome their fear of the stammer. The efforts will vary from kindness or fear to downright cruelty, very often, although at an unconscious level. The parent will be desperately anxious for somebody to abolish the symptom. In many cases the state of the parents' marriage will have to be examined.

This aspect of child psychiatry must be realised by the physician treating these cases. The mother's unconscious feelings towards her children will be ordained by her own emotional patterning. The first child can often be (unconsciously) seen as the gift to the father, i.e., not to the husband, as symbolising her love for her first sweetheart (her own father). The second child can represent a loved or hated sister or brother, and the third is where the poor husband comes into his own! It would appear to be a noteworthy fact that the woman finds herself unconsciously in competition with her mother or any woman who brought her up, to produce either the same number of children or one extra, in order to defeat the mother. In other words each child will represent unconsciously the emotions the mother played through her own parents and the siblings. If she has made adequate adjustments her attitude toward her children will be mature and adult, but so often these emotions will be released against or in favour of each child. For example, if she had a dominant brother and could never accept the father's aggression, the first male child can be incorporated in her fear of aggression and he will not easily be allowed to release his ordinary aggressive drives. It is possible that certain constitutional or genetic factors will now be included in the psychodynamic inheritance of the child, and psychosomatic phenomena may be released. The child who is not allowed to release his normal aggressive drives will be in danger.

A boy of eleven was treated for a stammer in 1954. Little attempt was made to probe at any significant level. Direct suggestions were used to the effect that he would worry less about the condition and that he would feel loved and understood by his parents. A deep state of hypnosis was achieved, and the child was finally discharged after two months' treatment, with the suggestion that within a year he would be speaking well.

Four years later the mother wrote to say that this child was cured, and would the therapist now treat a younger boy who had commenced to stammer. This child was seen in 1959, at the age of eight, and the same technique was employed. Little subjective improvement was seen in this case, and the analyst felt that deeper problems were to blame. On this occasion the mother was seen and showed obviously that she was closely associated with the child's stammer. Her attitude towards her husband was explored and tension and aggression were released. It was tempting to suppose that she had allowed the older boy to get well and then had shifted her unconscious fear of her husband's aggression to the younger boy. This was explained to her, and later reports suggested that the second child was losing his stammer.

One might postulate several theories in a case of this description and space only prevents one from doing so. It is unlikely that many stammerers will lose their symptom without some attempt at setting right the obvious parental problems. It would be so much easier if there were rules regarding those cases which might be treated by direct suggestions and those where some psycho-therapy must be given to the parents. Only the intuition, knowledge and experience of the therapist can be used to decide this matter.

TICS, NAIL-BITING AND THUMB-SUCKING

Most habit spasms acquired in childhood are the result of inner tensions. Undoubtedly some children display spasms which one of the parents will tell us they suffered from themselves. In fact it is almost a rule that nail-biters seem to have an hereditary background to their habit. Mothers will be able to remember that they suffered "peculiar" movements not unlike those of their children when they were young. It is difficult to decide how much psychogenic factors favour the tic or whether it can be laid at the door of a familial or constitutional background.

The tic seems invariably to be present in the anxious child. The introspective child will be more likely to develop a habit-spasm although this is not always the rule. That the tic is always of symbolic character is more accurate. The biting of the inside of the lip, shrugging of the shoulders, involuntary grunts—indeed any movement can be seen in this condition, but observation will often suggest the symbolic implication of the habit.

Many children suffering from tics will have fussy, perfection-istic parents. The tic itself becomes too important and sometimes seems to be the entire interest in the household. That tics follow unpleasant memories, shocks etc. will not be denied, although often no apparent reason can be found for their genesis. Constant eye-blinking can symbolise the desire to shut out unpleasant sights, rubbing movements may symbolise repressed masturbatory urges. There are few people in a community who will not show some form of tic.

The treatment of tics by psychotherapy is somewhat tedious. The approach by hypnosis offers a rational form of therapy. Direct suggestion has sometimes been remarkably successful and the older practitioners have written at length on the direct hypnotic treatment of these cases (3, 8, 12). To ensure, however, that the child does not exchange one symptom for another, these cases in quite young subjects offer a fruitful field of investigation and treatment by combined analysis and hypnosis. They are generally excellent subjects for deep hypnosis and advantage must be taken of this fact.

Recently, a girl of fifteen was seen on account of a constant desire to bite the inner part of the mouth. A portion of the mucous membrane was grasped between her pre-molars and continually rolled between these teeth. Analysis revealed that a dental surgeon had been consulted, who gave her the advice that if she continued the habit she might develop cancer! This only made matters worse. She was intensely aggressive toward her father and worried that something dreadful would happen to her mother. The child was unable to appreciate that her aggression toward her father covered her real love for him and that her fears for her mother's safety were indicative of her represssed death wishes against her. The parents were interviewed and certain problems were explained and accepted. The classical Oedipus situation was explained to the girl under deep hypnosis. A dream was asked for and she was told that in the dream would be the substance of her real fears, etc. As the analysis proceeded she was able to show far less aggression against the father and eventually realised that her real conflict lay with her mother. She went on with the tic to a lesser degree, but was gradually able to recognise its significance, particularly the masturbatory and other guilt fears in its genesis. She continued to become less tense and more relaxed, and later her parents wrote to say that whereas previously they had concentrated upon her tic, they now understood its significance and the entire family was much happier.

Thumb-sucking can lead to orthodontic problems after the

age of six. Hypnosis may often be used successfully in these cases, but care must be taken over analysing the situation in the home. Too much attention paid to the habit can sometimes ensure conditioning. Whether direct suggestions should be used in these problems, e.g: "You will not suck your thumb, for you want to be pretty like Mummy" or "You are a big boy now and you will be as big and strong as Daddy," is a question which is still engaging the attention of hypnotherapists. Where habits are causing temporary disruption in the home or additional emotional conflicts for the child, an attempt at explanation will have to be made with the parents, with emphasis placed upon the time which may be needed in order to break the habit. Parents are often looking for a magic wand where none exists.

OBESITY, ANOREXIA NERVOSA, ABDOMINAL MIGRAINE, SLEEP PROBLEMS

The "nervous" child can suffer from many psychosomatic problems from its mouth to its anus. Several years ago a syndrome of digestive problems, together with cyclic vomiting, headaches and intolerance to certain foods, were lumped together in the one diagnosis of "acidosis." These children were described as introspective, intelligent, perfectionistic, etc. As our knowledge of personality problems has grown it has become tempting to describe the "acidosis" child in more simple terminology.

Undoubtedly these children are often described to the doctor as: "She has always been difficult," or "he cried often as a baby," or again, "I cannot understand it, she was no trouble at all as a baby, good as gold and never a cry from her." For the purpose of pediatric problems and their treatment by hypnosis the author feels that the "acidosis" child should be described under a more general heading. Alimentary disturbances are usually the result of an inability to grow up, and can so often be traced to earlier problems in the first five years that treatment should be directed towards a correction of the mother-child relationship. It is revealing that when the family problems are analysed and resolved, alimentary disturbances can be more adequately controlled by the child.

If we can accept the statement that all illness has a gain factor it will be easier for the reader to follow the argument. The child seeks love in all its waking moments. If this need is satisfied, *in his own interpretation,* the baby and later the child will sleep and wake with the minimum of difficulty. There are undoubtedly children who will need greater reassurance and a more overt sign of being loved. These children will be more demanding and more grasping in their desire for a *demonstration* of love. Bodily contact in the first few months is a desperate need in most children. Sometimes, by reason of conscious and unconscious factors in the mother (and later in the father) this is not forthcoming. The baby's reasoning takes it as far as: "I love, therefore I must be loved, I don't feel love, therefore I am not loved, therefore I am unlovable, therefore I am hated, therefore I hate." This was neatly summarised by Stekel, who wrote: "If you my brother will not be I'll break your skull, you will see." Probably the baby's first hazard is its birth, but following this inconvenience it finds its haven at the breast of the mother. Pain following pleasure is the basic reasoning for Freud's pleasure-pain principle. The unconscious is not aware of time and the baby is hard-pressed to define the difference— indeed it cannot, and will substitute one for the other. If the mother is unaware of this fundamental principle she can make no allowance for the child's moods, behaviour, etc. The child will gradually find a haven of refuge in a temporary tummy-ache, fever or cold. If more *attention,* as opposed to a demonstration of love, is substituted at this point the child may become conditioned to temporary spasm or other psychosomatic manifestation in lieu of love. The so-called hysteric is about to evolve. If at this point erotic and later sensuous and sexual feelings cannot be tolerated or are inhibited by the child, in other words if the environmental factors become too difficult, emotion must be forced inwards and substitutes for erotic pleasure must be found. The substitutes are somatic problems, which the pediatrician will have to deal with and overcome. Temporary alleviation will be found in bottles of medicine and tablets, but symbolically these serve the purpose of "mother's milk"and are the very symbols of the need for the real thing.

If the basic dynamisms are understood, treatment by any

therapy is easier of accomplishment. Direct hypnotic suggestion will act as a temporary crutch or may tide the child over for a number of months or even years, until at puberty or adolescence the child will require greater adjustment and more adequate sublimation than he has been able to achieve up till that time.

Deep analysis of such problems is inevitably controlled to a great extent by material considerations. If every child who had insufficient breast-milk and resultant feelings of being unloved or unloveable is to be subjected to deep penetrating analysis, there will have to be a mushroom growth of clinics and doctors trained in the art of analysis. Fortunately many a harassed mother and her (sometimes) less over-emotionally orientated husband (the very fact that he is not at home as much and therefore has less contact with these problems gives him the ability of greater reasoning and less emotion), are quick to learn and often have considerable insight into their mistakes and interpersonal problems. If the hypnotherapist, by his suggestions, can temporarily alleviate the more pressing somatic manifestations of the problems of the psyche, he allows time for the acceptance of a more rational approach to the body's ailments.

The obese child is generally showing difficulties along the lines illustrated above. The child's fantasies, however, must be understood. For instance, the girl who is about to menstruate for the first time is bound to be assailed by fantasies, and it is these which can so often ordain the symptom. A fat child may not only be overeating because of a fear of not being loved.

A girl of fifteen was seen for obesity, which appeared to have commenced at the age of eleven. The mother was grossly neurotic and the family unit disturbed. The girl was an only child and had always realised that her father would have preferred a son. The mother was dominant, and her husband's work ordained that he left the home at 3:30 A.M. and returned at 6 P.M., when he would go straight to bed after a meal. They slept in separate rooms.

Analysis, using deep hypnosis, revealed that the child had commenced her periods at the age of eleven. The mother dealt with the problems of puberty by saying: "Now that you have started your periods you can have a baby, so be careful." The child said that at the time she did not understand this advice. Later she heard a girl at school say: "When you get a baby you stop your periods and get fat." Hypnosis was used at this point to try to bring into consciousness any fantasy or memory of the primal scene. She answered that she could remember sleeping with her mother when she had tummy pains. These were frequent when she was five or six years old. She would develop a fever and pain in the abdomen, feel sick and unable to go to school. She suffered a lot from constipation and both her mother and a nurse gave her enemas.

It was explained under hypnosis that fantasies of procreation would be commenced by this treatment. This was readily accepted by the patient. She began to see that her obesity might be the unconscious expression of her conflict about being the boy that her father always wanted but the girl she undoubtedly knew she was. She proved her understanding of the conflict by saying: "I wanted to be a girl with my conscious mind but a boy in the other mind, so I show this by eating too much ,stopping my periods, but wanting to be a woman having a baby."

Gradually she lost weight, left school and took a job where she lived in a hostel away from her parents. Later reports show her to be happy in her new work. Her obvious fear of the male became less and she went to dances and became interested in the opposite sex.

Obesity can be a symptom of making oneself different in order to avoid sexual fears, which adds greatly to an already existing conflict of childhood. Whenever a child presents a symptom, be it headache, constant abdominal pain of a functional nature, sleeplessness etc., the physician should be aware of the problems outlined above. It is of course taken for granted that these children will have been adequately investigated for evidence of organic disease and pronounced "psychosomatic" individuals.

SUMMARY

If we can accept a definition of the neurotic individual as a person who responds to the challenges of the present in terms of the obsessively remembered past, then as parents we must see that our children are not given "old erroneous notions fossilised into dogmas." (Aldous Huxley, "Borderlands of the Mind," Observer, Oct. 22nd 1961.)

The author has taken as his theme throughout the text that the child is the barometer of the parents. It is up to us to see that our children inherit from us not the dogmas of the past, but the rational understanding of the future. Neurosis and philosophy (rather the lack of it) go hand in hand. The child must be allowed to develop in his own image while we supply the love, security and guidance which are necessary to keep the child basically stable while allowing the personality free reign for expression. Every effort must be made to understand and tolerate the emotions, while destructive criticism, comparison with others, over-restrictive measures and the like are avoided. The physician is in the best position to correct obvious faults in the family unit, if and when encountered. It is an indictment of modern medicine if we as doctors can admit to ourselves that a few hours spent with the parents of a sick or neurotic child might have avoided a lifetime of misery for the young patient.

Hypnosis is not only a short-cut method for dealing with tension and anxiety in children, but it should be used for re-educative purposes.

Modern psychiatry may be likened to an overflowing trunk of clothes. In superficial psychiatry we put back the clothes as best we can and close the lid, hoping for the best. In deeper methods we open the lid and rearrange the top layers so that they fit more neatly. In psychoanalysis the object would be to take all the clothes out, shake them, refold and re-arrange them neatly before closing the lid. In child psychiatry we have an easier task. The trunk is small, the clothes few and the folding and repacking not so difficult.

The induction of the hypnotic state in a child is simple and will occasion no real difficulty. It will be found that many more children can be hypnotised than adults and their suggestibility is much greater. Bérillon (3), Wetterstrand (13), Liébeault (8), and Ringier of the old school all gave high figures for successful hypnosis in children. Of the modern school Moodie (9), Nichols (10), Newbold (2) and A. G. Davies have all had similar results. In particular, Solovey de Milechnin has written at great length in many papers on the ease of hypnotising children. The author wrote several years ago that group hypnotherapy, as practiced by Liébeault in 1889, should be re-commenced with children. This method would afford greater opportunity for more children to be treated whilst allowing the parents to be given understanding and insight in a separate room. Constant calls for research, however, have fallen upon deaf ears and little attempt has been made in this country to assess hypnotic techniques against other psychotherapeutic maneuvers in a clinical setting. It is this lack of research which has made the task of the child psychiatrist using hypnotic techniques more difficult of assessment. Many of us using hypnosis are clinically certain that in selected cases we have a powerful weapon to avoid continued ill-health in children, and are accomplishing valuable work for the future of adult psychiatry. The neurotic child is bound to grow up to be the neurotic adult. History has a habit of repeating itself and much more so has the family history. If we can cut across childhood neurosis we may prevent much misery and mental ill-health of the future.

The pattern of childhood neurosis was first outlined by Freud. His genius discovered the repetition of the first five year problems in puberty, adolescence and marriage. If the patient can be shown these patterns, something can be done to avoid the continuation of the patterning. If the psychiatrist is aware of the behavioural patterns much can be accomplished by suggestion and the giving of adequate insight, in order to avoid the pitfalls which lie in wait for the child, not only on account of his parents' mistakes but also because of his own interpretations. Hypnosis should be used to illustrate this patterning process. The child should see his faults and mistakes clearly as if on a screen. As treatment progresses so the screen becomes larger. Philosophical discussions should be encouraged. Many children seem more able to appreciate spiritual values than their parents. The hypnotist should not only be capable of breaking neurosis, but he must be aware that his patient might not only want something removed from his psyche, but something more to take its place. This something more might be a broader understanding and appreciation of what constitutes adequate good health and psychological insight.

The hypnotist should be aware of stress factors associated with the frustration of bottled emotions, so that he will not be able to rest content only with hypnotherapy in the child's treatment. The parents will have to be tackled and shown the error of their ways. Too high standards, emotional projection from one or both parents, inability to accept aggression and rage from their child, dogmas of religion and indeed any outmoded or outdated shibboleths must be corrected—and it goes without saying that the psychiatrist will unfortunately often find the parents a greater handful than their children.

It is true to say that for any psychiatric problem found in one parent, the other cannot be excluded from its patterning. Neurosis is produced overtly at marriage. If this is true, the children of the marriage will be endangered and it is up to modern psychiatry to embrace the family unit. The author has at times subjected an entire family to the hypnotic procedure at a group psychotherapeutic level. The family has even been able to voice its aggressions and interpersonal problems while in the hypnotic state, with subsequent benefit to all—but this is a technique of the future and requires greater research.

It is a sobering and helpful thought that the psychiatrist can only do his best—he cannot do better than his best. If his patient wants to get well and he acts as the catalyst in this process he is carrying out his duties to the best of his ability. In this respect it is considered that a psychiatrist using hypnotherapy, and in particular hypno-analytical techniques, should have faced a personal analysis himself. During this analysis he may find that he loses interest in hypnosis and may even lose his ability to hypnotise. But later, as he becomes more aware of his needs in using hypnosis, a subtle change comes about, a change difficult of precise explanation, but one which makes him more tolerant, more understanding and the better physician. It becomes easier to take a patient through a door which one has opened oneself, and during the actual hypnotic state an analyzed doctor can appreciate the wealth of material discharged by his patient. Not only does he recognise the material, but by his increased knowledge of fundamental dynamisms he can feed back to the patient the knowledge, understanding and forbearance which he will have achieved by a knowledge of his own psyche.

REFERENCES

1. AMBROSE, G.: *Hypnotherapy with Children.* 2nd Edition, London, Staples, 1961.
2. AMBROSE, G. and NEWBOLD, G.: *Handbook of Medical Hypnosis.* 2nd Edition, London, Bailliére, Tindall & Cox, 1958.
3. BÉRILLON, E.: Onychophagie, guerison rapide par la suggestion. *Rev. de l'Hypnotisme, 8:*15, 1896; and Les Applications de l'hypnotisme au traitment des enfants vicieuse. *Rev. de l'Hypnotisme, 2:*59, 1887.
4. FREDERKING, W.: Intoxicant drugs (mescaline and lysergic acid) in psychotherapy. *J. Nerv. Ment. Dis., 121:*3, 1955.
5. FRY, A.: The scope of hypnosis in general practice. *Brit. Med. J., 2:*1232, 1957.
6. KELSEY, D.: Phantasies of birth and prenatal experiences recovered from patients undergoing hypnoanalysis. *J. Ment. Sc., 159:*415, 1953.
7. KENNEDY, A.: The medical use of hypnotism. *Brit. Med. J., 2:*1317, 1957.
8. LIÉBEAULT, A. A.: Emploi de la suggestion hypnotique pour l'éducation des enfants et des adolescents. *Rev. de l'Hypnotisme, 1:*71, 1887.
9. MOODIE, W.: *Hypnosis in Treatment.* London, Faber & Faber, 1959.
10. NICHOLS, L. A.: Personal communication.
11. SANDISON, R. A. and WHITELAW, J. D. A.: Further studies in the therapeutic value of lysergic acid in mental illness. *J. Ment. Sc., 103:*431, 1957.
12. VOISIN, A.: Le traitment des habitudes vicieuses par la suggestion. *Rev. de l'Hypnotisme, 2:*364, 1887.
13. WETTERSTRAND, O. G.: Dritter Internationaler Congress für Psycologie in Munchen, Munich, 1897.

8

HYPNOSIS IN DENTISTRY

HOWARD W. MARCUS, M.D., D.M.D., DR.MED.DENT.

INTRODUCTION

Hypnosis in dentistry is at times referred to as "Hypnodontia" or "Dental Hypnosis." A too literal interpretation of these terms would imply that hypnosis when used in the dental office differs from the hypnosis used in medicine or psychiatry. In fact, it differs only in the manner and to the extent of its application, not in its basic nature. Obviously, the dentist who uses hypnosis for dental purposes, cannot use it without consideration of the total personality of his patient.

This undeniable fact has led some to deny the dentist's right to use hypnosis at all. Yet, as pointed out elsewhere (1), the modern dentist is not only concerned with the mechanical aspects of his profession. General medical, as well as surgical and psychological considerations form an inseparable and important part of his daily practice. Today's training of the dentist has incorporated general medical and surgical aspects within the framework of his dental education to such a point that they form an integral part of dentistry. As a result of this, it is unthinkable to consider modern dentistry as an art preoccupied with mechanical problems exclusively, rather than as a specialty within the general field of medicine.

Dentistry, as all other branches of medicine, has become more aware of the broader psychosomatic aspects to be taken into consideration in diagnosis and treatment of the patient. As a matter of fact, ever since Freud, special psychodynamic importance has been attributed to the oral region.

Importance of the Oral Region

The properly trained dentist of today is fully aware that modern dentistry is no longer confined to the mechanical aspects of his profession. He has learned to consider the tooth as part of a larger unit: the oral cavity with all its many tissues and functions. He has learned to consider the oral cavity as part of the human body, the body as part of the patient, and the patient as an inseparable unit of body and mind.

If we look at this oral cavity with which the dentist deals every day, a bit closer, we must realize that it is not only an assembly of incisors, cuspids, premolars and molars, plus perhaps some soft and hard tissues, tongue, lips and cheek, and some other anatomically interesting structures, but:

1. The oral cavity is the port of entry of life: Life begins with the first cry of the baby allowing air to enter through the mouth into the lungs and thus the cycle of rhythmic breathing begins and continues throughout life;

2. The oral cavity is also the organ with which the infant seeks his first contact with the outside world by touch of his mother's breast. Through this contact he derives warmth—comfort—food and security;

3. The oral cavity continues to serve the growing child as an organ of comfort as indicated by the use of the pacifier, the sucking of thumb, finger and other objects;

4. The oral cavity continues to serve as port of entry of life-sustaining air and food and thereby gives comfort and security throughout man's life;

5. The oral cavity takes on the vital role of communication with the outside world: as we speak—praise—scold—smile—cry and laugh;

6. The oral cavity becomes an organ of aggression, physical as we bite, verbal as we express anger and hate;

7. The oral cavity becomes an organ of love, physical and verbal;

8. The oral cavity is also a port of entry of disease-causing germs and disease-fighting medication. Many of the systemic diseases have their first manifestations in the oral cavity;

While the oral cavity has such vital functions which enables us to eat, drink, chew, talk, bite, suck, breathe, smoke, and to engage in many other pleasurable pursuits;

9. The oral cavity is also an organ of prime importance for our esthetic appearance: We think of the lips and teeth here, the well-known advertising smile on one hand, and anger, hate, dissatisfaction and unhappiness as expressed by contraction of the circumoral musculature on the other hand;

10. Finally, the oral cavity becomes an organ symbolizing aging whereby loss of teeth equals loss of power, physical and sexual decline with all its far-reaching psychodynamic ramifications. The numerous expressions which refer to the oral cavity in a symbolic way may further serve to illustrate the psychodynamic significance of this organ. We "swallow" our anger, "spit" into someone's face, use "biting" language, "sweet" words, feel "bitter," "eat up" our "honey," and refer to the oral cavity in many other symbolic ways.

Thus fully aware that the dentist deals day in and day out, whether he wishes to or not, with psychodynamically meaningful material, the question arises: is he then not entering the field of psychotherapy?

The logical sequence to this question is: should the dentist use psychotherapy? And where does psychotherapy begin? A slap on the back, an encouraging remark, our prescription, the relief of pain, the treatment proper of a painful or esthetically bothersome condition, or of a disturbed patient, especially if accompanied by a positive, suggestive, reassuring approach—all are psychotherapy.

The treatment of habits and symptom removal, regardless of what habit is involved—thumbsucking or bruxism or any other, and regardless of what method is employed, is psychotherapy.

Therefore, if we wish to or not, we cannot avoid engaging in and dealing with some aspects of psychotherapy, as long as we practice dentistry on living human beings.

However, if we begin to realize that the dentist's position with regard to psychotherapy is not different from his position with regard to borderline areas involving the field of medicine or surgery or anesthesiology, or others, then his actions in this particular area also should not be different from what they would be in any other field of activity in which the dentist's training and experience and competence are obviously confined to the framework of his specialty.

To make this point clear: It is not the dentist's place to administer psychotherapy as such anymore than it would be his place to open surgically and curet the antrum to recover a broken root tip. On the other hand, if the dentist could pick up the broken root tip while it is accessible from the oral cavity and all he had to do is to reach for it with a college plier, and if by such relatively minor intervention he could protect his patient from major surgical procedure later on, he would not only use good judgment, but stay well within the area of his competence.

The same criterion applies to the use of suggestion, hypnosis, the handling of habits, symptom removal or any other of the dentist's activities which reach over beyond their physical role into what can generally be classified as psychotherapy.

The more familiar the dentist is with the intricacies of his professional activities from a psychodynamic point of view, the more readily will he recognize his limits and limitations as dictated by his training, experience and competence. The more extensive his training, experience and competence, the readier will he be able to recognize those patients for whom referral to the psychiatrist for consultation or treatment is indicated (2).

There is, however, no reason why the dentist should not enlarge his horizon to enable him to deal with psychological problems that occur in his field in the same manner as he has learned to deal with medico-surgical problems which occur in today's practice of dentistry.

The evaluation and proper handling of psychodynamic factors involved in the dentist-patient relationship, including the use of hypnosis and suggestion, will enable the dentist to perform a more complete health service. It will enable a greater number of patients to benefit from modern dental services. It will lift the dentist's horizon and elevate dentistry from the mechanistic plateau of the past to a position of a truly respected and competent member of the healing arts.

The above outlined general position of dentistry with regard to hypnosis has been officially sanctioned by the Council on Mental Health of the American Medical Association as follows: (3) "The use of hypnosis has a recognized place in the medical armamentarium and is a useful technic in the treatment of certain illnesses when employed by qualified medical and dental personnel." And further: "General practitioners, medical specialists and dentists might find hypnosis valuable as a therapeutic adjunct within the specific field of their professional competence."

The American Dental Association followed the lead of the American Medical Association (4) and states as follows: "No physician or dentist should utilize hypnosis for purposes that are not related to his particular specialty and that are beyond the range of his ordinary competence. As an example, a trained and qualified dentist might use hypnosis for hypnoanesthesia or hyponanalgesia or for the allaying of anxiety in relation to specific dental work. Under no circumstances would it be proper for him to use hypnosis for the treatment of neurotic difficulties of his patient."

The emphasis of the editorial in the *Journal of the American Dental Association* is on proper training and limitation to the field of competence.

Training in Hypnosis

The importance of proper training of the dentist in the use of hypnosis and the psychodynamics of the hypnotic relationship is not only strongly endorsed by all serious workers known to the author, but has been stressed all along by many of them in their publications, in the printed constitutions of the most important societies to which dentists belong, by such training centers as the Institute for Research in Hypnosis and others (5-8). Recently, furthermore, an American Board of Hypnosis in Dentistry was formed. Its aims and purposes are best illustrated by quoting in part their circular dated October 4, 1960:

"STATEMENT OF POLICY

The American Board of Hypnosis in Dentistry was established in 1958 as a section of the American Board of Clinical

Hypnosis, Incorporated, and is incorporated in the State of New York.

This Board shall be developed as far as is possible in conformity with the rules and regulations of the American Dental Association, with allowances for differences in training measures and related technical considerations. It is our intention to cooperate with the Council on Dental Education of the American Dental Association and will refer to this Council for advice and guidance when necessary.

The purposes of the Board are (1) to certify trained or experienced dentists who use hypnosis in dentistry with a sufficient background of knowledge in the subject; (2) to support and uphold the utilization of dental hypnosis within the specific area of professional dental competence; (3) to alert itself against inadequate courses of instruction to maintain standards of proficiency in the clinical applications of hypnosis in dentistry which will safeguard the welfare of the dental patient.

Certification shall be based on training and experience, and examinations will be given as deemed appropriate and necessary by the Board."

At present the type of training most readily available to dentists consists of post-graduate courses given at various universities, dental schools and under the auspices of dental societies throughout the country. This basic training is especially valuable if followed by advanced training in the form of workshops as given periodically in different parts of the country, and membership in various professional societies and study groups, available to dentists, with lectures, discussions and periodicals.

The incorporation of basic courses in psychology, psychodynamics and hypnosis into the curriculum of our dental schools would be desirable. For practical reasons, the teaching of this subject will most likely have to be confined to the postgraduate level, as is done by some of our dental schools, although others have begun to include this subject in the regular undergraduate curriculum.

Historical Background

It is noteworthy, especially in consideration of the critical attitude of some with regard to the use of hypnosis by the dentist, that dentists were among the first in the United States of America to revive hypnosis after World War II. The Dental study groups and dental societies dedicated to the study and practice of hypnosis were founded all over the country, and as a result of this, there were for a long time many more practitioners of dentistry studying and using hypnosis than practitioners in other fields of medicine, including psychiatry and psychology. There is of course a reason for this. Historically speaking, dentists have always been in the foreground when pain had to be conquered. Horace Wells, a dentist of Hartford, Connecticut, used nitrous oxide in his dental practice as early as December 1844. William Thomas Green Morton, a dentist, demonstrated the use of ether as an anesthetic at the Massachusetts General Hospital in Boston on October 16, 1846. Elijah Pope, a dentist of Rochester, New York, used ether for the extraction of a tooth as early as January 1842 (9). Ever since, dentists have been most active in the further development and administration of general and local anesthetics. It is interesting to note that dentists engaged in the administration of general anesthesia have been exposed to similar criticism based on the same reasoning as those using hypnosis (10). Here too reference is often made to "dental anesthesia," if the general anesthetic is being administered by a dentist. At this point, it might be of interest to the reader that after the introduction of general anesthesia into medical practice, it was denounced as quackery by the *Philadelphia Medical Examiner* in December 1848 (9).

INDICATIONS FOR THE USE OF HYPNOSIS IN DENTISTRY

In spite of all technological advances regarding equipment and technics, premedication and the administration of local and general anesthetics, one is forced to admit that dentistry still represents a threat to the majority of our population, and the mere sight of the dental equipment still provokes a great deal of anxiety in a great many people. Therefore, it can easily be understood that historically there always has been such interest by dentists to find ways and means to cope with those factors which interfere with the administration of dental services and which cannot be controlled by all the physical and pharmacological means at the disposal of the dentists. Here is where the use of hypnosis comes into its rightful place, namely: to bridge the gap that exists between the dentist's ability to administer good dental services and the patient's inability to accept them for no other than psychological reasons.

Opportunities for the use of hypnosis and suggestion exist in every practice, regardless of the specialty involved. This does by no means imply that hypnosis should be used in a routine manner. Quite to the contrary, hypnosis should be used only if and when needed; if and when other standard procedures at the disposal of the dentist do not suffice; or if and when the desired results of treatment can be facilitated or improved by the use of hypnosis.

Hypnosis therefore is used in addition to, and not instead of, established dental procedures. In dentistry it can be used in a selective fashion for the following specific purposes:

1. It is used to reach those patients who do not submit to dental treatment, even the routine dental examination, under any circumstances. These patients generally are not seen by the practicing dentist. They are the patients who finally arouse the ire or the compassion of one of their close relatives, who then makes the appointment for them. They are the patients who usually do not keep such appointments. They are the patients who are referred to in the profession as "dental cripples." And let there be no misunderstanding by those in the profession whose activities are concentrated on the more mechanistic aspects of dentistry and who never see such patients: those of us who do see them know that they represent a much larger contingent than is realized generally.

2. Hypnosis is used to overcome fear and tension, to counteract previous unpleasant experiences or negative influences with regard to the dental situation; it is used to raise the threshold of pain, and to relax patients who are undergoing treatment.

3. Hypnosis is used for premedication in operative and surgical procedures, either in addition to or instead of chemical premedication, depending on need and circumstances.

4. It is used to allow for a reduction of chemical anesthetic agents such as procaine, nitrous oxide or others and to reduce the unpleasant after-effects of chemical anesthesia.

5. It is used to replace chemical anesthesia where the administration of such anesthesia is contraindicated for medical reasons, such as allergies, heart disease and others.

6. Hypnosis is used to overcome handicaps to the performance of proper dental service and to the normal dentist-patient relationship, such as gagging while roentgenograms are being taken; gagging while impressions are taken; gagging while dentures or other appliances are worn; gagging during the routine examination of the oral cavity for diagnostic purposes; gagging during routine dental treatment or during the routine use of the toothbrush at home.

7. It is used to overcome lack of proper cooperation during such procedures as bite registration, or in the wearing of appliances, such as bite planes or other orthodontic or prosthetic appliances (provided, of course, that this lack of cooperation is not due to faulty construction of the appliance).

8. Hypnosis may be used for the control of flow of saliva and capillary bleeding to some extent, if desirable, although its effectiveness in controlling capillary bleeding has been questioned.

9. Hypnosis can be used to neutralize the commonly encountered objections to the noise and vibration caused by the dental drill.

10. Hypnosis can be used further in the form of posthypnotic suggestion, for the control of postoperative sequelae, such as pain and bleeding. Reconditioning patients through posthypnotic suggestions to accept dentistry in the future without prejudice is one of the important and most rewarding applications of hypnosis in dentistry.

11. Finally, hypnosis can be used for the correction of habits which interfere directly or indirectly with dental treatment, and with the health, function or esthetics of the dental apparatus and the soft tissues of the oral cavity.

CONTRAINDICATIONS FOR THE USE OF HYPNOSIS IN DENTISTRY

The proper choice of any therapeutic device in medicine and dentistry must be based on evaluation of the advantages and disadvantages of its use in each specific and individual case. However, there are certain general considerations which apply to all cases. From such general point of view, the contraindications for the use of hypnosis in dentistry can be listed as follows:

1. Hypnosis is not to be used if the dentist lacks training in, and familiarity with the subject matter as a whole. Here the same limitations apply as in any other area of professional activity. It is at times as easy to hypnotize a patient as it is to put a patient to sleep with a bottle of ether—yet in order to use anesthesia or hypnosis in the dental office, the dentist should have acquired a thorough knowledge of, and background in all aspects which enter into the administration of either.

2. Hypnosis is not to be used if the dentist has emotional problems concerning his attitude toward the patient or toward hypnosis, or both. The dentist using hypnosis ought to have enough insight into his own emotions to enable him to desist from using hypnosis under circumstances which would not allow him to use it in an objective and professional manner. The same limitations apply here in the emotional area as would apply to the dentist who might be physically handicapped to perform certain mechanical functions.

3. Hypnosis is to be discouraged if the patient has emotional problems concerning his attitude toward the dentist or hypnosis, or both. The dentist using hypnosis ought to be able to recognize emotional problems in his patients which call for a "hands off" attitude on his part. Here again the same applies as in any other area of his activities. If the problem goes beyond the scope of the dentist's training and experience, referral to a competent specialist is the required procedure.

4. Any deep-seated or psychodynamically meaningful condition which the dentist may encounter in his area of contact with the patient should not be treated by the dentist. Referral to the psychotherapist is imperative.

5. Any manifestation of dependency on hypnosis ought to be recognized and counteracted promptly.

6. Hypnosis should not be used if the dental services required in the specific case can be equally well performed without the

use of hypnosis. Unless there are definite indications for the use of hypnosis, its use is contraindicated, as would be the use of procaine for the preparation of a devitalized tooth.

7. Hypnosis should not be used by the dentist to probe or explore the mind of his patient.

8. Hypnosis should not be used by the dentist on mentally aberrated persons, except with the consent and cooperation of a psychiatrist, and then all other conditions should be as given for any other patient.

9. Hypnosis should not be used by the dentist for any manipulation which is outside his sphere of interest and competency.

DANGERS IN THE USE OF HYPNOSIS IN DENTISTRY

A great deal of space has been devoted in the general dental literature of the past to stress the dangers of hypnosis. Whereas the authors of most of these articles appear to have no intimate personal experience with the subject matter under discussion, their motives should not be questioned. The main arguments brought forward against the use of hypnosis in dentistry can be summarized as follows: the danger of not awakening; the danger of improper posthypnotic suggestions or of posthypnotic suggestions being carried out by the inadvertent use of a cue by an outsider; the danger of causing mental aberrations through the use of hypnosis; the danger of using hypnosis in the schizophrenic patient; the danger of provoking a psychosis by the use of hypnosis and the danger of causing less desirable and more pernicious reactions after the hypnotically induced elimination of an undesirable habit. Finally, the training and competence of the dentist to deal with such reactions as might occur in hypnosis are being questioned.

Whereas there is no doubt that hypnosis can be dangerous and that these summarized reactions may follow the use of hypnosis, it ought to be emphasized that these dangers apply not as much to the hypnotic process as such, as to its improper use by the individual operator. In the hands of the untrained, inexperienced, unscrupulous or unethical practitioner, hypnosis can obviously be dangerous. The question arises however, why the properly trained and licensed dentist using hypnosis should not apply the same professional conduct, ethics and judgment to the use of hypnosis in his dental practice, as to any other professional service rendered by him. If applied under such conditions, it appears obvious that the potential dangers in the use of hypnosis in dentistry compare quite favorably with the possible dangers of the many other professional activities occurring in the everyday practice of dentistry, such as the administration of local or general anesthesia; the use of the surgical scalpel; the prescription of narcotics, antibiotics and other drugs; and the many other activities in which the modern dentist engages his patient and which are taken for granted. A comparative glance into the available literature will quickly convince the serious and objective researcher that hypnosis is actually far less dangerous from any point of view than the many other professional activities ever can be (11, 12). Many undesirable accidents have occurred and will continue to occur, in spite of all precautions. Some of these incidents are on record in the literature. In addition to this physical threat to our patient, no serious observer can deny the many psychologically threatening activities (from the patient's point of view) which occur daily in the dentist's office. One has to think only of the implied threat of the injection needle without consideration of the possible toxic reactions to the material injected; the loss of teeth with its many psychodynamic implications and accompanied by the loss of blood; the threat to the patient implied by his relative position in the dental chair; the threat as presented by the dental equipment in full view of the anxious patient, and finally the threat as implied in such commonly used terms as "operating room," "needle," "pull," "drill" and many others. Whereas such threats—be they of physical or psychological nature—can and at times do lead to unfavorable reactions, there is no question that every professional man, while fully aware of possible unfavorable reactions, at times has to take a calculated risk while serving his patient to the best of his ability.

While hypnosis can be dangerous if not used properly or in the schizophrenic or prepsychotic, it ought to be stressed that many other dental services can be equally or more dangerous if used under the same circumstances. As a matter of fact, an objective consideration of the dangers in hypnosis must come to the following conclusions:

1. The successful induction of hypnosis in mentally aberrated individuals is very difficult.

2. The average dental situation does not and should not lead to any probing and experimental conditions. The induction and depth to be reached should be clearly and definitely limited to whatever stage is required by the problem at hand. As a rule, no more than a light to medium stage is required for most conditions of concern to the dentist.

3. The generally well-trained dentist who uses hypnosis and who is properly trained in its use, will be able to recognize existing mental aberrations in his patient speedier and more clearly in the very beginning of and often before the induction procedure. This is due to various factors: The closer interpersonal relationship existing in hypnosis; the time spent in taking a proper patient history before induction; the information gained by the various tests; other conditions prevailing in the hypnotic situation, which allow for more insight into our patient's functioning and reaction than the ordinary non-hypnotic dental situation would. This early appearance of signs and symptoms allows for preventive steps to be taken then and there, such as the interruption of any induction procedure and referral for consultation, and if necessary for treatment, to a competent psychotherapist.

Upon careful consideration of the facts, it occurs that hypnosis used by the dentist is only dangerous if not used properly and even then possibly far less than other dental functions under similar conditions would be.

Avoidance of Dangers

The dangers which are inherent in the use of hypnosis can by and large be avoided if the dentist observes the following points:

1. Take proper case history before induction procedure;

2. Limit treatment under hypnosis to strictly dental problems;

3. Use hypnosis as an adjunct to, not replacement of other accepted dental procedures;

4. Use hypnosis, if necessary, to overcome the patient's refusal to accept dentistry for no other than psychological reasons;

5. Recognize that the light stages suffice as a rule to overcome the patient's resistance to dental treatment;

6. Use hypnoanesthesia alone only if other forms of anesthesia are contraindicated;

7. Exclude any form of hypno-psychotherapy;

8. Avoid suggestions of amnesia (if for no other reasons than it counteracts our goal to reeducate our patients to accept dentistry without prejudice, and hypnosis in the future);

9. Recognize that the patient, once amenable to treatment through the use of hypnosis as a rule, does not require repeated reinduction;

10. Avoid creation of dependency on hypnosis and counteract it if present;

11. Avoid the authoritarian approach, except in young children or other special situations;

12. Preferably use induction methods, whereby the patient is given to understand that the ability to enter the hypnotic state lies within him, and not the operator. The implication is that the operator merely guides the patient to the degree of relaxation required to overcome the problem at hand and which the patient is able and willing to reach;

13. Leave the implication that the patient may terminate the state of hypnosis any time he so desires;

14. Exclude any non-professional use or misuse of hypnosis in your patient by post-hypnotic suggestions, limiting the reinduction to professional men for treatment purposes only;

15. Consult with and refer the patient to a competent psychotherapist whenever there is any doubt.

PROCEDURE IN DENTAL OFFICE

Any induction procedure in the dental office should be preceded by a careful analysis of the indications for as well as the contraindications to the use of hypnosis in the specific case at hand. Such evaluation is only possible if a proper and thorough case history is taken first.

History Taking

It is imperative that the dentist who intends to use hypnosis spend some time with his patient first to gather all possible information which will be of interest and value to him in deciding:

1. If hypnosis should be used at all;
2. Which approach and method should be used;
3. If prior consultation with or referral to a competent psychotherapist is indicated. This first interview with our patient therefore basically is similar to the medical history taken before administration of a general anesthetic for oral surgery or other manipulations which go beyond the scope of what is generally considered routine dental service. However, in addition to the general information gathered here, we ought to elicit specific information from our patient, such as:

a) His previous experience with dentistry;
b) His previous experience with hypnosis;
c) His feelings about the use of hypnosis;
d) His reasons for the use of hypnosis in the present situation;
e) Any past or present psychotherapy for himself or his immediate family;
f) The existence of functional diseases including allergies, asthma, skin diseases and others.

This first interview session then serves at the same time to bring to the fore and correct where necessary any misconceptions with regard to hypnosis and its use for our patient. It gives the dentist an opportunity to correct in an indirect and casual way some of the most commonly encountered misconceptions.

In this first session the dentist may find it proper to stress or imply:

1. That hypnosis is a natural phenomenon;
2. That it is not sleep in the accepted sense;
3. That the patient will not be unconscious;
4. That no secrets will be elicited or revealed;
5. That no humiliating acts will be performed;
6. That the ability to enter the state of hypnosis is no indication of weakness or feeble-mindedness;

7. That there is no relationship to spiritualism, mysticism and other popular misconceptions;

8. That there is no danger if used properly;

9. That nothing will be done against the patient's will;

10. That the patient will be allowed to awaken easily and spontaneously, if he should so desire;

11. That he will be so comfortable and relaxed, he will prefer to stay in this relaxed state until the dental work is finished or the need for his being relaxed no longer exists;

12. That intelligence is a positive factor;

13. That the success depends on the patient, and the dentist merely serves as a guide;

14. That the patient's willingness and cooperation are essential.

All this incorporated into an informal interview session to the extent to which it seems proper and advisable, depending on the specific situation, will serve to insure our patient's cooperation, to lessen his resistance, to get acquainted with his psychological makeup and to establish rapport between dentist and patient.

Tests

If the result of this first interview with our patient is such as to convince us that hypnosis is indicated and no further consultation or referral is necessary, then only do we proceed to the next step, namely to test our patient for his degree of suggestibility and cooperation. The value of these tests is rightfully questioned by some dentists who prefer to omit them. It is true that these tests have no direct bearing on the success of inducing the hypnotic state in our patient. It is equally true that hypnosis may be induced in a patient, whose reaction to these tests has been a negative one. However, in practice these tests prove to be simple, consume little time, and are effective in showing the patient how suggestion actually works. It is not uncommon that the effect of a test on our patient is so profound as to lead right into hypnosis. The dentist, on the other hand gains some more insight into his patient's degree of suggestibility, his general attitude and reaction, and thus is able to adapt his future procedure accordingly.

Whereas this is not the place to describe these tests in detail, the most commonly used tests in the dental office may be listed here:

1. The postural sway test: a) forward, b) backward.
2. The hand clasp test.
3. The eyeball set test.
4. The picture test.
5. The circle test and others.

Methods of Induction

The next step is the induction proper. The various techniques of induction have been described elsewhere (13, 14). Here we intend to mention only the techniques most commonly used in the dental office:

1. The eye-fixation method.
2. The progressive relaxation method.
3. The picture visualization or imagery technique.
4. The hand clasp technique.
5. The arm levitation technique.
6. The eyeball set technique (rapid and authoritarian).
7. The direct stare technique.
8. The use of music.
9. The use of nitrous oxide or other drugs.
10. The placebo technique (suggestion only).
11. The use of magic (in children).
12. A combination of several of the above.

The method used should be adapted to each individual case and the experienced operator will at times change from one method to another and often use a combination of several techniques. It should preferably be non-authoritarian, permissive in nature, and should be adapted to and incorporated into our routine dental procedures as much as possible.

As dentists, we are most interested in having our patient sufficiently relaxed in the chair to enable us to do the necessary work without interference. At the same time, we like to see our patient in a cooperative frame of mind and free of unfavorable physical and mental reactions. All this can usually be achieved without going into the deeper stages of hypnosis. Therefore, we do not go any further with our induction than is necessary to accomplish our main goal which should always remain good dentistry and not deep hypnosis.

The properly managed patient generally enjoys the calming, relaxing effect of hypnosis and looks forward to its future application. However, we find that once the existing obstacle to the administration of our dental services has been removed by the use of hypnosis, it becomes unnecessary to employ hypnosis in the future. All our patients are prepared for this during the initial interview, while in the hypnotic state, through posthypnotic suggestions and by casual suggestions given during the waking stage.

The more familiar the dentist is with the techniques and principles underlying the use of hypnosis, the less he actually needs to employ rigid hypnotic procedures. He will often be able to achieve almost equal results with the constant and purposeful use of controlled suggestion which may then assume the character of what is commonly referred to as "waking hypnosis."

Deepening to Proper Level

Once hypnosis has been induced, various procedures to deepen the stage of hypnosis can be employed. As mentioned before, we, as a rule, do not try to reach deeper stages than are required by the problem at hand. The specific steps which lead to the deepening of hypnosis as well as the tests and challenges to establish the various stages reached, have been described elsewhere. As soon as our patient has reached the desired level of hypnosis, we begin with our dental work.

An alternate procedure consists of the posthypnotic suggestion that our patient accept the dental treatment while awake, without difficulty and prejudice. Local anesthesia may be administered while the patient is still in hypnosis.

The dental treatment is then administered on a fully awake patient who, once he has accepted the posthypnotic suggestion, does not resist the treatment any longer.

As previously stated, we consider it of importance to tie in all of our procedures with the dental situation. This means that we preferably use suggstions to induce, deepen and maintain the state of hypnosis, as well as posthypnotic suggestions and awakening procedures which apply to the position and surroundings of our patient. Specifically, this implies that we may suggest to our patient that he start to relax as he leans back in the dental chair; that he relax more as the towel is placed around him; that the sound of the saliva ejector helps him to go deeper; or, that the hum of the airconditioner helps him to relax further; that the sound of our voice will help him to relax still more, etc. We may suggest to our patient to visualize a trip by automobile or plane (provided our initial interview has not suggested otherwise), in order to tie in the commonly objected to noise and vibration of the dental drill with the noise and vibration of a car or plane. We avoid tests for depth and challenges which are extraneous to the dental situation by replacing for example the arm rigidity test by a jaw rigidity test. We merely suggest then that the patient's jaw will be wide open and remain in this wide open position until our work is done. If we wish to challenge our patient, we may do this here by suggesting that he cannot close his jaw even if he tries, and the harder he tries, the more difficult it will be for him to close it, etc.

Posthypnotic Suggestion

Before awakening our patient, we find it useful to employ some definite posthypnotic suggestions. Here again, we much prefer to use posthypnotic suggestions which are in line with the dental situation. Such posthypnotic suggestions may imply that our patient will reach the desired level of hypnosis very quickly the next time, as soon as he leans back in the dental chair, or the towel is placed around him, or the saliva ejector turned on, etc. Any posthypnotic suggestion will stress that our patient, after awakening, will feel normal in every aspect; it will remove any and all previous challenges if given; it will remove future fear and apprehension of dentistry; it will set a definite time limit to hypno-anesthesia if given, and it will prevent future use of hypnosis for other than treatment purposes by professional men.

Awakening Procedure

The awakening of our patient again can make good use of the dental situation. Our patient is told to awaken as soon as the saliva ejector is turned off, the light is switched off, etc. The implication always is, and it may be verbalized accordingly, that as soon as our dental work is finished there will be no need for the hypnotic state any longer, our patient will then be wide awake, alert and cheerful to know that the work has been completed.

Presence of Nurse

It is good practice for the dentist to have his nurse present when using hypnosis for the same reason as he would during the administration of a general anesthetic. The presence of the nurse during the induction procedure may work either way however. It may put the patient at ease, and thus facilitate the induction proper, or it may do the opposite by actually interfering with the self-conscious patient's ability to enter the hypnotic state in presence of an "outsider." In order to overcome this difficulty, the author has found it advisable to have the nurse in the adjoining room with the doors wide open, within hearing range but out of sight.

Operative Procedure

If we summarize the dental office procedure on a patient in hypnosis, we may make the following points:

1. Limit your dental work during the first session.

2. Use drug anesthesia where necessary, if in doubt, or to reinforce your hypno-anesthesia.

3. Set definite time limit for the termination of any hypno-anesthesia suggested.

4. Use the same technique as you would without hypnosis (water spray, etc.).

5. Announce any physical contact beforehand (insertion of the saliva ejector, other instruments, your hand, etc.).

6. Specifically exclude outside disturbances in your verbalization (such as street noises, the ringing of the doorbell, the typewriter, etc.).

7. Maintain an even depth of hypnosis throughout your procedure.

8. Use the monotony of sound of the saliva ejector or the hum of the air-conditioner to deepen or maintain the depth of hypnosis as required.

9. Be prepared to change your approach when necessary to overcome any resistance encountered.

10. Give your patient a reasonable metaphor (by attaching the sound and vibration of the dental burr to the sound and vibration of a car or plane or other mechanism).

11. After awakening, reinforce any suggestions given during the hypnotic state by positive remarks (such as: now that the work is done, you realize how easy it was for you, and how little you have to be concerned from now on).

12. Do not overhypnotize your patient.

The Child Patient

In order to deal properly with the child as a patient, we have to establish first how the child differs from the adult patient as far as his problems and their handling by the use of hypnosis and suggestion is concerned. We have to establish if the child patient presents special problems different from those of the adult and if there are special techniques and procedures to deal with them. If we consider these questions from a general point of view, we must come to the conclusion that the child patient for whom hypnosis is indicated, presents the same problem as the child patient in dentistry in general, that is the problem of adaptation of accepted and established and familiar procedures as used with adults to the child. In other words, basically we would use on our child patient the same procedures and techniques which we use on our adult patients with some minor modifications, just as we use the same basic techniques in filling cavities, extractions or in other dental manipulations regardless of whether the patient is an adult or child, with some minor modifications of technique and approach. As in dentistry in general, when dealing with a child patient, here in our particular area of reference the emphasis is on approach rather than technique.

Most of the techniques used on adults will be useful with some modifications for our child patient. The approach, however, will be quite different. It is obvious that one cannot approach the child patient on an equally rational, logical and intellectual basis as one might approach the sophisticated adult, if and when the subject of hypnosis is introduced to him. It is equally obvious that one cannot use the same permissive techniques which one might prefer to use on most adult patients. Therefore, there will have to be modifications of our interview and introductory procedure. There will also have to be modifications of our technique. The question arises, what then will determine the range and extent and nature of these modifications?

To begin with, we have to assume that there is a definite indication for the use of hypnosis in our child patient. Next, of utmost importance from a dento-legal point of view, as with all other procedures involving a minor, the parents' permission to use hypnosis ought to be obtained. Specifically, in dealing with the child patient, the following observations are of importance:

1. The child's age.

2. The limitations of communication between operator and child.

3. The level of intelligence and understanding.

4. The child's interests.

These factors should be established first and, while they somehow interrelate with each other, very often they vary from child to child. Yet, they will largely determine the specific approach to the child and also the technique most likely to succeed. The answer will have to be obtained in the interview session between dentist and parent and dentist and child. Generally speaking, we can say that the child is more suggestible than the adult. The specific technique used will have to be determined by the answer given to points one to four. We will select a technique which is basically:

a) Authoritarian, b) Permissive, c) A combination of a and b.

Our technique will be more authoritarian the younger the child, the more limited the communication between operator and child, the lower the level of intelligence, and also the more the child has been exposed and responds to authority in his home environment, as determined during the interview. Our technique will be more permissive the older the child, the more intelligent, the better he understands and reasons, the greater his interests. Our technique will therefore be built around:

1) A demonstration of magic.

2) The playing of games (including the playing of a sleeping game).

3) The arousal of the child's fantasies and stimulation of his imagination through the operator's suggestion.

4) The picture visualization technique.

5) All other techniques as used on adults.

We may utilize the child's own fantasies all the way: "Have a wonderful dream from beginning to end."

We may suggest the area of imagery and then leave the child to his own resources;

We may have the child relive a previous experience, as seen in the movies, on the stage, on TV, or as read in a book or as remembered from a story;

We may resort to the use of such devices as a revolving disk, a metronome, a colored marker on the engine belt, or to other methods of fixation of attention;

We may use the eye fixation method in its classical form or in its variation as a spot marked on the child's thumb as suggested by Aston, whereby the fact that the thumb goes down is used to reinforce the suggestion;

We may use the back count method;

We may use the progressive relaxation method (in older children only);

We may use a form of waking hypnosis, whereby the operator suggests a picture such as a trip by jet plane, which ties in the noise of our high-speed drill, and gets the child to participate by filling in parts of the picture not only, but also by assigning an active role to the child within the suggested picture. For example:

Operator: "Would you like to take a trip by jet together with me?" From then on say "you and I" (psychologically tying operator and patient together).

For the sake of simplification, we assume that the answer is always in the affirmative.

"Where shall we go?" patient suggests destination.

"I am the pilot" (meaning I am and intend to continue to be in control). "You are the co-pilot." (You have some responsibilities and obligations too. Children like to be active and in charge of things, not mere passive passengers.)

"Here we take off;" "Look out the window;" "See clearly;" "Hear the sound of the jet" (fixation of attention and utilization of various senses).

"We are in the air now." "Look at the people down there! Do you recognize some of your friends?" "See the houses." "Do you see your house?" "As we go up higher, the people and homes get smaller and smaller, the people look like ants now, the homes like toys and the cars like toy cars."

"There is a lake—boats—sailboats—motor boats—water skiers," etc.

"Now we approach mountains with snow." "See if you can see some people climbing and if you can recognize what kind of animals there are?" (Bring patient into the picture.)

"Now we go down to land, the people and houses are getting bigger; you can recognize them clearly; you can see your family and your dog at the airport waiting for you, and there we are, the plane is coming in for a landing and our work is done for today; I am sure you enjoyed the trip as much as I did, and the next time we may fly somewhere else together."

Habits

After having dealt with the child patient in general, there remains one aspect of concern and special significance which merits our consideration, namely, how should the dentist handle the many habits and symptoms which directly or indirectly interfere with the health, function or esthetics of the dental apparatus? Sorrin (15) lists 39 individual habits which are of interest to the dentist. Whereas many of these habits manifest themselves early in childhood, some persist over the years; others change their pattern and some occur later on in adult life. Among the most important habits of interest to the dentist are:

1. Sucking of thumb, finger, cheek, tongue, pacifier;
2. Biting of finger, nails, lips, tongue;
3. Chewing of pen, pencil, eyeglasshandle, etc.;
4. Bruxism;

5. Smoking (stain deposits, tar irritation, delayed wound healing, ulcers, leukoplakia, cancer of mouth, tongue, lips);

6. Tongue thrust;

7. Mouthbreathing and others.

If we consider just one of the above-listed habits, namely the sucking of the thumb, we note that there exists a definite shift of responsibility in dealing with this problem. As a rule, we find the following: The parent consults first with the pediatrician; the pediatrician advises non-interference and thus leaves the problem to the general practitioner of dentistry, who eventually sees the patient and the result of years of interference with the normal development of teeth, mouth and face. The general practitioner of dentistry then refers the case to the orthodontist. The orthodontist, more aware than any of the others of the practical importance of such habits in terms of malocclusion, lack of function and esthetic handicap, usually is the first one to interfere. He may attack the problem with one of the many ingeniously devised props, which are very effective in practice, because they administer some sort of punishment to the child each time he engages in the pursuit of his habit. Thus definite conditioned reflex patterns are established which avoid the punishment and the habit.

If we analyze the reasons for this status quo, we find that there is a widely held opinion among pediatricians and some dentists that a) the habit is harmless, and b) that the child will eventually outgrow the habit. This opinion is shared by many of the more psychologically oriented physicians and dentists who, in turn, consider the direct approach to the habit without consideration of the total personality and the psychodynamics of the individual case undesirable. Not only would these men consider the orthodontist's "miniature torture chamber" undesirable from their point of view, but it is their contention that any habit of long duration is a sign of underlying personality disorder; that unless the personality disorder is properly treated, the elimination of one habit will lead to the release of other, undesirable substitute outlets. If we share the opinion of these men, our thumbsucking girl should be referred for psychotherapy first, with all its implications.

In consideration of the above state of affairs, the following questions have to be answered:

1. Is it necessarily true that the removal of one habit *must* lead to other undesirable outlets?

2. Is it possible that a habit, once meaningful to the patient, may have lost the deeper meaning originally attached to it and continues to persist as a reflex pattern? If this is possible, the elimination of the habit could be achieved by establishing new reflexes which do not interfere with a) psychodynamically meaningful material, and b) the function or esthetics of the dental apparatus.

In our case, whereas the thumb may have meant to the infant a natural replacement for the deprived breast, it may now, in the ten-year-old, constitute a reflex pattern with no other meaning but pleasure and satisfaction associated with the act itself.

3. Assuming the validity of the objections to the direct approach of symptom removal as outlined above, can these objections not be overcome by selective substitutions of unquestionably undesirable habits with psychodynamically meaningful, yet more desirable substitutes? For example, the hugging of a favorite doll or a soft blanket by our thumbsucking girl would stand for love, warmth and cozyness; the clenching of the fist in bruxism would release tension, anger, aggression, etc.

4. Is it not true that a habit, if deeply rooted and meaningful to our patient, most likely will not be readily surrendered, if we are permissive and considerate of all other prerequisites as outlined in this chapter. The direct approach will be valueless in such case as a therapeutic tool, but may still be valuable as a diagnostic help. As a matter of fact, it ought to be mentioned that some therapists have pointed out that the removal of a symptom is often followed by the disappearance of other co-existing symptoms or personality disorders (16, 17, 18).

In full consideration of the above, what then is briefly and in general terms a practical approach to the subject of habits and symptom removal in the dental office?

1. The nature of the habit has to be determined. Questions to be answered are: How much does the habit interfere with the normal development, function and esthetics of the dental appara-

tus? How long does this habit exist? How deeply embedded it it? What is its psychodynamic significance? What is the extent of the patient's desire or lack of desire to get rid of the habit? What is the parents' attitude toward the habit and the child? Among others, a leading question that might be asked of our patient is: "What would happen, what would be different, if you would not engage in this habit?"

2. The child's and parents' general state of psychological equilibrium ought to be evaluated in separate interviews between dentist and parent, and dentist and child. Such evaluation will enable us to establish our general attitude toward the case before us to the same degree as thorough history-taking does, if taken prior to major surgical intervention. If our interview reveals that we are dealing with a severely disturbed child or parent; if there is a history of prior or present psychotherapy of child or parent or other member of the family; if the habit appears to be deeply embedded or very meaningful, we should insist on referral to a psychotherapist for at least consultation and possible treatment. If, on the other hand, we are satisfied that our thumbsucking girl has been the victim of a matrogenic or pediatrogenic disease, as is often the case; if the original meaning of the habit is lost and it continues to exist in the form of a reflex action, then we ought to explain to the parent, and if the case warrants it to the child, the disadvantages of a passive attitude from an economical, mechanical, esthetic and psychological point of view. That is, if our girl patient does not "outgrow" the habit in time, the correction of the deformity will take longer, be more difficult, perhaps less satisfactory and less permanent, cost more money and leave a definite psychological impact, the closer we approach the dating and mating time.

We will always call attention to a possible deeper meaning than is apparent and for the possible need for consultation or psychotherapy, if there is no response to our approach. The parent is asked to be a completely passive partner, to show no concern and not to interfere in any way with our procedure. The parent is directed to be outside the treatment room at all times; whenever possible, the child ought to come alone. Any questions that the parent might have are to be discussed over the telephone or whenever the child is not present. We inquire as to the child's preferred dolls, toy animals and their names, etc. Thereafter we see the child alone. After we have established some rapport, we pretend to examine the entire mouth without paying any attention to the deformity. As we "detect" an abnormality of the bite, we may ask: "Do you know that your teeth do not come together in front?" We may remark that it must be hard to chew and thus we may provoke a sympathetic response by our patient, since we understand why she is slow in eating, does not chew well and does not like certain foods. Next we may ask: "How come that your teeth are so far apart in front?" Since the thumb seems to fit the opening, there is generally complete agreement as to the cause of the trouble, especially if viewed through the handmirror and if there are tell-tale marks on the back of the thumb. Now we may imply that we too, when we were children, and probably mother and father and older siblings and many others used to suck their thumbs, that there is nothing wrong with this, and that everyone outgrows the desire to suck the thumb. We strongly imply that as people grow older, they learn to sleep better without their thumbsucking and as a result, their teeth grow better and more even; they can eat better, grow taller and stronger and stay healthier. We then dismiss our patient without leaving any doubt that she too will grow older and soon find out that she does not need the thumb any more and that she too will learn to sleep better, eat better and grow taller and look better and healthier. We suggest that our patient take her favorite doll, or, as the case may be, toy animal or soft blanket, to bed, hug her doll, keep her warm and cozy and watch whether possibly her doll sleeps with her thumb in her mouth. We ask our patient to return in a week and to bring her doll along. The outcome by then is one of three:

1. Our patient has stopped sucking altogether; 2. She sucks less often; 3. There is no improvement.

In any case we will reinforce our suggestion in subsequent visits at intervals of one week. The parent is asked to report on unusual developments.

If deemed advisable, either one of two procedures may be employed in addition to the above:

1. Hypnosis in the office. In using hypnosis, we limit ourselves to an entirely permissive approach, employing suggestions of growing up, no need or desire for the thumb, hugging of doll instead, etc. At no time do we set a *definite* time limit for the habit to be stopped or use any other authoritarian approach.

2. In recognition of the mother's natural position as a good hypnotist and if she appears suitable for the role, we may enlist her cooperation in the following fashion: In accordance with definite instructions given by us, but written out by the mother in her own words and then corrected by us, the mother is to read slowly in a soft and modulated voice, at a time when her child is just about ready to fall asleep, about as follows: "Mary is getting bigger and older every day; she is growing up; her babydoll wants to be hugged and kept warm; Mary will be a good Mommy. Mary is growing up, soon she will be old enough, then she will not need her thumb in her mouth anymore; she will then sleep better without the thumb, just as Mommy, Daddy, older brother and sister sleep now without their thumbs. The doll may put her thumb into her mouth if she wants to, because she is a baby. Mary is her Mommy, she is getting older every day. As soon as she stops putting her thumb into her mouth, her teeth will grow straighter, she will chew better, grow taller and look prettier," etc.

To summarize the cardinal points observed in the above-outlined procedure:

1. Avoidance of arousal of guilt-feelings.

2. Implication that the habit is natural and common.

3. Casual approach.

4. Permissive approach.

5. No setting of time limit, the patient is allowed to find his own timing.

6. Appeal to normal desire of growing up.

7. Appeal to esthetic and functional advantages.

8. Suggestion of harmless channels as substitute outlets.

9. Suggestion of psychodynamically meaningful channels as substitute outlets.

10. Avoidance of focus on taking a symptom away, rather than direction of the patient's needs and responses into desirable channels by positive and meaningful suggestions.

To elaborate on our last point, in the case of bruxism for example, instead of using the direct suggestion that the patient will not grind his teeth anymore, we would emphasize that he will learn to relax more and more, eventually be under less tension and then find no more need or desire to grind his teeth. If necessary, we give this patient a temporary, harmless outlet for his tension which is meaningful, such as clenching his fist.

In conclusion, we may say that if our patient is faced with certain physical, psychological and economic disadvantages in the future, it appears to be good practice to take the calculated risk of possible, but by no means certain, substitute outlets for the habit in question. If we are selective and use proper judgment and procedure, the danger of undesirable substitute outlets can be avoided by suggesting psychodynamically meaningful substitute outlets to begin with. If we are confronted with deeply rooted personality disorders, the habit will not disappear by the use of this procedure, yet it will have served as a diagnostic device and full-fledged psychotherapeutic procedures should be instituted by a competent psychotherapist.

REVIEW OF LITERATURE

No attempt is made here to give a complete and exhaustive review of the literature dealing with the subject of hypnosis in dentistry. We have attempted to show that fundamentally hypnosis in dentistry cannot be separated from hypnosis in other fields. On the other hand, it must be noted that specific contributions of merit written by and for dentists are very few. Therefore we will limit ourselves here to a brief review of some of those contributions which are worthy of consideration within the above-mentioned frame of reference.

To the reader who is interested in acquiring a broader background, the material contained in the chapter "Hypnosis in Dentistry" by Jules H. Weinstein in the first edition of *Hypnosis in Modern Medicine* (19) will be of value. Since this chapter differs in its entirety from the present one, the reader is referred to the original source.

Aaron A. Moss who introduced the term "hypnodontics" for

hypnosis in dentistry, lists in his book *Hypnodontics* (20) a number of case histories which illustrate the type of problem with which patient and dentist are faced in practice and describes his approach in detail. Of special interest to the practicing dentist is the author's description of how to deal with the gagging reflex by what the author calls "waking hypnotic suggestion" (21).

Stolzenberg, in his book *Psychosomatics and Suggestion Therapy in Dentistry* (22, 23) attempts to show the broader psychological and emotional aspects which enter into the dentist-patient relationship. Many of his case reports, contained in the book and elsewhere (24), go beyond what is generally considered the dentist's area of competence. One has to consider, however, that the book was written at a time when there were not too many professional men available who were competent to use hypnosis in their respective disciplines. Consequently, the dentist who was known to use hypnosis was often asked by his patients as well as by his colleagues in the dental and medical specialties to administer hypnosis for problems not strictly confined to his field. Very often such requests or referrals for treatment were preceded by the remark that everything else had been tried without result. The dentist faced with such a request for treatment, especially if coming from a physician or other dentist, was faced with some soulsearching and many times might have been inclined to submit to the dictates of his heart rather than to the objective consideration of his professional limitations. This era of conflict is reflected in some of the early writings on hypnosis in dentistry and has led to misunderstandings and misgivings on the part of those who interpreted what they read in the light of their own negative attitude toward the subject proper, and thus felt even more justification in their outright condemnation of the use of hypnosis in dentistry. This era of "conflict of interest" has passed by now. There are today competent professional men available in every branch of medicine who are able to administer hypnosis if and where indicated in their respective fields. This relieves the dentist trained to use hypnosis of the burden to choose between his professional competency and other considerations.

Reflecting this "new era," we quote Stolzenberg as follows: "Hypnosis may also be used to assist in conquering oral habits in patients where no basic emotional problem exists" . . . and: "Whenever possible, conscious suggestions are employed, but in stubborn or difficult situations hypnosis is utilized"; and: "It is significant that one who has been indoctrinated in the value of hypnosis in practice, finds a diminished need for its use" (25). The author implies here of course the existence of a dentist-patient relationship based on all factors which are considered of value in the hypnotic relationship, thereby eliminating the need for a formal induction of hypnosis.

Shaw, in his book, *Clinical Application of Hypnosis in Dentistry,* describes in detail the various techniques applicable to dentistry (26). His case reports are of interest to the reader who likes to become more familiar with the type of patient for whom the dentist uses hypnosis. Shaw makes the following statements: "Suggestions helpful to the timid dental patient can be successfully applied in the waking state, so that it becomes necessary to use hypnosis only with the extremely apprehensive and difficult patient (p. 112), and: "The conscientious dentist making use of hypnosis in his practice will only apply words and suggestions that relate to his patient's dental needs. When dental problems involve psychological factors (thumbsucking, bruxism, etc.) it is advisable to consult with the patient's physician for the purpose of referring the patient to a registered psychologist or psychiatrist" (p. 93).

With reference to the child patient, Shaw has this to say: "In many cases, the formerly apprehensive child patient actually asks to discontinue the "sleep game" or the "pretend game" because he is ready to accept dentistry and wants to see what is going on while he is in the dental chair. When this happens we know that the management of this particular child in hypnodontia has been decidedly successful" (27).

Here again, we notice the most significant trend of limiting hypnosis in dentistry not only to dental needs, but also to definite indications. This is the more significant in view of the fact that earlier writings by the same author decidedly go beyond the field of dentistry, reflecting the era of "conflict of interest" referred to above (28).

In discussing the dangers of hypnosis, Shaw compares hypnosis to the hypodermic syringe (12): "Just as the hypodermic syringe is a tremendously important instrument as a medium through which injected material enters into the physical part of the individual, so is hypnosis a most important vehicle for the injection of suggestions into the mental processes of the patient." He goes on to say that the qualified dentist makes use of a positive, permissive approach in *all* his patients and thereby avoids risks; that the hypnodontist avoids the use of deep phenomena and by doing so, the possibility of danger in the dental use of hypnosis is reduced to a minimum; that the properly trained hypnotist is psychologically oriented in his approach to the patient and has learned to recognize different responses which may be signs of disturbance or rejection by the patient.

Shaw then makes the following statement: "Reports of mental disturbances precipitated by the use of hypnosis at the hands of qualified hypnodontists are so rare that we can say, in spite of any claim to the contrary, that the properly trained hypnodontist who confines the psychodynamic approach of hypnosis to the dental patient, only within the realm of his own field of competence, never constitutes a threat to the welfare of his patient. In fact there is sufficient clinical evidence to prove that many thousands of dental operations have been performed successfully under hypnosis without any untoward effect on patients who previously were unable to accept dental work because of extreme anxiety and apprehension related to the mouth in connection with dentistry." And, "The danger that does exist in the application of hypnosis to dentistry lies in the hypnodontist with insufficient training to realize that there are certain risks to be considered, and the numerous courses of instruction given all over the globe by laymen and others offering a limited curriculum are daily adding to this danger."

Ament offers an interesting contribution by his introduction of the "as if" attitude (29). A thorough history-taking gives the dentist all information of value with respect to his patient's reactions, positive as well as negative, to a previous administration of chemical anesthesia. This allow the dentist to utilize the patient's own feelings by incorporating them into his verbal suggestions. At the same time, he can formulate his suggestions in such a manner as to exclude any previously experienced negative reactions.

Ament discusses in another paper (30) the significance of patients not seeing anything but color in spite of suggestions given to visualize scenery. Ament feels that these patients are actually in a deeper trance if they see only colors instead of the suggested scenery, and in a deeper state of trance yet if they see grey or black rather than colors. In still another publication (31) Ament describes his use of time distortion to make dental appointments of several hours duration more acceptable to his patients. He also uses time distortion for the purpose of getting his patient quickly used to a new prosthetic or orthodontic appliance by suggestions that the appliance has been worn for a long period of time and that the patient feels as if it were his own.

Kuhner (32) expresses a trend when he states: "The dentist should not enter the territory allotted to the psychologist and psychiatrist. He should not attempt to rid the patient of his bad habits or to solve his emotional problems under the influence of hypnosis," and ". . . the dentist should be cautioned against overstepping the bonds of dentistry. Any psychological help must relate directly to the immediate dental problem and not extend into the field of psychotherapy." Specifically he warns the dentist against the use of regression. He lists four case histories which are illustrative as to the problems encountered in dentistry and their handling by the selective dentist. He states: "The usual methods are tried first without hypnosis. Should they fail, hypnosis is added."

On the other hand, Singer refers to "dental psychotherapy" when he states: "The dentist who employs dental psychotherapy is attempting to solve a particular psychogenic problem which affects the mouth, such as gagging. If, in dealing with this particular problem, he should improve the patient's total personality, that is an incidental benefit, but not an intended one." Furthermore Singer says: "For selected patients, hypnosis may be the technique of choice for the removal of any psychogenic disorder which interferes with the proper carrying out and successful conclusion of dental treatment" (33).

In another publication entitled "Dental Psychotherapy," Singer states: "Already, far more psychotherapy than one might realize is in fact being practiced in dental offices by dentists who have made no special study of the subject, although they may be quite unaware that they are using it and it may be of a very haphazard type. Without psychological effectiveness, no dentist could maintain a practice. Thus psychotherapy of a sort is being practiced more or less by accident in every dental office now" (34). He describes his approach as based on Adlerian psychology. A questionnaire is handed to every new patient. Much valuable information is thus obtained even before any personal contact with the patient is made.

Singer states: "Following Adler's technique, every dentist would be able to understand his patient and perceive that patient's goals. Such understanding should be part of every examination, but in particular, it is necessary for the dental psychotherapy which every dentist should be able to carry out.

"A bad personal relationship between patient and dentist or resistance by the patient to dental treatment implies that the goals of dentist and patient are different. The only thing a dentist needs to do in psychotherapy is to bring the patient's goals into line with his own. In other words, in order to help a patient and know what his goals are, you must first understand him. In most serious cases, it is necessary to help the patient to understand himself, and eventually to change his outlook, his attitude, his movement toward life and others. Minor psychotherapy, which every doctor should practise, might be defined as the use of psychotherapeutic techniques to achieve immediate goals without intensive exploration or personality reorientation. All necessary means can be taken to achieve these immediate goals. This definition applied to dentistry means the treatment of a dental patient for a psychogenic disorder by the dentist as incidental to the dental service required of him."

He states further: "Hypnosis is a tool or technique and not itself a method of treatment. It is applicable to any method or form of psychotherapy. It acts as a catalyst, greatly speeding the rapport, contact or transference necessary for the successful outcome of any psychotherapeutic procedure." And, "For most patients, hypnotherapy is neither necessary nor recommended." However, he speaks of about 300 patients treated for dental reasons under hypnosis by him and says: "We consider it one of the safest techniques in all medicine."

Kornfeld (35) states that "the patient makes a poor subject for hypnosis immediately after an unsuccessful attempt to perform a dental service." He advises to defer induction to the next visit and before dental services are performed. Kornfeld states further that "The decision to employ hypnosis should be discussed with the patient in order to obtain the necessary consent for its use." Six case reports illustrate the author's procedure under varying conditions as they present themselves in the dental office. Of special interest is the case report of a thirteen-year old diabetic whose history showed a significant rise in blood sugar each time the patient had visited her dentist. Control of her hyperglycemia was apparently achieved by the use of hypnosis not only, but at the same time the patient was rehabilitated to the extent of not needing hypnosis and not fearing dentistry any longer (35).

Jacoby estimates the number of dentists who have had some instruction in hypnosis to be more than six thousand. He reports statistically on 308 patients in 1,214 appointment sessions, and favors the use of a tape recorder to condition his patients (36).

Papermaster makes the following statement: "Thumbsucking, nailbiting and bruxism should not be treated with hypnosis. These conditions are approached through psychiatry (37). He reports on "the harmful after-effects of a tactless suggestion" where a dentist regressed his assistant to age five "and created a state of conscious anxiety." On the other hand, the author resorts to age regression in order to obtain correct centric occlusion and vertical dimension. His case report of a four-year old is of particular interest to dentists who are concerned with the possibility of reaching small children through the use of hypnosis. Out of the total number of 1,840 patients treated by Papermaster, the age group of three to six years numbered thirty-seven out of which twenty were considered total failures by the author.

Staples stresses the importance of proper preparation and indoctrination of the patient prior to induction and presents two case reports which elaborate on this theme (38). He states further with reference to some of the habits of interest in dentistry: "The question as to whether these problems come within the jurisdiction of the dentist or the psychiatrist is a controversial one"; and "Many of these individuals can be taught, while under hypnosis, to become more relaxed, to lessen tension, and to be given the motivation for the stopping of the habit and for the forming of a new pattern of behavior."

Staples (39) says further: "A permissive type of approach should be continued when the subject is in trance. He can be told that he can react to a suggestion immediately, or more slowly in a minute or two, just as he chooses; that he can go into just as deep a trance as he wishes and thinks he needs to." He refers to relaxation through hypnosis as a learning process. He speaks of the benefits to the dentist who through the elimination of fear and tension in his patient becomes "a calmer, more relaxed person." He continues as follows: "I have been told by many dentists who have taken courses in hypnosis that, although they have never actually inducted a single patient, they find that they are putting into practice many of the psychological concepts and attitudes implicit in hypnosis; that they have a better understanding of human behavior and are able to render a better dental service."

Secter (40) goes further than most dentists in his approach to symptom removal as evidenced by the description of his dealing with the exaggerated gag reflex by:

"1. Authoritative waking suggestion.
2. Symptom removal by hypnotherapeutic suggestion.
3. Treatment of cause by brief hypnoanalysis."

In his discussion of the "treatment of cause by brief hypnoanalysis" he states: "Age regressions should be avoided by those untrained in the handling of repressed materials or by those who would be unable to cope with manifestations of strong emotion. Stimulating recall or revivifying the past, while keeping the patient in contact with the therapist and the present, is within the scope of the abilities and education of most physicians and dentists." He goes on to describe his "uncovering technique" and mentions that "Investigation of the mechanisms associated with other symptoms may be pursued in the same manner." However, he cautions: "If the symptom is one on which the patient relies for his adjustments to reality, or one associated with knowledge he cannot face at a conscious level, he should not be coerced into cooperation."

Secter suggests to replace the term "mind set," as often encountered in the dental literature with "patient orientation" (41). In describing the "case of Mrs. F." he mentions that this patient was "regressed to her childhood" and describes the difficulties that arose as a consequence of the psychological implications of suggestions of arm levitation for this particular patient. The absence of the author's comments on this case is remarkable. Secter exacts the promise from his patient, while under hypnosis, that he will "enter hypnosis only for proper purposes and only with properly qualified persons." He feels this approach to be more effective in protecting his patient from unqualified hypnotists than "an authoritarian prohibition." He describes as follows the "prayer technique" as a help in inducing hypnosis in children from religious background: "Now clasp your hands together, Johnny, and close your eyes and pray that Doctor Jones will be guided by the Lord to make his hands gentle and to keep you from being hurt."

Le Cron feels that extreme gagging as encountered in the dental setting is "almost invariably" associated with some childhood experience. He suggests that the cause can be brought to light under hypnosis and handled by the dentist who is sufficiently trained. He cites case reports. It ought to be stated that Le Cron is not a dentist (42).

Solovey and Milechnin (43) (also not members of the dental profession) recommend preparation of the dental patient outside the dental office for hypnosis and speak of the desirability of "a center for the preparation of patients for hypnodontic analgesia" in order to save the dentist's time. The authors make a number of statements which take issue with much of what has been published in the dental literature and with much that has been taken for granted in the past. These statements are made with great emphasis and, because of their nature and comprehensiveness, they may be of interest to the reader. The authors state as follows: "There are still some residues from the period of decadence of hypnotism, when hypnosis was understood as the domination of a supernatural quality of one person over another, and it was thought that suggestion had a magical and invincible power and could bring about organic changes. Among such residues are certain completely superfluous suggestions, alien to the nature of the hypnotic state, that are still given in various clinical applications of hypnotism, including hypnodontia. Such are the suggestions to arrest the bleeding after dental extraction, to have amnesia for dental work, to have no post-operative discomfort, for healing rapidly, and even for entering the hypnotic state more rapidly in the following interview.

"When a direct suggestion of this nature seems to be carried out, this is due, as has been indicated by Gorton and others, not to the direct suggestion in itself, but to the psychophysiological characteristics of the emotional state in which the subject finds himself.

"The hypnotic state induced by relaxation procedure brings about per se, and with no suggestion whatever, a decrease in the adrenalin in the blood with a lower blood pressure and a decrease in the loss of blood from small vessels. We have already insisted on the relationship between the emotional condition of the subject and the amount of blood lost after dental extraction.

"Similarly, the reduction in the flow of saliva is not produced by direct suggestion, but by the emotional condition or by certain associations which the person may have in relation to salivation. If the flow of saliva is not reduced spontaneously in the hypnotic state, it becomes necessary to create a psychological situation which will lead to this effect.

"The case of hypnotic amnesia is to a certain point different, since this phenomenon corresponds to a personal trait that is revealed in a deep hypnotic state. The subject who has this peculiarity may forget temporarily, for minutes or hours, what happened to him under the hypnotic state, even though no suggestion was given in this respect. The apparent fulfillment of the suggestion is, in these cases, a mere coincidence.

"The absence of post-operative pain and a more rapid healing are not produced by suggestions either, but result from the emotional condition of the patient after the operation.

"When we find a certain post-operative analgesia and a greater speed in healing, these are not caused by the corresponding direct suggestion received under the hypnotic state, but by a favorable emotional condition following the hypnotic experience. Such a favorable emotional condition may be reactivated by personal contacts between the patient and the operator during the post-operative period, even over the telephone. Similar reactivation may be caused by other people who have, or can establish, constructive interpersonal relationships with the patient, giving him rationalizations and even appropriate suggestions.

"Suggesting to a patient that he will enter a deeper hypnotic state in the next interview is also groundless, because the deepening of the hypnotic state in the following session will not result from this suggestion, but will depend on the patient's readiness.

"When the hypnodontic session has been finished, it is not necessary to state formally: 'Now you will come out of the hypnotic (or relaxed) state!' Normally, it is enough to let the subject understand that the work is finished, giving him at the same time those rationalizations that will help him to maintain a favorable emotional condition during the post-operative period."

The dentist who uses hypnosis may wonder after reflecting on Solovey and Milechnin's emphatic assertions how valid in fact some of the things he has done routinely are. On the other hand, he may also wonder how valid the authors' statement is when "the decrease in the adrenalin in the blood" resulting from the relaxed state achieved by hypnosis is given as the reason for "a decrease in the loss of blood from small vessels." He may find that not only some of his beliefs as acquired by reading of the dental literature on hypnosis are severely shaken, but also some of his beliefs as acquired in his training in physiology, pharmacology and in clinical experience.

Barnett, in the *British Dental Journal,* states that "deliberate hypnotic suggestion is merely a scientific development of a good chairside manner" (44).

Ecker (45) stresses "the psychic needs of the doctor or dentist applying the hypnotic technique" and says "as the doctor enters this interpersonal relationship, he must have his own neuroses under control." He feels that "hypnosis is of particular value in surgery about the head and neck, especially when a general anesthetic would be hazardous or contraindicated. Patients requiring (as a result of accidents) extensive suturing of facial lacerations or intermaxillary wiring of fractures of the mandible and maxilla do not have airway problems under hypnosis." He also states that "plastic procedures about the face are made much easier by developing a relaxed patient" and goes on to say: "The physical changes obtained by such surgery are completely acceptable on suggestion."

He reports on two patients with abdomen-hand flaps who kept their hands in situ for four or five weeks with the suggestion that their hands were "stuck" to their abdomen and could not be moved (45).

Heron, a psychologist, in discussing the role of hypnosis in dentistry, makes the following statement (46): "In addition to the above categories there are some other kinds of dental situations which are amenable to control by means of hypnotic suggestion. Some of these would be thumbsucking in children, tonguethrusting and bruxism. The latter condition, however, may be considered to be on the borderline between a dental problem and a psychological one. In these borderline problems it is, of course, preferable to get at the etiology of the condition. In other words, bruxism is thought to be a symptom of some underlying difficulty. To simply terminate the symptom, as can be done in some cases through hypnotic suggestion, may only mean that the individual will develop some substitute symptom. However, in both dentistry and medicine sometimes the only thing that can be done because of various circumstances is to give symptomatic treatment."

Heron and Secter (47) state: "Most thumbsucking is held to be on a habit rather than a neurotic basis. Hypnosis is a practical aid for control or elimination of thumbsucking which is not neurotic in origin."

Levbarg, a physician, describes his method of combining inhalation anesthesia with hypnosis as follows: "Experience has taught me that in difficult cases, the use of a combination of Neurolene and hypnosis proves most satisfactory and, once the patient is conditioned, I find it no longer necessary to start hypnosis with a drug of any kind" (48).

Raginsky, a physician, speaking of hypnosis, states (49): "Its use in dentistry is restricted to only two minor purposes: to allay apprehension and anxiety, and occasionally to produce anesthesia. Broader use of hypnosis by the average dentist may lead to difficulties." He states further: "It appears that psychotherapy will have a place in dentistry of the future." In another publication, Raginsky concludes: "The future of psychotherapy in dentistry, skillfully applied, appears to be bright and fruitful" (50).

Again in a different place, one finds Raginsky making the

following statement: "A sick person is not only a body attacked by disease, but also a mind disturbed by worry. Yet, in most cases, the former receives all the care. Focusing one's attention on the physical lesion, the dentist may not always see the person behind it. Judging by the enormous increase in the number of articles dealing with dental psychosomatic problems, dentists are realizing that regardless of the pressure of work and the wear of routine, he must become more conscious of his patients' complexity and more attentive to the psychological processes that precede or accompany physical derangements." Further on Raginsky states: "No medication has yet been discovered that can replace the powerful force that lies in the patient-doctor relationship." And speaking of hypnosis, he says: "Sophisticated use of this modality is so subtle and gentle that the procedure should be barely perceptible."

He speaks of three general attitudes toward hypnosis by dentists:

1. "The attitude of relative skepticism."
2. "The attitude of intense interest."
3. "The attitude of balanced judgment." (51)

Raginsky, again, in a different publication has this to say: "Hypnosis can be a useful tool in the dentist's kit. With its use, however, goes a serious and unavoidable responsibility for understanding human behavior, the significance to the patient of hypnosis, and the significance of its use to the dentist himself" (52).

Rosen, a psychiatrist (53), who has repeatedly warned about the dangers of hypnosis, feels that a routine history taking of all dental patients for whom hypnosis is considered, is essential and that the patient should be asked whether or not he is under psychiatric treatment. Permission should be requested from the patient to contact his psychiatrist. Rosen is particularly outspoken against teaching the patient autohypnosis and against the use of hypnosis for symptom removal by the dentist. He also objects to such seemingly harmless suggestion to dental patients: "that they will feel happy" and states: "such suggestions frequently take effect; they nevertheless frequently can cause trouble." He cites various case reports to emphasize his point. On the other hand, Rosen states: "The dentist who rigidly limits his use of hypnosis to the area of his actual professional competence will not and cannot run into difficulties of this type."

Rosen is also outspoken against the use of recordings for the purpose of inducing hypnosis in patients and cites a case report to illustrate the dangers of this procedure. He recommends a screening procedure of applicants for instruction in hypnosis similar to the procedure in use for psychiatrists and psychologists in training.

With reference to autohypnosis, Rosen states: "Unfortunately, there is little in the whole field of psychodynamics with so great a potential for harm," and "It would therefore seem indicated never to recommend self-hypnosis, except for therapeutic reasons. This falls within the province of the psychotherapist, not the dentist."

Under "Precautions and Recommendations" Rosen has this to say: "No dentist would administer nitrous oxide without knowing, not only its potentialities and value, but its contraindications as well. No dentist would allow himself to be taught how to use nitrous oxide—or, for that matter, any other anesthetic—by a non-dentist, by a non-physician, by a non-professional. But a fairly large number of dentists make use of hypnosis as an analgesic or anesthetic, with some knowledge of its potentialities but with no knowledge of its dangers, and some of these have found themselves precipitated into rather serious trouble. Suicidal depressions have come to the fore, emergency psychiatric consultation has had to be arranged even from the dentist's office, and psychiatrists have occasionally had to take care of overt psychotic reactions which had been unleashed by inept or untrained handling, although not purposely so, of the hypnosis."

And further on Rosen states: "With a meaningful knowledge of these (dangers), with competent instruction under the aegis of your dental schools of your city and county dental societies, I see no reason why dentists should not utilize, to a progressively larger degree, hypno-anesthesia in their attempt to control the severe pain from which their patients suffer. If you do not try to suggest away symptoms that are neurotically or psychotically based, but instead restrict your use of hypnosis to the induction of analgesia or anesthesia, remembering not to hypnotize patients who show anxiety reactions during the induction process, remembering also to suggest to those patients whom you do hypnotize that after they leave your office, they will not be able to hypnotize themselves, I can see no contra-indication to its use on your part."

Meares, a psychiatrist, states the following (54): "The use of hypnosis in dentistry involves many techniques which only the dentist can really appreciate. But dentists run a grave risk if they isolate themselves from the psychodynamic insights of the psychiatrist and psychologist. And this applies to others who work with hypnosis. There can be no hypnosis just of the mouth for the dentist, or of the pelvis for the obstetrician, or hypnosis that is only skin deep for the dermatologist." It appears that this statement is of great importance and similar thoughts have been expressed by the author of this chapter here and elsewhere (1: p. 1150).

One would be amiss without mentioning one of the earliest and most comprehensive reviews of the use of hypnosis in dentistry by F. L. Marcuse, a psychologist. The interested reader is referred to the original (55) because of the unique combination of an objective appraisal of the literature as it existed up to then (1947) and an extensive list of references. Apart from the strictly dental references, the historically interested reader will find a description of the attitude toward hypnosis by the Roman Catholic Church and by Mary Baker Eddy, founder of the Christian Science Movement.

SUMMARY

The review of the literature on hypnosis in dentistry is significant insofar as it shows very distinctly a most common trend among the various authors in question. This trend very clearly reveals the increased interest and concern of these authors with the psychological aspects of the ordinary dentist-patient relationship, and the psychodynamics of the hypnotic relationship. It seems that the interest in hypnosis and the closer dentist-patient relationship as it exists during hypnosis have opened up broader vistas and interests on the part of the dentist. It is perhaps significant that many among those who have been using hypnosis for a great number of years, express or imply that they can at times achieve almost equal results by incorporating the essential ingredients of the hypnotic relationship into the ordinary dentist-patient relationship.

Thus it appears that what may have been originally merely an interest in a technique which promised results in cases that resisted treatment by any other means, has led gradually to an interest in the patient as a whole. It has led to a better realization and understanding of the patient's actions and reactions before and during the stressful dental episode, and it has led to an appreciation of and an increased quest for knowledge of the psychodynamics not only of the hypnotic relationship, but also of the everyday dentist-patient relationship.

This development is of interest because it shows perhaps better than any elaborate interpretation of the dentist-hypnotist's personality with all its shortcomings of approach, of limited material, questionable interpretation and questionable selection of material (56, 57) that the dentist-hypnotist indeed must have certain characteristics that differ in some way from those of the dentist who is primarily concerned with the mechanistic aspects of his profession. It would be difficult to conceive that such differences should not exist (58-60). It stands to reason that the personality characteristics of the average dentist would differ in many respects from those of the professional man engaged in the practice of surgery or obstetrics or psychiatry or other specialties. It also stands to reason that personality characteristics differ in dentists engaged in the different specialties. One can assume that the prosthodontist differs somewhere from the oral surgeon and the dentist-anesthesiologist. As far as the dentist-hypnotist is concerned, it appears that his sensitivity and concern for his patient has led to a greater understanding of the patient's role in dentistry. It has also led to an ever-increasing demand for a broader instruction of dentists in general psychology, psychodynamics and psychopathology (61). It is noteworthy that this demand originates from the rank and file of the practicing dentists interested in the broader aspects of the dentist-patient relationship (62). One can only hope that future dental school curricula will allow for the proper incorporation of such subjects into the undergraduate program. Postgraduate courses, as they are given at present under different auspices, varying in length and depth of instruction, can at best be considered poor substitutes. It is to be hoped that the dentist in the future will be able to receive proper instruction in his dental school in psychology, psychodynamics and psychopathology, in addition to the mechanics of hypnotic induction techniques. Such instruction will not only prepare the dentist better to understand and deal with the various personality factors which he is bound to encounter in his practice, but it will also serve to relegate hypnosis to its proper frame, that is the broader aspects of the dentist-patient relationship and the proper management of the patient.

Once the dentist is adequately trained in "patient management," which should include the use of controlled suggestion and hypnosis with all its indications and contraindications, then there will be no need to be any more concerned about the "dangers" of the use of hypnosis in dentistry, than there is need to be concerned about the dangers of oral surgery or general anesthesia or any other "dangerous" activity within the field of dentistry. The danger will then shift from the subject matter to the subject proper, that is from hypnosis to the dentist who uses it. All conditions being equal, the dentist who uses hypnosis ought to compare quite favorably with the dentist who engages in any other "specialty."

Once hypnosis is used in dentistry as it should be used, and not as it is envisioned in the minds of many of its critics who show complete lack of awareness of the essential difference between their prejudiced concept of hypnosis and its actual use by the properly trained and responsible dentist (63-70), many of the other aspects which have encountered strong criticism within the profession and from the outside will lose their importance. Then even such critical and sensitive areas as the dentist's role in dealing with habits which interfere with the function or esthetics of the dental apparatus, by the use of hypnosis or suggestion, will be appraised by logic and reason and no longer by emotion and prejudice. Then even our colleagues within the field of psychotherapy who speak of their preference for a "malocclusion of the mouth rather than a malocclusion of the personality" will accept the fact that very often by not dealing in time with the malocclusion of the mouth, they are bound to end up with both a malocclusion of the mouth and of the personality.

Then those within and outside our profession who warn the dentist against the use of hypnosis in dealing with habits, will see very little difference between the accepted mechanical interference by the use of appliances, as commonly used by the orthodontist, and the psychological interference as used by the hypnodontist. It will be readily understood that these mechanical devices also have a psychological effect which by necessity is far more forceful and direct, and lends itself to far less control than hypnosis and controlled suggestion which can and ought to be permissive, casual, gentle and administered in doses graduated according to age, type and circumstance. It will become apparent that whatever the dentist's specialty or inclination, he cannot avoid dealing with psychological problems as long as he deals with patients. It will be obvious that the problem presented by the use of hypnosis and suggestion in dentistry is solved far better by a positive approach, which places emphasis on proper instruction and training within the framework of undergraduate training, as is the case in such other borderline subjects as oral surgery and anesthesiology which on one hand are confined in their practical application by the dentist, and on the other hand cannot be clearly separated from the broader field of general medicine and surgery.

Recognition has been given to the need for training of the practitioner of medicine in general psychiatry as evidenced by the many officially sponsored postgraduate courses in this area. The time has come to equally recognize and train the practitioner of dentistry in the principles of psychology, psychodynamics and psychiatry. Hypnosis and suggestion may then form part and parcel of this broader training and cease to be a "specialty." The dentist thus trained will be able to deal better with all his patients. He will become a member of the healing profession whose special mechanical skills are combined with a broad medical and psychological background.

The dentist's contribution to the health and welfare of his patient is a most important one from many points of view. His professional activities are concentrated in an area which has been generally recognized as a most sensitive one, physiologically and psychodynamically. The dentist therefore should be neither a mechanic nor a hypnotist, but rather a professional man trained in all the basic sciences and arts which are of importance in the practice of dentistry.

Principles of mechanics and esthetics, medicine and surgery, psychodynamics and psychopathology, are part of the foundation on which modern dentistry rests. Hypnosis and suggestion are part of this broad foundation and should not be separated from it.

REFERENCES

1. MARCUS, H. W.: The role of hypnosis and suggestion in dentistry. *J.A.D.A.*, *59*:1149-1154, 1959.
2. MARCUS, H. W. and BOWERS, M.: Hypnosis and schizophrenia in the dental situation. *Int. J. Clin. & Exper. Hyp.*, *9*:47-52, 1961.
3. A.M.A. Council on Mental Health: Medical uses of hypnosis. *J.A.M.A.*, *168*:186, 1958.
4. Editorial: The therapeutic use of hypnosis. *J.A.D.A.*, *57*:704-705, 1958.
5. WALD, A. and KLINE, M. V.: A university program in dental hypnosis. *J. Clin. & Exper. Hyp.*, *3*:183-187, 1955.
6. KLINE, M.: Hypnosis in dental medicine: educational and clinical considerations. *J.A.D.A.*, *54*:797-807, 1957.
7. DORCUS, R. M.: Training in hypnosis for therapy. *J. Clin. & Exper. Hyp.*, October, 1958.
8. A.M.A. Council on Mental Health, Committee on Hypnosis: Training in Medical Hypnosis. 1961.
9. A History of Medicine in Pictures. *Therap. Notes, 68*:15-22, January, 1961, Parke, Davis & Co., Detroit.
10. FIERSTEIN, M.: Limitations of the dentist anesthesiologist. *New York State D. J., 26*:163, 1960.
11. MOSS, A. A.: Hypnodontics today. *Dent. Items of Interest,* July, 1952.
12. SHAW, I. S.: The dangers of hypnosis as applied to dentistry. *Int. J. Clin. & Exper. Hyp., 9*:53-57, 1961.
13. MARCUS, H. W.: Dental applications in hypnosis. In Bowers, M.: *Introductory Lectures in Medical Hypnosis.* New York, Institute for Research in Hypnosis, 1958.
14. MARCUS, H. W.: The use of hypnosis in dentistry. *J. Dent. Med., 12*:59-65, 1957.
15. SORRIN, S.: In Miller, S. C.: *Oral Diagnosis and Treatment.* Second edition, Philadelphia, Blakiston Co., 1946.
16. WOLBERG, L. R.: Current practices in hypnotherapy. *Progress in Psychotherapy.* New York, Grune & Stratton, 1956.

17. CONN, J. H.: Preparing for hypnosis in general practice. *Roche Report on Medical Progress, 3*:No. 2, January, 1961.

18. FOX, J.: The systematic use of hypnosis in individual and group psychotherapy. *Int. J. Clin. Exper. Hyp., 8*:110, 1960.

19. WEINSTEIN, J. H.: In Schneck, J. M.: *Hypnosis in Modern Medicine.* Springfield, Thomas, 1953.

20. MOSS, A. A.: Hypnodontics or hypnosis in dentistry. *Dent. Items of Interest,* pp. 226-227, 1952.

21. MOSS, A. A.: The confident dentist can eliminate gagging. *Dent. Survey, 26*:198-199, 1950.

22. STOLZENBERG, J.: *Psychosomatics and Suggestion Therapy in Dentistry.* New York, Philosophical Library, 1950.

23. STOLZENBERG, J.: *Dental Hypnosis Handbook.* Hollywood, Calif., Wilshire Book Co., 1961.

24. STOLZENBERG, J.: Case reports on bruxism and periodic hysterical trismus. *J. Clin. & Exper. Hyp., 1*:67-70, 1953.

25. STOLZENBERG, J.: Hypnosis in orthodontics. *Am. J. Orth., 45*:508-511, 1959.

26. SHAW, S. I.: *Clinical Applications of Hypnosis in Dentistry.* Philadelphia, W. B. Saunders, 1958.

27. SHAW, S. I.: A survey of the management of children in hypnodontia. *Am. J. Clin. Hyp., 1*:155-161, 1959.

28. SHAW, S. I.: *Hypnotism Can Help.* Philadelphia, David McKay Co., 1948.

29. AMENT, P.: The "as if" attitude in illusions of anesthetics with hypnosis. *J. Am. Soc. Psychosom. Dent. & Med., 4*:52-56, 1957.

30. AMENT, P.: The significance of positive visual illusion in clinical practice. *J. Am. Soc. Psychosom. Dent. & Med., 6*:October, 1959.

31. AMENT, P.: Time distortion with hypnodontics. *J. Am. Soc. Psychosom. Dent. & Med., 2*:11-12, 1955.

32. KUHNER, A.: Evaluation of hypnosis in dental therapeutics from the dentist's viewpoint. *J.A.D.A., 54*:789-796, 1957.

33. SINGER, R. M.: Should dentists shun hypnosis? *J. Canad. Dent. A., 26*:705-710, 1960.

34. SINGER, R. M.: Dental psychotherapy. *J. Canad. Dent. A., 26*:203-209, 1960.

35. KORNFELD, B.: Hypnosis as applied in modern dental practice. In *Lippincott's Handbook of Dental Practice,* Third ed., Philadelphia, 1958.

36. JACOBY, J. D.: Statistical report on general practice. Hypnodontics. Tape recorder conditioning. *Int. J. Clin. & Exper. Hyp.,* 3:115-119, 1960.

37. PAPERMASTER, A. A.: A clinical application of hypnosis and hypnoanesthesia in dentistry. *Dent. Digest,* April, May, June, 1959.

38. STAPLES, L. M.: A psychological approach through hypnosis to certain psychosomatic problems in dentistry and medicine. *Am. J. Clin. Hyp.,* 2:116-121, 1960.

39. STAPLES, L. M.: Relaxation through hypnosis, a valuable adjunct to chemo-anesthesia. *J. Am. Dent. Soc. Anesth.,* October, 1958.

40. SECTER, I. I.: Some notes on controlling the exaggerated gag reflex. *Am. J. Clin. Hyp.,* 2:149-153, 1960.

41. SECTER, I. I.: *The Practical Application of Medical and Dental Hypnosis.* New York, Julian Press, 1961.

42. LeCRON, L. M.: The relief of gagging by hypnosis. *J. Am. Soc. Psychosom. Dent.,* 2:13-15, 1955.

43. SOLOVEY, G. and MILECHNIN, A.: Some points regarding hypnosis in dentistry. *Am. J. Clin. Hyp.,* 1:59-77, 1958.

44. BARNETT, S.: Hypnotic suggestion in dentistry. *Brit. Dent. J., 88:* 96-101, 1950.

45. ECKER, H. A.: Medical hypnosis in maxillofacial and plastic surgery. *Am. J. Surg., 98:*826-829, 1959.

46. HERON, W. T.: Hypnosis and psychology in patient control. *J. Mich. State Dent. A., 35:*131-135, 1953.

47. HERON, W. and SECTER, I.: Clinical applications of hypnosis in dentistry. *Dent. Survey, 30:*331-333, 1954.

48. LEVBARG, J. J.: Hypnosis—a useful therapy to physicians and dentists. *Dent. Items of Interest,* October, 1952.

49. RAGINSKY, B. B.: Preanesthetic management of the dental patient. *J.A.D.A., 49:*672-683, 1954.

50. RAGINSKY, B. B.: Psychosomatic dentistry. *J. Canad. Dent. A.,* September, 1954.

51. RAGINSKY, B. B.: A consideration of new tranquilizing drugs and hypnosis for the dentist. *New York J. Dent.,* 27:297-306, 1957.

52. RAGINSKY, B. B.: Psychosomatics, pharmacology, premedication and hypnosis. *Ann. Dent.,* 27:No. 1, March, 1958.

53. ROSEN, H.: Hypnosis, mental hygiene and the dentist-hypnotist. *J.A.D.A., 54:*808-818, 1957.

54. MEARES, A.: *Newsletter, Soc. Clin. Exper. Hyp., 4:*No. 2, May, 1961.

55. MARCUSE, F. L.: Hypnosis in dentistry. *Am. J. Orth. & Oral Surg.,* 33:796-809, 1947.

56. BORLAND and EPSTEIN: Psychological evaluation of hypnosis in dentistry. *J.A.D.A., 62*:68-79, 1961.
57. SECTER, I. and TREMAINE, D.: Hypnosis and the personality of the operator. *J.A.D.A., 63*:106-108, 1961.
58. RAGINSKY, B. B.: The dentist as a person. *J. Canad. Dent. A., 20*: 72-79, 1954.
59. RAGINSKY, B. B.: In Schneck, J. M.: *Hypnosis in Modern Medicine.* Second edition, Springfield, Thomas, 1959.
60. BERNSTEIN and BALK: Common diseases of practicing dentists. *J.A.D.A., 46*:525, 1953.
61. SHAW, I. S.: A consideration of personality factors in the use of hypnosis in dentistry. *J.A.D.A., 62*:49/675—53/679.
62. ATTERBURY, R. A.: Chicago Academy studies psychology. *J. Hyp. & Psych., 1*:25, 1957.
63. Editorials: *New York J. Dent.,* June-July, 1953; November, 1953; March, 1954.
64. BODECKER, C. F.: Hypnosis in dentistry. *New York State Dent. J., 22*:226-227, 1956.
65. BODECKER, BORLAND, MILLER, SCHEMAN: Use of hypnosis in dentistry. *New York State Dent. J., 24*:165-172, 1958.
66. Editorial: Hypnosis in dentistry is extremely impractical. *J.A.D.A., 40*:590-591, 1950.
67. Editor's Note: *North-West Dent., 29*:182, 1950.
68. Editorial: Psychosomatic sleep. *North-West Dent., 28*:101-108, 1949.
69. Editorial: *North-West Dent., 28*:164-165, 1949.
70. KUEHNER, G.: The role and scope of psychosomatic dentistry. *North-West Dent., 30*:245-293, 1957.

9

HYPNOSIS IN CLINICAL PSYCHOLOGY

MILTON V. KLINE, M.A., ED.D.

The modern history of scientific hypnosis may be divided into three somewhat distinct periods. The first, starting in the latter part of the nineteenth century and continuing into the twentieth, rotates around the developing interests of psychoanalytic thinking and concern with the nature of psychodynamic functioning in relation to personality theory and concepts. Therapeutic and case history investigations as well as phenomenological observations of hypnotic behavior, such as those reported by Liébeault, Bernheim, Prince, Janet, Sidis, Freud and James highlight this period which placed great emphasis upon clinical observational data, essentially of a descriptive nature and oriented towards emerging dynamic concepts of psychopathology.

Following this period, and beginning shortly after World War I, a somewhat more obscure approach to scientific hypnosis was characteristic of interest and investigation. Influenced by psychoanalytic dynamics, there continued to evolve the utilization of hypnosis essentially as a therapeutic tool in relation to the psychotherapy of neuroses with particular emphasis upon hysterical and allied dissociative disorders. Some attention continued to be given, as earlier, to the use of hypnosis as an anesthetic modality and as a means for experimental investigations into psychophysiological functioning. The work was largely fragmentary, with little unification, and theoretical constructs were virtually nonexistent.

The third period begins with the significant experimental approaches of Clark Hull (16) and his associates during his period at Wisconsin and continuing through his distinguished stay at Yale University. Here, for the first time, well controlled experimental investigations into basic psychological mechanisms and behavior organizing processes were undertaken systematically and in an integrated manner. There are to be found in Hull's studies, observations, conclusions and implications, meaningful references to the use of psychological evaluations and testing procedures largely operational in nature and essentially consistent with the need to measure psychomotor functions, aspects of learning mechanisms and, to some extent, personality functioning characteristics.

This latter period merged into the renaissance of scientific hypnosis which we are currently witnessing. Beginning with the period following World War II, clinical psychological studies of hypnosis, hypnotherapy and the many complex variables that go into the structuring of hypnotic behavior began to be reported (8, 9, 20, 21, 27, 62).

For the greater part, the use of clinical psychological procedures which have become increasingly more sophisticated and highly developed as devices of measurement for personality and mental functioning are to be found in experimental and clinical studies of hypnosis and its therapeutic applications from the period in the early 1940s to the present time (1, 3, 5, 6, 10, 15, 19, 24, 32, 33, 34, 35).

Clinical psychology has, since World War II, moved rapidly into the area of psychotherapy and as this field has become a specialty within professional psychology a good deal of the work reported during the past decade bears essentially on the therapeutic process and the integration of hypnotic procedures in relation to treatment approaches, problems and goals (21, 24). Inasmuch as this material is in this volume included in the chapter on Psychiatry, it will not be reported in any detail here, but this chapter will focus essentially upon the use of clinical psychological procedures for the evaluation of the hypnotic process, the behavioral organizing mechanisms that have been studied in relation to personality dynamics, and the relationship of these findings to such provocative aspects of behavior as perception, learning theory, psychodynamic formulations, psychophysiology and the broader, more holistic aspect of personality functioning (26, 27).

The general significance of studies in this area during the

past decade has been to shed light on the motivational as well as the structural processes involved in both the induction of the hypnotic state and the development of the hypnotic transference and its relationship both theoretically and operationally to emergent behavior as a natural sequence to hypnotic intervention with its parallel and integrated relationship to behavior on non-hypnotic levels.

A number of experimental investigations dealing with the nature of hypnosis and its general implications for theoretical constructs have not necessarily involved the dynamic techniques and approaches of clinical psychology and are, therefore, not comprehensively incorporated in this review but may be found meaningfully in a number of recent contributions to the literature (20, 21, 49).

DIAGNOSTIC PSYCHOLOGICAL TESTING

The use of hypnosis in connection with psychological testing both of a projective and standardized nature tends to extend the use of such devices significantly both in relation to clinical evaluations and the amplification of diagnostic pictures relating to therapeutic considerations, as well as to the possibility of developmental and evaluative studies of personality apart from therapeutic considerations. Such applications have clarified the nature and meaning of hypnosis as well as delimiting some of the mechanisms of psychological test functions themselves (17, 24).

A number of studies report data which emphasize the use of psychological testing procedures for the evaluation of hypnotic age regression as well as related alterations in chronological and temporal variables. Tests that have been employed include, among others, the Wechsler-Bellevue Scale, The House-Tree-Person Test, the Minnesota Multiphasic Inventory, the Rorschach and the Thematic Apperception Test (11, 25, 28, 29, 31, 39, 44, 47, 50, 56, 65).

Although hypnotic age regression continues to be a somewhat controversial problem in relation to its validity, studies with the changes brought about through the use of hypnotic age regression Wechsler-Bellevue have particularly tended to indicate that age tend to be functionally more fact than artifact, and that they may well reflect valid alterations in the level of perceptual structuring and affective response for some subjects. In this respect studies with figure drawings, the Thematic Apperception Test, the Rorschach, as well as such tests as the Glasser-Watson Critical Thinking Test and the Vernon-Lindzey Scale of Values reflect consistent changes with self-image as it relates to age identification, and suggest that the behavior which emerges is dynamically consistent with alterations in body image and the nature of the interpersonal contacts and encounters that the subject develops, rather than representing a more mechanistic chronologic regression on a sensory-motor or psychomotor level alone (25).

Psychological test findings certainly indicate that there are selective aspects to the nature of regressive experience and that intellectual functions maintain the same level of adaptability and creativity,* or in a simpler sense, the same power elements in intellectual operations persist in regression. However, the manner in which associative functions are utilized and emotional responses to critical observations take place becomes altered and are more consistent with an image of earlier age levels to which the subject has been regressed.

One series of studies dealing with hypnotic age regression utilizing the Terman-Miles Masculinity-Feminity Test indicated that with a perceptual image of advanced age there was for the subject evidenced changes in self-attitude, response mechanisms, affective displays and the general arousal of anxiety and defenses against anxiety consistent with that which on this scale is normatively related to actual changes in aging. Simulation attempts in this direction were statistically quite different and much more consistent with waking levels (17).

Despite certain conflicting evidence which, at the present time, would appear to be related more to the nature of the hypnotic involvement and the transferance characteristics, the general hypothesis appears to be that hypnotic age changes that are

---

*Creativity and psychological productivity constitute a provocative area of increasing study at the present time with considerable suggestion that ego regressive aspects of hypnosis may lead to adaptative creativity on a level that transcends nonhypnotic functions (21).

measurable are essentially dynamic in nature and have particular and significant relationship to wide areas of psychological concern (25). For if hypnotic changes represent changes in perceptual organization and structuring, the extent to which manipulation and alteration of such determinants of percept response can play a role in altering patterns of behavior is of great pertinence to therapeutic approaches.

The use of psychological tests in studying changes in anxiety and the utilization of defenses against anxiety constitutes an important and significant area for future research. Recent evidence that the induction of hypnotic emotion constitutes genuine emotionality akin to that which can be experienced in normal behavioral involvement emphasizes the value of developmental studies of the role of emotions in relation to personality as well as physiological variables which can be designed and controlled with the use of hypnotic procedures (22, 28, 42).

Earlier study with the use of word association techniques and hypnosis indicated that the utilization of the hypnotic process itself in relation to such testing tended to produce a marked increase in the incidence of associative alterations and an increase in the percentage of more rapid reaction times, as well as a decrease in the slow reaction times during the hypnotic process (33). It was also reported that there was an increase in the percentage of serious disturbance reactions for both patient and control groups when hypnosis was used. This is consistent with the idea that hypnosis itself constitutes a state of increasing, though fluctuating decline in self-awarenes which, as Bellak (2) pointed out, involves some degree of self-exclusion.

Similar results have been obtained with the use of the Rorschach and Thematic Apperception Test in studies involving hypnosis and non-hypnotic evaluations with comparable groups. While such techniques find their greatest utilization in relation to hypnotherapy, they certainly can also be used for comprehensive personality investigations and as diagnostic procedures in relation to non-hypnotic therapeutic approaches as well. Although the results of additional studies of hypnosis with diagnostic testing procedures involving associative as well as other projective phenomena do not necessarily produce direct insights to the nature of unconscious ideation or affect, there are indications that the addition of hypnosis facilitates imagery activity and a certain degree of spontaneous sensory response which may often produce meaningful data for both therapeutic application and, as mentioned before, for personality investigation.

For many subjects, the hypnotic process is one which is akin to dreaming and frequently brings forth responses from projective devices which are elaborated more than usual, which tend to become somewhat more agglutinated and, for the greater part, more vivid, producing at the same time from the clinical point of view, more direct evidence of emotional involvement and less rigid ego controls.

Wilkins and Adams (64) in an early report on the use of the Rorschach under hypnosis found that this technique was particularly useful in the inaccessible patient, cases where there was a paucity of response or where there was a great deal of anxiety. This has been substantiated in other studies which show that coarctated and highly restricted individuals tend, either spontaneously or with relatively simple suggestions, to be more productive both on a verbal and imagery basis, through the use of hypnotic intervention in relation to the testing procedure.

The study of Wilkins and Adams indicated that under hypnosis, Rorschach protocols tended to show an increase of percentage of responses, particularly to cards VIII, IX and X. They also found that the total number of rejections was greatly reduced, usually to zero. Sum C generally was noted to decrease and M and FM to show marked increases. The findings, which are typical of the way in which patients respond clinically to Rorschach under hypnosis, point not only to the development of this examining procedure as a specialized technique for the study of difficult patients, but also as a technique for the study and validation of what it is that goes into a projected test response. The determinants of such response formation and the ability perhaps to isolate some of the variables that help determine such percept formation continue to be of great interest in relation of psychodynamic concepts.

In this connection, Lane (34) had reported on an interesting validation study of the Rorschach movement interpretations. Investigation of the validity of these M score interpretations comprised inducing productivity and introversive mechanisms by hypnosis and noting results and changes in M scores and experience type on the Rorschach. The results indicated that hypnosis *per se* tends to produce a slight, though positive, increase in introversive tendencies beyond the normal state, while the gross effects of hypnosis with specific suggestions intensifies the introversive tendencies far beyond the level of hypnosis itself. Lane found further that the qualitative analysis of movement responses indicated that subjects were responding with movement interpretations to suggestions that were allied to this reaction.

Bergman, Graham and Leavitt (3) in their study of Rorschach changes during consecutive hypnotic chronological age regressions found the test changes to parallel closely the clinical life data of the patient. The appearance of new interpersonal relationships which produced anxiety and unconscious hostility were noted along with the expression psychometrically of defense mechanisms designed to cope with these new developments.

Spiegel, Shor and Fishman (56) utilizing such test techniques as the Stanford-Binet Intelligence Test, the Kohs' Block Test, the Rorschach Test, the electroencephalogram as well as the Thematic Apperception test, the Shor Completion Blanks and the Tendler Projective Sheets also confirm the general results from projective testing in relation to the hypnotic process: that hypnosis tends to bring about a more productive psychological state within the patient or subject, which may result in certain responses reflecting less ego control and marginal fluctuations in reality testing.

These alterations are not pathological changes for the greater part but constitute the same kind of alteration in the handling of consciousness that takes place in states of daydreaming, fantasy and nocturnal dreaming, with the development of more vivid imagery. There appears to be a wider lattitude of associative functions, a more direct incorporation of emotional response for both thinking and perceptual mechanisms and a tendency towards a feeling of more direct involvement in the experiential process of the testing process.

Studies utilizing tests of vocational interest and attitude with a variety of hypnotic procedures which varied from the use of the hypnotic state *per se* to the use of hypnotic age regression have been utilized in studying both the nature and genesis of occupational interests and have emphasized the extension of visualization procedures similar to dream sequences induced by hypnosis as a means of extending and clarifying the nature of response to vocational interests and attitudes (19, 31, 32, 49). Reports in this area emphasize that the intensification of imagery in relation to these tests are meaningful in studying further the personality motives and dynamic processes which lead to the development of occupational interests. It was found that significant scene visualizations could be obtained from patients in extremely light states and that additional hypnotic and therapeutic techniques could be employed in the interpreting and analyzing of the productions from these visualizations. In many instances, it was possible to undercut the conscious motivations for specific vocational ideas and to get at some of the more symbolic unconscious origins of these identifications (53).

In sum, findings from a variety of studies utilizing projective and standardized psychological tests with hypnosis have tended to indicate that hypnosis facilitates productive response to testing procedures, permits the expansion of test responses and makes available much greater material for diagnostic clarification and for eventual inclusion in therapeutic approaches.

The findings tend to be consistent with the idea that hypnosis involves varying but increasing degrees of decline in self vigilance and a type of self-exclusion process similar to that encountered in nocturnal dreaming, fantasy formation and the general movement toward more direct unconscious incorporation into consciousness.

It is particularly noted that the addition of hypnosis leads to greater involvement with the testing procedure and the development of a good deal of spontaneous behavior both in terms of test response and handling of the testing relationship. As such, it extends the diagnostic utility of such approaches as well as lending itself to more extensive research approaches into both the nature of the elucidated material and some aspects of the nature of hypnosis itself.

From those studies which are reported in literature, particular techniques relating to the use of psychological tests have been elaborated upon and perhaps can be summarized.

HYPNODIAGNOSTIC TECHNIQUES

The clinical use of hypnosis in relation to diagnostic psychological testing to some extent will be influenced by the manner in which the psychological examination is conducted as an overall clinical procedure. In some settings hypnosis may be utilized from the beginning with patients who present coarctated and unproductive responses in the initial interview. Techniques for this approach have been described and its extension into projective testing reported (18). In other instances, hypnosis may be utilized as a means for specifically elaborating on certain types of projected test responses. For example, following the administration of a Rorschach, patients may then be asked, during the inquiry, to elaborate not only on the determinants of the response under hypnosis but to allow for spontaneous visual associations as well as ideational associations in connection with the original response formation.

Figure drawings may be obtained under hypnosis and, as reported in a series of studies, hypnosis may be utilized to conduct parallel and comparative examinations, one in the waking state and one in the hypnotic state. Schneck and Kline (51, 52, 54) in a series of studies relating to clinical psychiatric status and psychological test alterations both in connection with diagnostic procedures and evaluations of psychotherapy describe the use of these procedures in intensive studies of all forms of hypnotic therapy ranging from the most simple methods in hypnotherapy to the most involved forms of hypnoanalysis. While well-aware of the frequently introduced questions regarding the presence or absence of meaningful personality changes, it was possible to determine and to clarify the nature of certain objective aspects of clinical improvement in relation to test performance with and without hypnosis. In this respect, it is frequently found that drawings given in the waking state following a period of therapy reflect the clinical improvement which is to be observed and reported by the patient and through therapist evaluation. On the other hand, when examined under hypnosis, frequently it is found that psychological test data approaches that which were obtained during the initial contact at the diagnostic period prior to therapy. This does not in any way mitigate against the fact that therapeutic gain was involved but reflects, rather interestingly, on the type of defenses and changes in defensive structuring in connection with ego activities that have allowed for therapeutic and adaptive change. In this respect, it would seem that hypnosis permits more direct access to some of the basic and fundamental aspects of personality which may not be greatly influenced at certain levels of therapeutic progress.

In addition to comparative hypnotic and waking evaluations, projective tests frequently can be administered in hypnosis with the patient given specific instructions to visualize scenes relating to the presenting test stimuli rather than to simply report their associations. For example, in connection with the Thematic Apperception tests, patients are frequently told that when shown a card they will then become aware of a scene very much like a dream sequence and are then asked to describe this material. Likewise, in connection with the Rorschach, they are shown the Rorschach plates and then asked to describe what associations may occur on a scene-like basis.

Material of this sort can frequently be utilized during the course of psychotherapy rather than just in diagnostic periods or as part of a diagnostic examination and can be utilized following the routine administration of the tests.

Depending upon circumstances and the need for such relatively complex procedures, the use of age and time regression procedures for psychological testing can also be utilized.

In addition to its diagnostic use, hypnosis in connection with psychological testing has been employed to study aspects of personality functioning and dynamics and to examine the nature, effect, as well as impact of hypnosis upon many facets of behavioral reaction.

Arluck and Balinsky (1) report a study of possible shifts in functioning through hypnotic suggestion. The study concerned the possible effects of the way individuals function in roles suggested during hypnosis. The two main points in question were the extent and kind of changes that could be attained in the subjects and the manner in which the particular individual perceived the suggested role.

Pertinent earlier studies go back as early as that reported by Breuer and Freud (4) indicating changes in personality through the use of hypnotic suggestion and, of course, changes in psychodynamic levels of activity and induced neurotic symptoms as reported by Sweetland (57, 59). More recently Levine, Grassi and Gerson (35) utilized hypnotic suggestion to induce mood changes noted by means of the Rorschach. While they indicated that hypnosis itself did not appreciably alter the Rorschach record, induced changes in personality apparently did. Arluck and Balinsky (1) found that the effect of suggestion in the trance state brought about changes in the way the individual functioned. The manner and extent of change varied from subject to subject. The greatest degree of change apparently took place between the waking and trance suggestion state. Their impression also was that there was no necessary relationship between the depth of hypnosis and the extent to which personality was involved. Generally, they found that changes in functioning occurred during the trance state and further changes during the trance-suggestion state. In many instances the changes as measured by the Rorschach and sentence completion test shows a significant difference between the responses of the two states. It was also interestingly noted that the changes reported varied considerably from subject to subject in terms of the personality characteristics of the subject.

Schneck (48) in a paper describing hypnoanalysis and hypnotherapy and card 12M of the Thematic Apperception Test used this technique to reveal what was reported about the meaning of hypnosis, hypnotherapy, hypnoanalysis and the hypnotic interpersonal relationship for patients in therapy. He found that a variety of aspects of hypnoanalytic and hypnotherapeutic contacts are reflected abundantly in stories offered to card 12M by patients in therapy. In many ways the material availed itself of exact and ample confirmation of data obtained in therapy. Particularly significant was the fact that there appeared to be revealed important clues regarding transference phenomena and an evaluation of the treatment process in general. On the basis of this investigation it would appear that Card 12M might be administered serially from beginning to end of hypnotic therapy both in analytic and non-analytic approaches in order to maintain some objective evaluation of progress or lack of progress and particularly of changes in transference phenomena.

Ventur, Kransdorf and Kline (60) report later studies utilizing card 12M in investigating attitudes and feelings about hypnosis generally, and the meaning of hypnosis to a group of amputee patients and control subjects. The results of the TAT material revealed rather striking differences in certain projective trends. The amputee patients appear to be more hostile and resistive to a therapeutic interpersonal relationship. They avoid and perceptually mask the issue of hypnosis more frequently and more deviously than do the control subjects.

It would seem that the element of transference and specifically the element of transference anxiety, is more centrally involved in the patient protocols. Although manifest anxiety is to be found in both the patient and subject records, the handling of this anxiety and the meaning attached to the anxiety appear different. In the control group, the greatest degree of anxiety is related to the problem at hand, and the likelihood of its resolution. Among the patients, anxiety is predominantly related to the relationship, and the inherent characteristics of the hypnotist figure.

This difference in the direction of anxiety and the nature of the anxiety-producing stimuli may have much to do with the difference in hypnotizability. The patient group appears to be more responsive to the perception of a dependency element in the transference relationship. It assumes a threatening characteristic for many of them and they express conflict as to how such a relationship might be accepted and handled. The dependency factors appear less intense for the subjects, somewhat subliminal in nature, as one element in a perceptual pattern which is essentially problem centered rather than interpersonally centered.

On the basis of clinical experience utilizing hypnosis with samples of both of these populations, as well as the data from the

Thematic Apperception Test, it becomes strongly suggested that the prevalence of dependency anxiety and the unconscious reactions it produces may play a significant role in limiting the extent and depth of hypnosis in a patient population as compared with a non-patient population.

Thus one of the factors that has to be considered in the therapeutic use of hypnosis is the role in which the patient perceives himself, and the psychological reactions to this role. Card 12M of the Thematic Apperception Test would seem to offer a rapid and penetrating technique for evaluating this aspect of the treatment relationship in those medical and psychotherapeutic situations where hypnosis is to be considered.

In those patients where patient role and dependency reactions are conflicting in nature, resistance to hypnosis in the treatment setting might be anticipated even before induction is considered. This knowledge on the part of the therapist may permit him to restructure the treatment relationship so as to avoid or overcome the latent resistance to hypnosis as a therapeutic activity.

Hammer (15) in a study of the effect of posthypnotic suggestion upon certain aspects of psychological functioning utilized a number of tests determined to measure many facets of mental functioning and in a study of nine subjects during normal waking and posthypnotic activities in areas of motor capacities, attention and perception, association, learning, memory, speed of reading comprehension and the application of abstract ability, found that hypnotic techniques tended to produce better test results.

Rather significant in studies of personality function was Glasner's (13) experimental approach in connection with modification of attitudes. He utilized Thurston's "Study of Nationality Preferences." He found the responses on an attitude test can be altered by hypnotic prestige suggestion. He did find however, that repeated prestige suggestion was no more effective than a single suggestion in altering social attitudes but that the results tended to remain longer.

Sweetland and Quay (58) working with a number of college students in an evaluation of their hypnotic dreams in relation to "ego involving stimuli" found that ego involvement was believed not to have affected reaction time, dream duration or symbolization. Recall was affected primarily as a function of recency.

Shapiro and Kline (55) in studying the use of hypnosis in the evaluation of physiological and psychological components in the functional impairment of patients with multiple sclerosis utilized hypnosis in a case of multiple sclerosis for one goal only. This was made very clear to the patient. Hypnosis was being employed simply for the purpose of improving muscular coordination and control over bodily movements. It was thus considered to be an aspect of physiological therapy rather than psychotherapy and in no instance was there any attempt to involve the patient in a psychotherapeutic process in a formal sense. Psychological testing and evaluation was done prior to the hypnotic procedure and afterwards in order to determine what changes if any did occur in relation to this therapeutic experience. From the test data there appeared to be significant changes in self-confidence both in relation to the specific aspect of physiological equilibrium and the corresponding decrease in general emotional stress. The tests utilized in the evaluation of the patient's response to this form of simple hypnotherapy included the Wechsler-Bellevue Scale, the House-Tree-Person Test, the Rorschach and the Bender-Gestalt.

The results were as follows: (a) While the general overall pattern of intellectual functioning was essentially unchanged, there was some indication that memory and concentration were not as effective in the hypnotic state as in the waking state. (b) Anxiety levels in hypnosis appeared to be considerably reduced. (c) Sensory-motor coordination, special perception and general handling of small muscle activity was distinctly improved in hypnosis. (d) The hypnotic Rorschach was more expansive than the waking test protocol. There appeared to be much less constriction and general inhibition of affect. Response to color was noticeably increased and there was likewise an increase in movement response. In general, the Rorschach differences suggested that the effect of hypnosis for this individual was to increase his emotional spontaneity, permitting the emergence of greater expression of aggressiveness and of hostility. As this emotion was expressed, anxiety indicators appeared to decline significantly and to assume a less important role in the total Rorschach configuration. (e) The Bender-Gestalt and the House-Tree-Person Tests revealed better control of hand movements in hypnosis. The drawings in hypnosis were better positioned, more stable and more mature in form. There was freer expression of sexuality and less distortion of body imagery. From the test data there was gained the impression that the effect of hypnosis for this particular patient was to release a good deal of feeling and ideation that usually were withheld with much self control. With this release there seemed to be less fear of losing control of the self and a tendency to project more stable feelings about the self. There was less morbidity than in the waking state and the very real projection of depression was almost completely obliterated. Thus it would seem that hypnosis *per se* had a significant effect upon the way in which this patient viewed himself. To a great extent the alterations reported may best be described as ego alterations and were largely unconscious. Thus, for this patient the utilization of hypnosis, though limited to a physiologically and paramedically oriented therapy had, nevertheless, all of the inherent components of effective psychotherapy. This approach in many ways illustrates the variability and complexity of hypnosis in relation to human behavior both as an aspect of its clinical use in diagnostic and treatment situations and as a device for the investigation of many aspects of personality and behavior organizing procedures generally.

While the literature contains many references to the use of psychological tests in connection with hypnotic experiments, hypnotherapy, and specific phenomenological aspects of hypnotic response, certain general conclusions can be drawn from data available at the present time:

A. For some individuals, it would appear that the presence of hypnosis in and of itself does not bring about significant or even noticeable changes either in clinical behavior or psychological test findings.

B. For other individuals, significant changes may occur in clinical behavior without significant changes in psychological test findings as well as the reverse of this in which no apparent clinical change occurs but very significant changes may be observed on psychological examination. In other instances, demonstrable changes both on a clinical and on a psychometric basis may be recorded.

From the vast range of research currently available, it would certainly seem that hypnosis cannot be considered as a unitary phenomenon which has a generalized effect or produces generalized reactions in subjects, but that the nature of such reactions will be determined largely by the personality characteristics and needs of the subjects or patients involved and the nature of the interpersonal relationship within which the hypnosis may be experienced.

In this connection, it would appear that mental functioning components may vary considerably between waking and hypnotic levels depending upon the circumstances, and that the frequently expressed statement that what can be produced on a hypnotic level can also be produced on a non-hypnotic level has limited validity so long as absolute determinants of the hypnotic state and hypnotic relationship still remain largely descriptive, and highly fluctuating and variable.

The degree to which hypnotic experience produces fluctuation and changes in mental functioning varies in subjects from being very significant in some to non-existent in others. Therefore, therapists and investigators who have worked with patients for whom the hypnotic experience constitutes no fundamental change psychologically between waking and trance levels may very well be able to report similar phenomenological reactions at both levels.

As previously reported and as increasingly confirmed, the so-called depth of hypnosis may have very little or nothing to do with response formation, but the nature of the interacting process and many of the spontaneous alterations in consciousness relating to this process will be the primary determinants of the degree to which mental functioning components will reflect change.

In this respect, inferential concepts about the nature of hypnosis from psychological test changes as reported in clinical and experimental investigations tend to emphasize the fact that hypnosis as a phenomenon is closely related to the basic determinants of consciousness and perception, and to those complex elements of creative psychological experience which include such constructs as self awareness, body image, personality functioning and the entire range of adaptive defensive and integrating mechanisms.

In connection with these rather basic issues as to the theoretical nature of hypnosis and its effect upon human behavior, Faw and Wilcox (10) in an experimental study of the personality characteristics of susceptible and unsusceptible hypnotic subjects report an interesting study in which the susceptible subjects were compared with the unsusceptible in connection with the Minnesota Multiphasic Personality Inventory and the Rorschach. They found that the susceptible had better overall adjustment scores on both the MMPI and the Rorschach as well as clinical assessment of personal diaries. However, there were among the more poorly adjusted of the susceptible a small group with a very high HY score on the MMPI indicating that they had responses similar to patients who had developed conversion hysteria. Their susceptibility was attributed to two factors: first, on the items of the HY scale the responses indicated rather optimistic cooperation attitudes which would make their initial reaction to hypnotic suggestions favorable; secondly their tendencies to translate psychological stress into bodily symptom tendencies which have a great similarity to the criteria of hypnotic behavior, would indicate a common response mechanism for the expression of hysterical symptomatology and hypnotic behavior.

This, of course, rather interestingly highlights the somewhat controversial issue of whether hypnosis constitutes a normal or pathological process and whether or not it intensifies or stimulates pathologic elements in those subjects who are more responsive.

The unsusceptible tended, in this study, to have poorer overall adjustment scores and they particularly had poorer scores on the D scale, the MF scale and the SC scale indicating a greater tendency towards depression, less security in regard to sexual status and more bizarre thoughts and feelings.

In a further investigation by the same investigators (63) they tested the hypothesis that hypnotic susceptibility is significantly related to the way in which a hypnotic subject perceives or characterizes fundamental aspects of his social and environmental milieu. In order to do this they compared susceptibility with unsusceptibility in relation to how subjects perceived or characterized the following areas: a. their parents, b. personal worries and problems, c. social activities and interests as a group or individually oriented, d. participation in social events in school, e. physical care. Interpretation of results afforded the hypothesis that the susceptible perceived their social and environmental milieu in more positive terms than did the unsusceptible. The susceptible perceived their parents in significantly stronger affection and supportive relationships than did the unsusceptible. The susceptible were less concerned about adjustment to the opposite sex, not so worried about personal appearance, more group oriented and likely to engage in social activities than were the unsusceptible.

Wagner (61), in studying attitudes towards hypnotic induction, found that in spite of a supposed interest in hypnosis, less than one quarter of fifty-three psychiatric residents were willing to volunteer as subjects in a research project in hypnosis. Immediate impression of a general attitude of anxious hesitancy was confirmed through subsequent projective testing as well as by clinical interviews and hypnotic experiments.

MEASUREMENT OF ALTERED STATES OF BEHAVIOR EXPERIMENTALLY PRODUCED THROUGH HYPNOSIS

Starting with the work of Sweetland (57, 59) in the measurement of induced forms of experimental behavior disorders, there has been increasing emphasis upon the use of hypnosis as a modality for bringing about alterations in functioning on psychological and physiological levels, and in recent years increasing studies utilizing psychological tests as a means of evaluating this effect.

Gidro-Frank and Bull (12) have reported on a clinical technique for the elucidation of emotions on a hypnotic level which permits a degree of standardization necessary for adequately controlled experiments. Eichhorn and Tracktir (9) used a modification of this procedure in a study reporting significant changes in gastric functioning following the induction of hypnotically developed emotion with single word stimulus.

Counts and Mensch (5) in an interesting report of personality resulting from hypnotically induced hostility used a method based upon previous interaction between subject and experimenter. Significant psychological changes and their relationship to psychosomatic evidences of hostility are discussed.

Hypnosis can be utilized as a productive process for the arousal and expression of genuine emotion through single stimulus techniques which permit a high degree of standardization and through more complex "interaction" procedures. It would now seem possible to contemplate comparative psychological test evaluations of these techniques in order to clarify the meaning and nature of induced emotion and their behavioral correlates.

Kline, Guze and Haggerty (30), in studying the effect hypnotic deafness in relation to auditory feedback, utilized a test of reading skill and comprehension in order to measure the effect of speech disturbances. They found that whereas hypnotic deafness does not produce a level of freedom from auditory feedback akin to that produced by actual organic deafness, nonetheless the masking effect of the hallucinated experience was such as to bring about significantly better functioning clinically in connection with speech, and particularly with regard to objective measure of speech from a standardized reading test.

Kline (20) and Kline and Guze (29) have reported on the use of psychological tests to evaluate not only regression but also the experience of hypnotic age progression as well as responses to hallucinatory experiences. Significant changes in psychological test data have been reported and the nature of these changes have rather strikingly pointed out the degree to which the subject interprets his experience and the effect upon his feelings of self consistency and the nature of defenses that he has to create against the induced anxiety and overall stress.

It has been found that hypnotic removal of the perception of weight produces an immediate loss of equilibrium on a physiologic level (22), and emotional reaction beginning with giddiness may range in some individuals into manic and somewhat schizophrenic expression. Reality appraisal on the Rorschach and TAT appears to be radically altered. On a clinical level observations of behavior are consistent with this and at other times, not so. It would appear that in the experimental induction of altered states of behavior the use of psychological tests may serve as a guide to the degree of involvement in the suggested experience hypnotically, and may help to separate those subjects who are actually involved on an intensive level with the experience as contrasted with those whose performance may be much closer to role playing.

This distinction which is very hard to make on a clinical level appears to be much more likely to be made from psychological test data and may be the most useful in the selection of subjects for experimental work and the separation of the "role players" from non-role players. This may, in future research, clarify some of the confusion with regard to paradoxical findings in connection with many aspects of hypnotic behavior.

Levitt and Grosz (37) have reported on a comparison of quantifiable Rorschach anxiety indicators in hypnotically induced anxiety and normal states. The basic design of the study was to compare the Rorschach records of normal S's as they would be obtained under ordinary circumstances with those in a hypnotically induced anxiety state. In order to control for the effects of the hypnotic state itself on test performance, a record in hypnosis without anxiety was also obtained. Appropriate analyses of twenty-five quantifiable Rorschach factors indicated that decreases in W and F+ and increases in sum Y and the reaction time of first responses as well as the incidence of M reflect the anxiety state. An increase in FM was found to characterize the hypnotic state *per se* but not the anxiety state. This study interestingly reflects observations obtained in other studies and clinical observations, namely that in some instances hypnosis *per se* appears to significantly affect the nature of psychological productivity and personality functioning itself and that hypnosis may be used as an experimental technique for bringing about specific states of emotion which are then quantitatively capable of being measured with psychological testing techniques.

In a later study, Levitt, den Breeijen and Persky (36) studied the induction of clinical anxiety by means of a standardized hypnotic technique. Tests used include the Manifest Anxiety Scale

(MAS), the Ad Check List (ACL) and the TAT. In addition, physiologic variables that were used to assess anxiety included systolic blood pressure, diastolic blood pressure, pulse rate and plasma hydrocortisone. Of the seven measures, only the plasma hydrocortisone failed to show a significant change from the hypnosis (pre-anxiety base line) to the hypnotically induced anxiety state. The clinical anxiety rating along with the MAS and the ACL show sharp increases with anxiety. The ACL consisted of twelve anxiety plus adjectives, like afraid, nervous, shakey, etc. and twelve anxiety minus adjectives like calm, contented, secure, etc. Subjects checked those which applied to them and their score was the number of anxiety words plus the number of anxiety words not checked. These words are taken from a larger group on the basis of their ability to significantly differentiate normal individuals from patients in severe anxiety states. Of the twenty-four adjectives, twenty-one significantly differentiated the hypnotic state from the hypnotically induced anxiety state in this study. This is perhaps one of the most dramatic illustrations of the degree of correspondence between hypnotically induced anxiety and actual psychopathological anxiety.

Levitt and Persky (38) also studied the relation of Rorschach factors and plasma hydrocortisone levels in hypnotically induced anxiety. In this study, plasma hydrocortisone was determined under hypnosis and following a hypnotically induced anxiety state in twelve normal subjects. At the same time Rorschach tests were administered. A change in level of PHC was significantly correlated with three of the twenty-six factors scored on the Rorschach test. The three factors were responses determined by color (Pure C), popular response (P) and percentage of good form response (F + percentage). Correlations were in the predicted direction, pure C being positive and the other two negative. Five other Rorschach factors known to be significantly elevated following a hypnotically induced anxiety state and which are indexes of neurotic anxiety did not achieve a significant correlation with the change in hormone level. It was suggested that the appearance of the three prepsychotic indicators was dependent on an increased level of circulating hydrocortisone. In another study, it was found that hydrocortisone levels were not significantly affected by induced emotion (43). The absence of a significant difference in the latter study was unexpected but was possibly explained by the fact that the elevated levels in the pre-anxiety state may possibly influence the result.

These studies interestingly reflect the degree to which specific personality factors may be involved in an emotional response as well as the fact that certain defenses may be created which serve to create in turn a movement toward homeostatic functioning on physiologic levels and on clinical behavioral levels though this may be more easily detected by the dynamic changes observable on psychological test protocols.

In a study of the effects of various hypnotically induced emotions on blood glucose levels, it has been found that significant changes occur at times in clinical behavior, at other times in spontaneous descriptive verbalizations by the subjects and in virtually all instances, psychological test functions indicate significant emotional stress and at times acutely disturbed behavior, with no effects of significant nature noted on blood glucose levels both in diabetic patients and normals*. This is somewhat contradictory to general clinical observations and some clinically oriented experimental studies particularly of diabetic patients in which blood glucose levels have been known to be affected by emotion. This is particularly true since the administration of adrenalin will effect blood glucose and an adrenalin related stress reaction would theoretically bring about blood glucose changes. However, it was noted that a movement towards homeostatis in experimentally induced emotions may be brought about because of the nature of the transference involvement but that this homeostatic aspect is more pronounced on physiologic than on psychologic grounds. Further evaluation of this, particularly through this use of intensive psychological testing under hypnosis and in various altered states of hypnotically induced functioning are now in progress.

Gebhard (11), in a review of hypnotic age regression, brings together the results of various psychological tests that have been used to recover remote memory. He summarizes the work of

*Kline, M. V., Weller, C., Linder, M. and Nuland, W.: Unpublished research.

Sarbin (47), Young (65), Kline (20, 21), Reiff and Scheerer (44) as well as the work of Orne (39) and Crasilneck and Mitchell (6). While the conflicting results do not sharply clarify the chronological validity of hypnotic age regression, it does reflect upon the selective characteristics of meaningful recall and emphasizes the multiple characteristics of hypnosis itself as an experimental modality and the multivariant process that is involved in behavior elucidated through the hypnotic process.

Orzeck, McGuire and Longenecker (41) initiated a study designed to evaluate the hypothesis that two distinct selves occur when moods are varied. Utilizing an empirical definition for the term "self," the study was designed to produce two distinct self-concepts by the induction of moods of depression and elation. Memory was controlled hypnotically. The statistical analysis for the twenty subjects involved in the experiment revealed that fourteen subjects apparently shifted orientation while six did not. It was speculated that there was considerable similarity between these induced value orientations and actual case recordings. In a later paper, Orzeck (40) drew some implications for personality theory based upon these observations. In keeping with his observation that personal values shifted because moods shifted, it was hypothesized that the essential aspect of personality theory should be the moods or the emotions of people and not their specific belief behavior system. From such a beginning theory, a system of psychotherapy was proposed that would emphasize the individual's moods and would strive to bring about a positive or healthy mood system.

Kline (28), discussing differences between induced behavioral reactions in clinical and experimental settings within which hypnosis is utilized, emphasized the fact that subject and patient roles can very strongly affect the type of hypnotic relationship, and that due to variations in transference phenomena, experimental observations can not be considered to be equivalent to those derived from therapeutic situations unless specific approaches are incorporated in the experimental design to provide for a parallel type of emotional involvement. These considerations appear to be increasingly significant in the design of experimental studies with hypnosis in areas of personality functioning and dynamics.

Kline (23), in reporting on sensory imagery techniques in hypnotherapy, describes its use not only as an induction technique but as a diagnostic procedure using modified versions of the House-Tree-Person and Thematic Apperception Tests.

This particular approach in which a visual imagery technique is fitted into a projective hypnodiagnostic approach can be used initially in patient assessment and then may offer a basis for comparative material when either of these tests is given in more complete and conventional form as part of the diagnostic examination.

With a visual imagery induction technique, both the House-Tree-Person and TAT visualizations are obtained first in the waking state and then as part of the actual hypnotic induction, offering a comparison with the initial test, in which the differences very often prove to be provocative.

The following case material illustrates response differences with this technique for a 26 year old married woman who was seen diagnostically because of intense depression and a variety of somatic symptoms: *Waking visualization*: "This is a pretty house. Right near it there is a rose arbor which is very nice to sit under and relax. It has a pretty cobblestone path and it's a cute little house. It has flowers and is generally associated with good things and good weather and prosperity." *Hypnosis:* "This is a witch's house. It's very old and musty and very bad. It's a very unhappy house and it keeps people locked inside. But in the meanwhile it has a lot of windows so that people can look inside and criticize you. Everything around the house is dead. There's only rocks and a dead tree and a cold moon."

Kline (25) in a study of hypnotic age regression in psychotherapy, reports on the use of age regression in connection with experimental forms of psychotherapy in which patients were seen in therapeutic sessions, both on a hypnotic and a non-hypnotic level, within which psychological testing was performed for comparative purposes. In addition to a wide range of standardized and projective tests, this experimental procedure also utilized a polygraph pneumatically operated to record changes in blood pressure, pulse and respiration, supplemented with a unit for recording the GSR.

The results of this study which went on for more than two years indicated the following observations:

1. Subjects in age regression examined by the polygraph reveal little evidence of deception or its equivalent characteristic of simulation when questioned rigorously as to the reality of the regressed state.

2. The same subjects, however, in both waking and hypnotic states, show definite evidence of deception or lying when confronted with material that they have either been instructed to or have spontaneously denied. Hypnosis itself did not appear to permit a subject to lie more easily in connection with material which he was reporting as being untrue without showing some evidence of change in the polygraph recording.

3. Within the regressed state, intensive attempts to confront subjects with logical and empirical evidence of their actual chronological status failed to alter polygraph tracings significantly.

These data, along with results from projective and standardized testing, indicated that in age regression, reality appraisal as it exists in the waking state is temporarily disrupted. Associative links with temporal, sensory and motor cues are either dissociated or so effectively blocked or masked as to permit the emergence of reality appraisal on a newly structured hypnotic basis which is relatively uninfluenced by the externalized perceptions of either the waking state or the chronological state within hypnosis.

Subjects in age regression believe in the essential nature of the hypnotically induced reality not through suggestions but through the natural utilization of more primitive mechanisms of reality appraisal and prelogical reasoning. These are essentially the regressive structures of cognition and the internalized process of perception which may be described under a variety of headings ranging from dissociation and subliminal functioning to infantilism and dependency. The interpretation of such a process and its thorough understanding must await a more exacting measuring of this experience and its appropriate role in the hierarchy of the development of human behavior and mental functioning.

Schneck (50) in a study of hypnotic regression and revivification, presents evidence which interestingly relates to these observations by emphasizing the fact that the transference elements in revivifications have been given attention and when observed seem to be consistent with the proposed concept of dynamic hypnotic age regression in contrast to a chronological hypnotic age regression.

Increasingly, the evidence seems to be that age regression, like all other hypnotic phenomena and behavior induced through hypnosis must be evaluated in terms of its meaningfulness to the subject and within the context of the hypnotic transference which has been created. Otherwise, comparative studies between ob- servations in clinical and experimental settings tend to create an invalidity based upon this discrepancy.

Kline and Haggerty (31), in a study dealing with the genesis of occupational interests and choice, utilized hypnotic age regres- sion and the Thematic Apperception Test in which, in alternating hypnotic and waking states, TAT cards were administered with instructions to identify the occupation of the major figure and to explain why that particular occupation seemed indicated. The TAT was administered at hypnotic regressed ages of seven, ten, thirteen and nineteen with alternating administration and waking simulation ages of seven, ten, thirteen and nineteen, during which the subject was asked to "Make believe you are seven," ten, thirteen or nineteen years of age and to react on this basis.

Two techniques for quantitative analysis in addition to clini- cal evaluations were utilized in the treatment of the data: 1) A word count method, and 2) A language usage quotient. The language usage quotient is a technique for computing the relative percentages of differing parts of speech in a subject's language usage. Norms are available for various age levels. The results from this study indicated that the subject, in regression, used lan- guage more nearly like that of children and that the usage range in hypnotic age regression was considerably different from in waking simulation. As an experimental means for studying the development of interests and attitudes, hypnotic age regression would appear to offer a means for comparative investigation.

Dittborn (7) reports on a clinical investigation with a forty-six year old patient undergoing psychiatric examination. His study had to do with the use of dehypnotization and associated words utilizing a word association test. The most significant finding from this experiment was that of two words that produced dehypnotization according to the suggestion given during the trance, only one, "thief," fulfilled the accepted requirements of conflict-provoking words. Thus, it appeared that with the subject involved in hypnosis, dehypnotization was used as a new method to investigate the conflict-provoking quality of certain stimulus words in an association word test.

Sweetland (59) found that scores on Maslow's Security-Insecurity test moved in the direction of improved adjustment when compared with the waking state and the change approached statistical reliability. There have been other studies which also reflect on the possibility that hypnosis *per se* alters psychological test functioning to some degree and this must be taken into account in studies dealing with the induced emotion and attitudes either in relation to studies of hypnotic psychopathology or measures of psychological functioning derived through hypnosis procedures.

Grosz and Levitt (14) report an interesting study of the effects of hypnotically induced anxiety on the Manifest Anxiety Scale and the Barron Ego-Strength Scale. Significantly, this study emphasizes the degree to which hypnotically induced reactions are measurable and quantifiable.

The area of experimental psychopathology and the use of hypnosis in studying it is becoming an increasingly more provocative area for study, particularly with emphasis upon the elucidation of stress and those defenses and reactions against stress which can be experimentally isolated and evaluated. Earlier studies of a more clinical nature in this area are those reported by Luria. The recent studies extend the range of applicability from that of experimental psychopathology to the study of psychodynamic functioning in relation to induced alteration in perception, consciousness, and the many variables of personality. These studies have emphasized both the spontaneous response to hypnosis *per se* and the problems involved in induced reactions by simple suggestion and those produced by more complex conflict involvement for the subject.

Kline (22), in commenting on this aspect of hypnosis in relation to psychodynamic theory and experimental investigation, indicates that hypnotic alterations of consciousness fall into two major categories:

a. That which is produced by the particular level of hypnosis achieved by the subject, and

b. That which is produced by the hypnotic instrumentation being employed and this includes particularly the nature and meaning of the hypnotic transference.

Hypnosis is most clearly neither a singular nor a simple reaction, but rather a compactly agglutinated state within which stimulus function may become radically altered and reality regulating mechanisms more flexible and capable of multifunctional transformation. Perceptual constancy may be replaced by a multiplicity of perceptual organizing devices. For this reason, present day findings and observations with hypnosis in areas of personality functioning may produce seemingly paradoxical and, at times, conflicting results.

The problem still to be resolved involves that of clearly differentiating between the hypnotic and non-hypnotic involvement and the differences not only in stimulus awareness and stimulus response, but in self awareness and self response which, from a dynamic point of view, appears to be one of significance not only in relation to personality theory generally, but in relation to the use of personality constructs in experimental studies with hypnosis and its implications for behavior theory.

Glasner (13) in discussing the social-psychological aspects of hypnosis, has reported on provocative experimental studies of his own in relation to attitude and its alteration through hypnotic procedures. Earlier, H. H. Remmers (45) in connection with a discussion on the effects of propaganda, briefly reported on two experiments in which he had attempted to change his subject's attitude by means of hypnosis. In one instance, a student with a highly favorable attitude towards Jews was hypnotized. During the trance, a number of rather general suggestions regarding alleged undesirable characteristics of Jews were given. Following the trance, the student was instructed to fill out the second form of an attitude scale that had been used in the original evaluation of his favorable attitude. The score showed an extremely negative attitude. There was an apparent spontaneous amnesia for the hypnotic experience.

Glasner (13), in the more recent study, conducted two very carefully controlled experiments involving sizeable numbers of subjects to test the effect of single and repeated hypnotic and waking suggestion in the modification of racial and nationality preferences, both positively and negatively. Using a modification of L. L. Thurston's compared comparisons, "A Study of Nationality Preferences," he tested somewhat over 160 students. The test was scored in terms of total number of deviations from the anticipated responses in all choices involving Negro, Turk, Hindu or Chinese as scaled by Thurston's subjects. Both qualitative and statistical results indicated significant and marked effects that were produced by both waking and hypnotic suggestions. In evaluating and interpreting the results of this experiment, certain new questions arose: Would any greater effect have been produced in repeated hypnotic sessions than in just a single session with a single suggestion? In other words, is there a factor of learning in this type of personality modification? Were the changes noted on one test in response to direct suggestion limited to the test or would they have represented a more fundamental change in attitude if evaluated even more intensively? A second study was designed to attempt to answer these questions. Glasner concluded that repeated prestige suggestions produces no more marked effect than does a single suggestion in changing social attitudes. He also reported from his second experiment that whereas waking suggestion had some effect, hypnotic suggestion was considerably more effective.

This observation coincides with a more recent study by Salzberg (46) on the effect of hypnosis on psychological functioning contrasted with waking suggestion. Again, the results seem to be significantly clear that hypnotic procedures can produce changes that transcend those reported on a waking suggestive level.

Current research with hypnosis in clinical psychology ranges on one hand from rather well defined experimental investigations of such variables of personality as consciousness, attitudes, reality testing and perceptual constancy to more fluid and dynamic considerations as self, body image, and ego defenses. There is an increasing movement toward the integration of experimental and clinical approaches with hypnosis in the study of all behavioral mechanisms ranging from aspects of hypnotic analgesia to the meaning and nature of hypnotic age regression. The gulf between experimental and clinical approaches and findings appears to be narrowing as the essence of hypnosis becomes more conceptualized and understood as a dynamic process. This includes the recognition of learning theory mechanisms as well as intrapsychic factors in the production of the hypnotic state and relationship.

Recent investigations using clinical psychological approaches have emphasized the nature of hypnosis as a productive modality and have extended the parameter of understanding of this phenomenon of behavior. In addition, it has extended in a meaningful way specific procedures and techniques for the utilization of hypnosis in the diagnostic appraisal of personality characteristics and functioning and the incorporation of this material into psychotherapeutic approaches both of an hypnotic and a non-hypnotic nature, ranging from supportive psychotherapy to analytic methods.

As the dynamic considerations for the elucidation and maintenance of the hypnotic relationship become clearer, many of the paradoxical results apparent in the literature in the past may be better understood and clarified as we become more aware that results from hypnotic experiments and hypnotic approaches may not always represent hypnosis at all but one of the multivariables of consciousness that, in certain respects, parallel hypnosis but in effect do not constitute it. This appears to be one of the most significant areas for further research and it not only will lead to the conceptualization of the nature of hypnosis as a major mechanism in ego functioning, but will significantly contribute to its extension and utilization in a variety of therapeutic and investigative areas.

REFERENCES

1. ARLUCK, E. W. and BALINSKY, B.: Possible shifts in functioning through hypnotic suggestion. *J. Proj. Tech., 4*:447, 1953.
2. BELLAK, L.: An ego-psychological theory of hypnosis. *Int. J. Psycho-Anal., 36*:6, 1955.
3. BERGMAN, M. S., GRAHAM, H. and LEAVITT, H. C.: Rorschach exploration of consecutive hypnotic chronological age level regressions. *Psychosom. Med., 1*:20, 1947.

4. BREUER, J. and FREUD, S.: *Studies In Hysteria*. New York, Nerv. & Ment. Dis. Monograph., 1947.

5. COUNTS, R. N. and MENSH, I. N.: Personality characteristics in hypnotically induced hostility. *J. Clin. Psychol.*, 6:325, 1950.

6. CRASILNECK, H. B. and MICHAEL, C. M.: Performance on the Bender under hypnotic age regression. *J. Abn. Soc. Psychol.*, 54:319, 1957.

7. DITTBORN, J.: Dehypnotization and associated words. *J. Clin. & Exper. Hyp.*, 2:136, 1954.

8. DORCUS, R. M.: *Hypnosis and Its Therapeutic Applications*. New York, McGraw-Hill, Blakiston Division, 1956.

9. EICHHORN, R. and TRACKTIR, J.: The effect of hypnotically induced emotions upon gastric secretion. *Gastroenterology*, 29:432, 1955.

10. FAW, V. and WILCOX, W. W.: Personality characteristics of susceptible and unsusceptible hypnotic subjects. *J. Clin. & Exper. Hyp.*, 2:83, 1958.

11. GEBHARD, J. W.: Hypnotic age regression: a review. *Am. J. Clin. Hyp.*, 3, 1961.

12. GIDRO-FRANK, L. and BULL, N.: Emotions induced and studied in hypnotic subjects. Part I, method. *J. Nerv. & Ment. Dis., 111*: 91, 1950.

13. GLASNER, S.: Social psychological aspects of hypnosis. In Kline, M. V.: *Hypnodynamic Psychology*. New York, Julian Press, 1955.

14. GROSZ, H. J. and LEVITT, E. E.: The effects of hypnotically induced anxiety on the Manifest Anxiety Scale and the Barron Ego-Strength Scale. *J. Abn. Soc. Psychol.*, 59:281, 1959.

15. HAMMER, E.: Post-hypnotic suggestion and test performance. *J. Clin. & Exper. Hyp.*, 2:178, 1954.

16. HULL, C. L.: *Hypnosis and Suggestibility, An Experimental Approach*. New York, D. Appleton-Century Co., 1953.

17. KLINE, M. V.: Hypnosis and diagnostic psychological testing. *Personality*, 3:243, 1950.

18. KLINE, M. V.: The application of hypnosis to non-directive psychotherapy. *J. Clin. Psychol.*, 3:383, 1951.

19. KLINE, M. V.: An hypnotic experimental approach to the genesis of occupational interests and choice: II. The Thematic Apperception Test. *J. Gen. Psychol.*, 48:79, 1953.

20. KLINE, M. V.: *Hypnodynamic Psychology.* New York, Julian Press, 1955.

21. KLINE, M. V.: *Freud and Hypnosis.* New York, Julian Press, 1958.

22. KLINE, M. V.: Societ and western trends in hypnosis research. *Int. J. Parapsychol., 1*:89, 1959.

23. KLINE, M. V.: Sensory-imagery technique in hypnotherapy: psychosomatic considerations. *Topic. Probl. Psychother., 3*:161, 1960.

24. KLINE, M. V.: Hypnosis and clinical psychology. In Abt, L. and Riess, B.: *Progress in Clinical Psychology.* Vol. IV, New York, Grune & Stratton, 1960.

25. KLINE, M. V.: Hypnotic age regression and psychotherapy. *Int. J. Clin. & Exper. Hyp., 8*:17, 1960.

26. KLINE, M. V.: The nature of hypnotically induced behavior. *Psychol. Rep., 6*:332, 1960.

27. KLINE, M. V.: Hypnotherapy. In Roback, A. A.: *Present-day Psychology.* New York, Philosophical Library, 1954.

28. KLINE, M. V.: Hypnotic age regression, clinical and theoretical considerations. *J. Nerv. Ment. Dis.* (in press).

29. KLINE, M. V. and GUZE, H.: The use of drawing technique in the investigation of hypnotic age regression and progression. *Brit. J. Med. Hyp., 3*:10, 1951.

30. KLINE, M. V., GUZE, H. and HAGGERTY, A. D.: An experimental study of the nature of deafness: effects of delayed speech feedback. *J. Clin. & Exper. Hyp., 2*:145, 1954.

31. KLINE, M. V. and HAGGERTY, H. D.: An hypnotic experimental approach to the genesis of occupational interests and choice: III. Hypnotic age regression and the Thematic Apperception Test—a clinical case study in occupational identification. *J. Clin. & Exper. Hyp., 1*:18, 1953.

32. KLINE, M. V. and SCHNECK, J. M.: An hypnotic experimental approach to the genesis of occupational interests and choice. I. Theoretical orientation and hypnotic scene visualization. *Brit. J. Med. Hyp.,* Winter, 1952.

33. KLINE, M. V. and SCHNECK, J. M.: Hypnosis in relation to the word association test. *J. Gen. Psychol., 46*:29, 1952.

34. LANE, B. M.: A validation test of the Rorschach movement interpretations. *Am. J. Orthopsychiat., 2*:292, 1948.

35. LEVINE, K. N., GRASSI, J. P. and GERSON, M. J.: Hypnotically induced mood changes in the verbal and graphic Rorschach: a case study. *Rorschach Res. Exch.*, 7:130, 1943.

36. LEVITT, E. E., DEN BREEIJEN, A. and PERSKY, H.: The induction of clinical anxiety by means of a standardized hypnotic technique. *Am. J. Clin. Hyp.*, 4:206, 1960.

37. LEVITT, E. E. and GROSZ, H. J.: A comparison of quantifiable Rorschach anxiety indicators in hypnotically induced anxiety and normal states. *J. Consult. Psychol.*, 24:31, 1960.

38. LEVITT, E. E. and PERSKY, H.: Relation of Rorschach factors and plasma hydrocortisone level in hypnotically induced anxiety. *Psychosom. Med.*, 3:218, 1960.

39. ORNE, M. T.: The mechanisms of hypnotic age regression: an experimental study. *J. Abn. Soc. Psychol.*, 46:213, 1956.

40. ORZECK, A. Z.: Some implications for personality theory and for psychotherapy based on research employing hypnosis. *Am. J. Clin. Hyp.*, 3:189, 1961.

41. ORZECK, A. Z., McGUIRE, C. and LONGENECKER, E. D.: Multiple self concepts as effected by mood states. *Am. J. Psychiat.*, 115:349, 1958.

42. PATTIE, F. A.: The effect of hypnotically induced hostility on Rorschach responses. *J. Clin. Psychol.*, 10:161, 1954.

43. PERSKY, H., GROSZ, H. J., NORTON, J. A. and McNURTRY, M.: Effect of hypnotically induced anxiety on hydrocortisone level of normal subjects. *J. Clin. Endocrinol. & Metab.*, 19:700, 1959.

44. REIFF, R. and SCHEERER, M.: *Memory and Hypnotic Age Regression.* New York, International Univ. Press, 1959.

45. REMMERS, H. H.: Propaganda in the schools: do the effects last? *Pub. Opin. Quart.*, 2:197, 1938.

46. SALZBERG, H. C.: The effects of hypnotic, posthypnotic and waking suggestion on performance using tasks varied in complexity. *Int. J. Clin. & Exper. Hyp.*, 8:251, 1960.

47. SARBIN, T. R.: Contributions to role-taking theory. I. Hypnotic behavior. *Psychol. Rev.*, 57:225, 1950.

48. SCHNECK, J. M.: Hypnoanalysis, hypnotherapy and card 12M of the Thematic Apperception Test. *J. Gen. Psychol.*, 44:293, 1951.

49. SCHNECK, J. M.: *Studies in Scientific Hypnosis.* Baltimore, Williams and Wilkins, 1954.

50. SCHNECK, J. M.: Dynamic hypnotic regression. *Am. J. Psychiat.*, 113:178, 1956.

51. SCHNECK, J. M. and KLINE, M. V.: Clinical psychiatric status and psychological test alterations following hypnotherapy. *Brit. J. Med. Hyp.*, Autumn:1, 1950.

52. SCHNECK, J. M. and KLINE, M. V.: A control study relating to H-T-P testing and hypnosis. *Brit. J. Med. Hyp.*, Autumn:1, 1951.

53. SCHNECK, J. M. and KLINE, M. V.: Hypnotic scene visualization and the word association test. *J. Gen. Psychol.*, *46*:29, 1952.

54. SCHNECK, J. M. and KLINE, M. V.: Hypnodiagnosis and evaluation of therapy in psychiatry and clinical psychology: a report of a case involving the H-T-P. *Brit. J. Med. Hyp.*, Autumn, 1953.

55. SHAPIRO, A. and KLINE, M. V.: The use of hypnosis in evaluating the physiological and psychological components in the functional impairment of the patient with multiple sclerosis. *J. Clin. & Exper. Hyp.*, 5:69, 1957.

56. SPIEGEL, H., SHOR, J. and FISHMAN, S.: An hypnotic ablation technique for the study of personality development. *Psychosom. Med.*, 5:273, 1945.

57. SWEETLAND, A.: Hypnotic neuroses: hypochondriasis and depression. *J. Gen. Psychol.*, *39*:91, 1948.

58. SWEETLAND, A. and QUAY, H. C.: An experimental investigation of the hypnotic dream. *J. Abn. Soc. Psychol.*, *47*:678, 1952.

59. SWEETLAND, A.: Experimental psychopathology. In Kline, M. V.: *Hypnodynamic Psychology*. New York, Julian Press, 1955.

60. VENTUR, P., KRANSDORF, N. and KLINE, M. V.: A differential study of emotional attitudes toward hypnosis with card 12M of the Thematic Apperception Test. *Brit. J. Med. Hyp.*, Winter:3, 1956.

61. WAGNER, F. F.: A clinical study of attitudes towards hypnotic induction. *Int. J. Clin. & Exper. Hyp.*, 1:3, 1959.

62. WEITZENHOFFER, A. M.: *Hypnotism, An Objective Study in Suggestibility*. New York, John Wiley & Sons, 1953.

63. WILCOX, W. W. and FAW, V.: Social and environmental perception of susceptible and unsusceptible hypnotic subjects. *Int. J. Clin. & Exper. Hyp.*, 3:151, 1959.

64. WILKINS, W. L. and ADAMS, A. J.: The use of the Rorschach test under hypnosis and under sodium amytal in military psychiatry. *J. Gen. Psychol.*, *36*:131, 1947.

65. YOUNG, P. C.: Hypnotic regression—fact or artifact? *J. Abn. Soc. Psychol.*, *35*:273, 1940.

10

PSYCHOPHYSIOLOGY OF HYPNOSIS

Eugene E. Levitt, M.A., Ph.D. *and* John Paul Brady, B.A., M.D.

INTRODUCTION

Earlier studies on the physiology of hypnosis have been reviewed by Gorton (78, 79), Crasilneck and Hall (37), and Barber (8, 9). In this survey, emphasis has been placed on the more recent work and on experimental investigations. Clinical studies are presented in support of experimental data, in areas where experimental findings are rare or entirely absent, or where the nature of the area is such that clinical evidence can carry more than its usually limited weight.

We will make use of the expression "neutral hypnosis," as suggested by Crasilneck and Hall (37), to denote a state of hypnosis without specific suggestions intended to induce any effect beyond hypnosis itself.

The investigator into the nature of hypnosis faces, in addition to the usual problems of research design, certain special design problems. These involve a series of factors whose effects the investigator must seek to control, measure, or at least consider in drawing inferences from his data.

1. *Hypnotic Capacity of the Subject:* Individual differences among subjects are not eliminated by hypnosis. Ability to behave and react in various manners under hypnosis—so-called "depth" of hypnosis—varies considerably among subjects. Obviously, such differences can affect experimental results. A study using "good" subjects may yield quite different data from one employing "poor" subjects.

2. *Expectations of the Subject:* It is entirely possible, though not yet clearly demonstrated, that the subject's preconceptions about hypnosis and its effects may influence his behavior under hypnosis. Behavior which the subject believes can be induced hypnotically may be obtained more easily in that subject. The skeptical individual may make a "poor" subject, apart from other considerations.

3. *Sophistication of the Subject:* It is usually assumed that most hypnotic subjects, especially "good" ones, are motivated to please the experimenter by behaving in a requisite fashion. Research results may thus vary, depending upon whether or not the subject actually knows how the experimenter wishes him to react. A demonstration of hypnotically induced color hallucination, in which the criterion is the unsuggested perception of the appropriate after-image, would be more convincing if it is known that the subjects were ignorant of color vision dynamics. Even then, it may sometimes be possible that the investigator's intent is communicated to the naive subject by subtle, unintentional cues.

4. *The Meaning of Hypnosis to the Subject:* Being hypnotized may have a variety of personal meanings to different individuals, some conscious and some unconscious. To some, it may represent an act of dependency; to others, a sexually toned submission. It may be perceived as an opportunity to obtain surcease from tension, or as a novel and exciting adventure. The subject's perception of hypnosis, his feelings and attitudes toward it, may affect not only his reactions to specific suggestions, but his **physio**logical state in hypnosis itself.

5. *The Induction Procedure:* The physiological state of the subject, and his readiness to react to specific suggestions, may be influenced by certain suggestions used to induce hypnosis, e. g., suggestions of sleep or of bodily heaviness.

6. *The Relationship Between Subject and Experimenter:* An hypnotic subject may be skeptical or credulous, anxious or relaxed, or motivated to varying degrees, depending upon his relationship to the hypnotist. Dyads like doctor-patient, professor-student, and male-female, may produce differing experimental results.

7. *Baseline Control Levels:* A satisfactory demonstration of an hypnotic phenomenon usually requires that the subject's experimental performance be compared with some baseline performance. The nature of the baseline performance depends upon the investigator's purpose. It might be the waking state, neutral hypnosis, ordinary sleep, or the waking state under special conditions such as relaxation instructions, incentives, or other factors motivating performance.

8. *Mediation of Autonomic Response by Voluntary Acts:* It should not be assumed in the absence of appropriate controls, that an autonomic response to an hypnotic suggestion is involuntary. For example, holding the breath, a response under voluntary control, produces changes in heart rate, blood pH, etc.

It is evident that some of these factors are not independent of others. Hypnotic capacity may be partly a function of expectation, of the significance of hypnosis, etc. Expectation may be related to the relationship of subject and experimenter, and so forth. These interdependencies serve to complicate the problems of experimental design.

It is not surprising, therefore, to find that many, if not most, of the studies concerning the physiology of hypnosis are methodologically deficient in one way or another. The space available for this survey does not permit a detailed and critical review of each article, calling attention to defects in design in each case. The reader may surmise, however, that those reports that are reviewed in more detail are among those with minimal methodological shortcomings.

The review will proceed by physiological systems, with separate sections dealing with hypnotically induced lesions, manipulation of physical symptoms, and physiological changes in hypnotic age regression.

NERVOUS SYSTEM

Electroencephalography

Neutral Hypnosis: Interest in the electroencephalographic correlates of neutral hypnosis has centered around two issues. First, the possibility of finding characteristic EEG changes in hypnosis which might serve as a test of whether or not a subject is hypnotized. Second, the possibility that EEG tracings in hypnosis might resemble those described in sleep, thus adding credence to the view that hypnosis and sleep are closely related states.

The majority of careful studies report no EEG changes specific to hypnosis (e.g., 50, 65, 122, 123, 176). The EEG changes which other investigators have reported are indeed similar to those seen in sleep, thus suggesting a similar physiological mechanism underlying the two states. Franck (67) reported "random delta activity" characteristic of deep sleep during hypnosis and Marinesco *et al.* (137) reported decreased electrical potentials in both hypnosis and sleep. Similar changes have been reported (163) in persons in a self-induced hypnotic state. Diamant *et al.* (45) reported that sleep activity EEG's occur in subjects in light hypnosis more often than in deeper states. The major methodological pitfall in studies of this kind is that hypnotic subjects may, in fact, fall asleep. Further, the EEG changes of sleep do not occur abruptly. They begin gradually with drowsiness and light sleep and then progress, in a more or less orderly fashion, as has been recently delineated by Dement and Kleitman (43). Thus, some deeply relaxed and drowsy hypnotic subjects might be expected to show EEG changes suggestive of light sleep. For example, Barker and Burgwin (13) found that the repeated suggestion of sleep in hypnotized subjects did bring about a disappearance of alpha waves which were replaced by the characteristic slow waves of sleep. During this time, communciation with the subjects still seemed possible. However, communication was not possible in the presence of C-waves and larger random slow waves characteristic of deeper sleep. They concluded that "suggestions which minimize sensory stimuli and insure maximal muscle relaxations are associated with change in the brain wave pattern toward that of sleep." The subtlety of the relationship of EEG patterns to contact with the hypnotist is further illustrated by a related study of Barker and Burgwin (12). They reported that the word "sleep" spoken as part of the induction of a deeper hypnotic state was frequently associated with the onset of EEG patterns suggestive of sleep. However, the word "sleep" spoken with the subject in light sleep broke the silence and reestablished contact with the hypnotist and was associated with a return of alpha patterns.

Darrow *et al.* (39) reported an increased parallelism or synchrony between frontal and motor EEG activity in hypnosis. They reported further (40) a similar increase in frontal-motor parallelism during drowsiness and early stages of sleep. Here again, however, it is likely that relaxation and drowsiness obtained in early stages of sleep and in hypnosis under some circumstances was the common denominator.

In conclusion there is little evidence of EEG changes accompanying hypnosis that cannot be ascribed to the drowsy state often present. The persistence of clear EEG changes characteristic of sleep in a subject who has been hypnotized suggests that the subject has, in fact, entered a state of light sleep and may be no longer hypnotized. It might be possible to use the onset of such changes as an indication that such a change has occurred.

Effects of Hypnotic Suggestion: Many investigators have used EEG changes, such as alpha blocking, to test the genuineness of hypnotically induced blindness and visual hallucinations. Thus, Blake and Gerard (23) reported alpha blocking in subjects with eyes opened or closed with the suggestion of a light shining in the eyes when no light was present. Barker and Burgwin (13) point out, however, that the "mental effort" of trying to see the light in these instances may be responsible for the desynchronization of alpha since changes in set and attentiveness alone can produce alpha desynchronization in the wake state. In this regard it is interesting to note that Barker and Burgwin (13) produced alpha blocking in hypnotized subjects with auditory as well as visual hallucinations. Efforts to prevent alpha blocking by having subjects open their eyes in a lighted room following a suggestion of blindness or total darkness has been largely unsuccessful (e.g., 12, 65, 128). However, Loomis *et al.* (123) point out that opening and closing the eyes alone can produce alpha blocking. Again, the act of "trying to see" may itself cause abolition of the alpha pattern. To get around these methodological difficulties, Loomis *et al.* (123) suggested blindness in a lighted room to subjects whose eyes had been taped open. Under these experimental conditions alpha patterns were found to reappear. With one excellent hypnotic subject whose eyes were kept continuously open with adhesive tape, the alpha pattern remained intact despite photic stimulation. The experiment was repeated 16 times with the same results. The alpha rhythm disappeared only when he was told he could see again. It must be remembered, however, as Barker and Burgwin (13) have pointed out, that some individuals exhibit an alpha pattern with the eyes open in the wake state, which indicates that the phenomenon is not unique to hypnotically induced blindness. Guze (85) was unable to replicate the findings of Loomis *et al.*, however.

Schwarz *et al.* (171) demonstrated suppression of alpha activity with hypnotically induced visual hallucinations. Lambda waves were obtained in five of 11 subjects when visual images were seen but no such waves occurred during waking control sessions during which subjects imagined visual scenes. In the same study it is reported that the wicket rhythm did not change in five subjects with hypnotically induced phantom hands.

Hypnotically induced dreams have been the subject of recent EEG studies. Sirna (176) found no EEG changes to accompany normal day-dreams or hypnotically induced dreams. Schiff *et al.* (170), using one subject, studied ocular movements and the EEG in hypnotically induced dreams. They found a waking EEG in hypnotic trance, whether the subject was dreaming or not, and in post-hypnotically induced dreams. However, the dreams of natural sleep, whether hypnotically suggested or not, have an EEG characteristic of light sleep.

Finally Davis and Davis (41) reported changes in EEG in hypnotically induced emotional states similar to those observed in the wake state with changes in psychological set.

Reflex Activity

The Galvanic Skin Reflex: Despite the early report by Estabrooks (60) of a decrease in the GSR in hypnosis, the accumulated weight of evidence now indicates that in general, the GSR is unaffected by the hypnotic state *per se*. Studies reporting no change include those of Levine (117), Dynes (49), Sears and Beatty (173), Barber and Coules (10), and Ulett, *et al.*, (186).

The nature of the hypnotic induction technique, and specific suggestions given to the subject, may alter the GSR. Davis and Kantor (42) reported that a lethargic state (possibly a plenary trance) decreased skin conduction, while activity in the hypnotic state increased it. A similar finding was reported by Barber and Coules (10), though the decrease was minimal. In both the Barber and Coules, and the Ulett *et al.* studies, termination of the hypnotic state resulted in a sharp drop in skin resistance, despite the fact that there had been no increase during hypnosis. The former report that the conduction remained high, while the latter found that it returned rapidly to normal.

The possibility of a sex difference is suggested by the investigation of Sears and Beatty (173). Over their total sample of twelve male and twelve female subjects, no GSR differences between the waking and hypnotic states were found. This was also true for the males alone, but not for the females, who manifested less conductivity.

Conditioned Reflexes and Responses: Scott (172) and Leuba (114, 115) report that conditioned responses are easier to obtain under hypnosis than in the waking state. There are similar reports in the Russian literature reviewed by Crasilneck and Hall (37) and by Gorton (79). Fisher's work (63) suggests that conditioning under hypnosis does not really correspond to classical conditioning, but depends instead on post-hypnotic suggestion. That is, the association of stimulus and conditioned response is not based on repetition, but on a suggestion given under hypnosis. This would account for the apparent speed of conditioning.

The Patellar Reflex: An early report by Bass (14) claimed that the patellar reflex was unaffected by the hypnotic state. Since the patellar reflex is retarded in sleep, Bass suggested that it could be used to differentiate hypnosis from normal sleep. However, it is a well-established, neurophysiological fact that tendon reflexes are reduced not only by sleep, but by any relaxed condition. One might therefore infer that Bass' subjects were not actually hypnotized, or were in a very light trance, or that hypnotized persons who engage in activity are no more relaxed than in the waking state, as suggested by Barber (4, 8). The need for an alternative explanation of Bass' data is emphasized by Koster's (105) replication of Bass' study, which yielded contrary results. Koster found that the patellar reflex was diminished in both hypnosis and sleep as compared to the waking state.

Other Reflexes: Lundholm (126, 127) and Dorcus (46) found that hypnotically suggested blindness did not inhibit pupillary contraction to bright light, but Schwarz *et al.* (171) reported that the pupillary reaction was sluggish. Lundholm (127) also reported that hallucinating a bright light does not result in pupillary contraction. On the other hand, he found that blinking in response to light stimulation, and general avoidance responses when the eye is threatened, are inhibited by induced blindness.

In a clinical report, Secter (175) claims that an "authoritative approach" under hypnosis and "breathing instructions" will control exaggerated gag reflex in 90 per cent of the cases. Gwartney and Krikes (86) report on a case in which a cough which had persisted for seventy-two hours and was refractory to chemical therapy was inhibited and then eliminated by direct suggestion under hypnosis.

CARDIOVASCULAR SYSTEM

Neutral Hypnosis

Reports of cardiac effects of neutral hypnosis are inconsistent and reflect some of the methodological problems outlined earlier. Most investigators report no change in heart rate (e.g., 18, 210). However, both a decrease (180) and an increase (15) in heart rate have been reported. The latter author observed that his subjects were excited and restless after the induction of a trance.

Most authors report no appreciable change in blood pressure in neutral hypnosis (e.g., 38, 111) although Bier (21) reported a small decrease in some subjects. In a plethysmographic study of one subject, Walden (193) reported vasoconstriction in neutral hypnosis. Bigelow *et al.* (22) found greater fluctuations in finger volume during hypnosis than in the wake state. They attributed this finding to a lessening of cortical inhibition of the autonomic nervous system. Plethysmographic measurements of peripheral circulation are reported to be identical in the waking state and in hypnosis (47).

Effects of Hypnotic Suggestion

Hypnotically induced strong emotions causing arousal of the individual, such as anxiety, anger, pain or wrath, cause an increase in pulse rate (17, 21, 207). Contrariwise, hypnotically induced states of peace of mind, tranquility, etc. bring about a fall in pulse rate (e.g., 18, 44, 72). Similar effects, although less marked, have been reported on blood pressure: an increase in blood pressure following the induction of emotional states of anxiety and anger, and a decrease following induced states of calm and peace of mind (e.g., 21, 206, 216).

EKG changes have also been described in hypnotically induced emotional states. Berman *et al.* (20) reported various T-wave changes in seven out of fourteen normal subjects. One normal subject showed depression of the ST segment in precordial leads. Hypnotically induced anxiety also produced T-wave alterations in four of eleven cardiac patients (coronary sclerosis and angina pectoris). The changes produced were not identical to those seen with exercise and typical anginal attacks in these patients. Nevertheless, the experiment demonstrates the point that observed electrocardiographic changes may be more related to emotional factors than "organic changes" in the myocardium under some circumstances.

Bennett and Scott (18) reported similar EKG changes in hypnotically induced states of anxiety and anger. They found a lowering of T-1 and a flattening of T-2 and T-3 within a matter of two or three minutes with reversion to normal sixty to ninety seconds after the subjects were reassured. Two experienced electrocardiographers, who were unaware of the experimental conditions used, interpreted these records as characteristic of acute rheumatic fever or coronary artery disease. The same authors produced similar EKG changes in one of their previous subjects by the subcutaneous administration of epinephrine. They suggest that the mechanism of EKG changes induced by hypnotically suggested emotions may be sympathetic stimulation and the release of epinephrine from the adrenal medulla. Some authors (35, 161) have reported failure to produce EKG changes in this manner.

Other changes reported to follow hypnotically induced emotional states include an elevation in venous pressure which was apparently independent of changes in muscle tonus, breathing, etc. (19), and slight cardiac enlargement as revealed by x-ray (35).

Cardiovascular changes have been reported also to follow hypnotic suggestions other than those involving specific emotional states. Thus, Berman et al. (20) reported an increase in heart rate following the suggestion of hard physical work. The increase was not as great as that which followed actual mild work performed by the same subjects. Deutsch and Kauf (44) report similar results. It is possible that some degree of emotional arousal akin to anxiety or apprehension was induced in these studies and that these emotional responses were responsible for the changes observed. Another mechanism, equally likely, is that the subjects voluntarily tensed their muscles, breathed more deeply, and emitted other behavior under voluntary control in an effort to stimulate hard work which in turn produced increased heart rate.

Raginsky (158) gives an interesting case report of temporary cardiac arrest induced under hypnosis. The patient had been surgically treated with removal of the carotid sinuses because of episodes of fainting related to cardiac arrest. In a medium to deep hypnotic state he was instructed to visualize with great clarity his worst attack of faintness. The patient became pale and limp, his pulse unobtainable, and an EKG showed complete auricular and ventricular standstill for a time interval of four beats. Ten minutes later the experiment was repeated with comparable results. It is possible, of course that the same results may have been obtained by having the patient visualize his worst attack in the wake state. It is possible also that cardiac standstill may have resulted from inducing any powerful emotional reaction under hypnosis, such as visualizing a serious automobile accident. These controls were not done, however. In any case, the experiment does demonstrate the powerful effects obtainable by hypnotically suggested states.

Stern et al. (179) instructed hypnotized subjects to assume mental attitudes in an emotionally charged interpersonal situation which they believed were typical of patients suffering from essential hypertension, hives and Raynaud's disease. In the "hypertensive" attitude the greatest rise in diastolic blood pressure was seen whereas the "hives" attitude was associated with the greatest rise in skin temperature following an initial fall seen in all conditions.

Vasomotor changes have also been reported to follow hypnotic suggestions. Talbert (183) reported vasoconstriction in the arm to follow hypnotically suggested cold, and McDowell (132) and Von Eiff (192) reported vasodilation of arm vessels to follow hypnotically suggested warmth. Doupe et al. (47) reported transient vasoconstriction on suggestion of cold but could not demonstrate changes in digital circulation with suggestions of warmth. Norris and Huston (146) failed to induce vasospasm in a female patient suffering from Raynaud's disease during a remittive phase of her illness when extreme cold was suggested. Immersion of the finger in cold water during this same remittive period also failed to produce vasospasm.

The older hypnotic literature abounds with reports of successful alteration of heart rate by direct suggestion (e.g., 66, 213). Most of these studies have many methodological short-comings. Other reports, on the whole more carefully conducted, report a failure to show this effect (e.g., 99, 180).

Two studies throw particular light on this problem. Van Pelt (188) recorded a continuous EKG on one subject, first with the induction of hypnosis alone, then with the suggestion that the heart would beat faster, but that she would remain calm, and finally, in an induced emotional state. With the induction of hypnosis, a slight increase in heart rate was seen without visible signs of emotion. With the direct suggestion, the heart rate rose from 78 to 135 without there being other evidence of emotion (no change in respiration, facial expression and no somatic tremors were seen on the EKG). However, with the induction of the emotional state, an increase in rate, but to a less degree, was seen, and there was overt evidence of strong emotion (increased respiration, apprehensive facial expression, and somatic tremors on the EKG). Van Pelt concluded from the greater rise in heart rate with direct suggestion, as well as the absence of evidence of an emotional state,

that the heart rate can be manipulated by direct hypnotic suggestion. However, the measures taken to rule out an emotional state
in the case of directly suggested heart rate increase were crude.
Also, there was no control study to ascertain whether or not the
subject was able to suppress tremor, respiratory changes, and
changes in facial expression in the wake state in an emotionally
disturbing situation.

Perhaps more light is shed on the problem by an experiment of
Solovey and Milechnin (177). A change in heart rate was seen in
two of twenty-three hypnotized subjects in response to direct suggestion. When these two subjects were carefully questioned about
their subjective feelings during the experiment, both reported an
emotional experience. One stated he imagined himself looking
down from a height and with someone pushing him on the shoulder
and the other reported "vague distress." Although it is possible that
the accelerated heart rate occurred first and that this occasioned
the disturbing emotional experience, the reverse seems equally
likely. That is, on the suggestion of accelerated heart rate,
the subjects experienced an emotional state which in turn brought
about an increase in heart rate. This raises the question as to
whether or not an intervening emotional state is always present
in those instances in which increased heart rate followed direct
suggestion.

RESPIRATION

Neutral Hypnosis

Reports of the effect of neutral hypnosis in respiration are
also inconsistent. Most investigators report a general slowing in
respiratory rate (e.g., 193, 221) but some do not (e.g., 99).

Effects of Hypnotic Suggestion

Respiratory rate is easily influenced by hypnotically induced
emotional states (e.g., 30, 72). Reiter (161) studied respiratory
changes by means of a pneumograph and found alterations with
such divers suggestions as pain, anxiety, delight, wrath, and grief.
All but the last produced an increase in both frequency and depth.
The suggestion of grief caused shallow and irregular breathing

with occasional sighs and pauses. Reiter also reported increased respiratory movements with the suggestion of bodily effort. Astruck (2) reported an increase in respiration with the direct suggestion that the respiration would increase. These effects are real, but the possibility that they are mediated by volitional changes in an effort to comply with the wishes of the hypnotist cannot be excluded.

GASTROINTESTINAL SYSTEM

Neutral Hypnosis

Luckhardt and Johnson (125) reported a rise in volume of gastric secretion following the induction of hypnosis. However, the subjects had been given the suggestion of ingesting food in a previous experiment under hypnosis. Eichhorn and Tracktir (53) sampled the gastric contents of 24 naive subjects at 15 minute intervals before, during and after hypnosis. No differences were found for bile or consistency. However, there was a tendency for gastric free acid, total acid, volume, and pepsin to fall during hypnosis and recover partially post-hypnotically.

Effects of Hypnotic Suggestion

Hypnotically induced emotional states exert profound effects on GI activity. Thus there are clinical reports of relief of bowel spasticity and constipation by suggestion of a pleasant, relaxed state (95), and experimental studies (213) which reported an increase in bile flow with hypnotically induced delight, fear or grief, and a decrease in bile flow with anger or annoyance. Eichhorn and Tracktir (55) reported a tendency toward increased total and free acid, volume, and pepsin levels of gastric secretion in hypnotically induced contentment, and a tendency toward a decrease in these measures with fear or rage. Recognizing the complexity of the situation, however, they attempted to study the interaction of factors such as anxiety with the gastric response to suggested emotions (54). They reported, for example, that high anxiety subjects show a greater increase in free acid and total acid than do low anxiety subjects. However, the low anxiety group showed higher free acid and total acid on hypnotically induced anger than did the high anxiety group.

Many studies have focussed on the effects of the suggestion of eating various kinds of food on GI activity. Heilig and Hoff (89, 91) reported hyperacidity to follow the suggestion of eating a food which the subject liked, and hypochlorhydria to follow the suggestion of a disliked food. Heyer (94) reported quantitative differences in gastric secretion following the suggestion of various kinds of foods. Similarly, Pronko and Hill (156) hypnotically suggested reversal in sweet and acid stimuli and brought about reversals in salivary content appropriate to the two stimuli. Suggestions of sweet or acid when water was actually given is reported (24) to have similar effects.

Glaser (74) reported a leukocytosis to follow the hypnotic suggestion of eating a meal. It was of the same order of magnitude as followed the actual ingestion of a meal by his subjects.

None of these findings are entirely surprising, however, since similar effects can be demonstrated with suggestions without hypnosis. It is well known that the smell, sight, or even thought of food produces alterations in GI activity, probably on a conditioned reflex basis.

There are also a few clinical reports such as that of Heyer (95), who relieved a spastic bowel syndrome by the suggestion of relief from abdominal discomfort. Here the role of hypnosis in facilitating general relaxation and freedom from anxiety might play a part.

Frick et al. (68) reported cessation of hunger contractions on suggestion of food and the absence of such a response with suggestion in the waking state. Scantlebury (168) also reported inhibition of hunger contractions on suggestion of food under hypnosis but failure of this effect with suggestions in the waking state.

Finally the possibility of altering GI activity by direct suggestion is illustrated by a report of Zikmund (220) who induced vomiting by directly suggesting to the subject that he would vomit.

METABOLISM

Neutral Hypnosis

Reports of the effects of neutral hypnosis on the basal metabolic rate (BMR) are inconsistent. Thus Von Eiff (191) reports an average decrease of 7 per cent in hypnosis, whereas Fulde (69) reports no change. Two methodological problems might account for these inconsistencies. First, it is essential that a subject be completely relaxed when a control baseline is obtained in the wake state. The BMR is often elevated with incomplete relaxation or minimal anxiety. Secondly, it is important to ascertain that the subject has not fallen asleep when "hypnotic" measurements are made, since the BMR is reduced in sleep. Thus, Whitehorn *et al.* (209) reported a 10 per cent decrease in BMR during sleep. However, there was no difference in BMR during hypnosis as compared to the waking state, provided that precautions were taken to have subjects sufficiently relaxed in the waking determinations. Wallis (195) reported that hypnosis caused a fall in BMR in restless and agitated patients but a rise in BMR in emotionally composed, control subjects. It may be that in the first instance hypnosis had a calming, relaxing effect and in the second, with subjects maximally relaxed, a slightly anxiety-provoking effect.

Although it would seem parsimonious to account for changes in BMR with neutral hypnosis entirely on the basis of relaxation, a careful study by Goldwin (77) suggests otherwise. Goldwin insured that his subjects were maximally relaxed, both physically and mentally, when wake control BMR's were taken. Each of his eighteen subjects did show a reduction in BMR with hypnosis, the average decrease being 3.88 per cent.

Schazillo and Abramov (169) reported no change in the potassium-calcium ratio with neutral hypnosis and Goldwin (77) reported no change in a variety of metabolic determinations (blood MPM, urea, sugar, and creatinine).

Lovett Doust (124) reported changes in oxygen saturation of the arterial blood in peripheral arteries with neutral hypnosis. He suggested that oxygen saturation as determined with spectroscopic oxiometry could be used as an index of the depth of hypnosis, the depth varying inversely with oxygen saturation. However, it is known that oxygen saturation decreases also with increasing relaxation and drowsiness, and is appreciably depressed in sleep. Thus the oxiometric variation may be associated with the drowsiness and sleepiness *per se* rather than with hypnosis.

Finally, Wheeler *et al.* (205) reported a decrease in circulating eosinophiles in neutral hypnosis. Again, these changes may have been the result of increased relaxation and freedom from anxiety. Wittkower (214) reported no changes in leucocytes counts in neutral hypnosis. Goldwin (77) reported no changes in white and red blood cell counts.

Effects of Hypnotic Suggestion

Suggestions of anxiety, fear, or excitement are particularly powerful in elevating the BMR (80, 208). Less marked changes in BMR have been recorded with hypnotically induced pleasurable states (81). Fulde (69) reported increased pulmonary ventilation, O_2 consumption and CO_2 production following hypnotically induced excitement. Related to these studies, Lovett Doust (124) reported a relative anoxemia following hypnotically induced unpleasant emotions and an increased oxygen saturation of peripheral blood with hypnotically induced pleasant emotions. In all these studies, however, changes in respiratory rate, to which the BMR is very sensitive, might account for the differences observed.

Several investigators have focussed on the serum calcium level in hypnotically induced emotional states. Kretschmer and Krürer (106), using three patients with elevated baseline levels, reported an increase in serum calcium levels following suggestions of excitement, and a decrease following quieting suggestions. They reported that patients with normal resting serum calcium levels were unaffected by suggestions. Glaser (75) reports similar results in reducing abnormally high serum calcium levels in an agitated patient by quieting suggestions. He reported that the effect could be reproduced by suggestions in the wake state, however.

Weller *et al.* (200) reported no change in continuously monitored blood glucose levels following hypnotically induced emotional states.

In a controlled study using a balanced design, Levitt and Persky (120) studied the relationship between hypnotically induced anxiety, plasma hydrocortisone levels, and Rorschach factors. They reported elevated plasma hydrocortisone levels in induced anxiety and a statistically significant positive correlation between plasma hydrocortisone level and pure C response on the Rorschach, and a significant negative correlation between the plasma level and popular responses, and plasma level and percentage of good form responses. It was suggested that the appearance of these three pre-psychotic indicators is dependent on an increased level of circulating hydrocortisone.

Wittkower (214) reported a leukocytosis following hypnotically induced emotions but no change in the differential count. Similar results are obtained with post-hypnotically suggested emotions, and in the waking anxious state. Finally, Duncan *et al.* (48) reported the circulating eosinophile count to be raised in hypnotically induced anxiety. This change is probably secondary to adrenocortical stimulation associated with the hypnotically induced anxiety, an effect which has been repeatedly demonstrated by Persky and his co-workers (120, 153).

Several investigators have reported changes in O_2 consumption, CO_2 production, and apparent changes in pulmonary ventilation in subjects in whom the suggestion of doing work was given (e.g., 145). Levin and Egolinsky (116) reported increased pulmonary ventilation and O_2 consumption on suggestion of work, but no reduction in these measures in subjects who were actually working but were told under hypnosis that they were at rest.

A number of investigators have sought to demonstrate changes in blood sugar level on hypnotically induced hallucinations of eating. Povorinskij and Finne (155) reported an elevation in blood sugar in two subjects who were given the suggestion of eating sugar and honey. A similar elevation was produced in one of the subjects when given the same suggestion in the waking state. However, the possibility of emotional arousal or excitement induced by the suggestions cannot be excluded as the mechanism. Marcus and Sahlgren (136) reported no change in blood sugar level in subjects who were given water to drink but were told they were drinking a sugar solution. The same four "deeply hypnotized" non-diabetic subjects showed a hyperglycemia following the ingestion of glucose when told, under hypnosis, that they were drinking water. Similar negative results are reported in a well controlled study by Nielsen and Geert-Jorgensen (144).

Grassheim and Wittkower (82) attempted to manipulate the

specific dynamic action of protein (SDA) by hypnotic suggestion. They reported that a protein meal did produce a typical SDA curve even though the subjects were told that they had received no test meal and did report a sensation of hunger. A non-protein test meal accompanied by suggestions of protein intake, on the other hand, did not yield a protein type SDA curve. The authors concluded that the specific dynamic action of protein cannot be manipulated by hypnotic suggestion.

Finally, several experimenters have attempted to manipulate pancreatic secretion of insulin by the direct suggestion that "your pancreas will secrete insulin and your blood sugar level will decrease" (73, 178). These studies report positive results, but they were poorly controlled and involved small numbers of subjects, chiefly diabetics. The role of relaxation *per se* in producing a decrease in blood sugar level in diabetics was not ruled out.

NEUROMUSCULAR SYSTEM

Transcendence of Muscular Capacity

A popular belief concerning hypnotic suggestion is its ability to improve muscular strength, endurance or steadiness. The earlier experimental studies appear to leave the issue unresolved. Manzer (134), Nicholson (143), Wells (202) and Williams (211) have reported such transcendence, while Williams (212) and Young (218, 219) found no differences between waking and hypnotic states. Roush (165) and Mead and Roush (139) reported transcendence as measured by the arm dynamometer, but not the hand dynamometer or in length of time hanging by the arms. Eysenck (61) also reports no improvement on the hand dynamometer task, but did find an increase in endurance under hypnosis. Investigations of Roush (139, 165) suggest that hypnotic improvement of muscular performance is maximally obtained when suggestions of anesthesia of the muscle are given.

The idea that manipulation of the subject's motivation to perform can affect experimental findings was suggested long ago by Hull (97). Much anecdotal and clinical evidence seems to indicate that muscular capacity is widely variable within an individual as a function of motivation.

Orne (147) suggested further that the hypnotic state itself has a "motivating nature" for the subject which affects his performances. If the subject was properly motivated in the waking state, the advantage of hypnosis would be neutralized. To investigate this possibility, Orne hypnotized nine subjects by a hand levitation technique, (which does not employ suggestions of bodily heaviness) and then had them hallucinate a table. The subject was instructed to place a weight on the "table" but to continue to hold it in his hand. Suggestions of lack of fatigue and pain were given. Prior to performance in the waking state, each subject was told that female subjects had succeeded in holding the weight for an amount of time which was the same as the subject's performance under hypnosis (a datum of which the subject was otherwise unaware) and that male subjects could achieve a half-minute more.

Under hypnosis, the subjects held the weight for 5.76 minutes on the average, and for 6.75 minutes in the waking state. Seven of the nine subjects did better in the latter state. When the remaining two subjects were given a second chance, they, too, exceeded their hypnotic performances, with the group mean scores changing to 5.73 minutes and 7.81 minutes. This difference is now significant beyond the 2 per cent level ($t = 3.10$), while the original means did not differ significantly ($t = 1.10$).

It would appear that Orne has demonstrated not only that hypnosis offers no facilitation beyond a motivated waking state, but that, in fact, the latter is more efficacious.

The Orne study was a test of the presumably inherent motivation of the hypnotic state against deliberate, calculated motivation in the waking state. If Orne's view is correct, then it is conceivable that deliberate motivation would be facilitated by the hypnotic state as compared with the waking state. A study by London and Fuhrer (121) failed to verify this point. However, it did point up another causal variable which could account for the confused and conflicting results, not only in the area of muscular activity, but in many other hypnosis studies.

London and Fuhrer identified two groups of female subjects —the "tranceable" and "untranceable"—on the basis of performances on the Stanford Hypnotic Susceptibility Scale (198). These would correspond roughly to "deep state" or "good" hypnotic subjects, and "light state" or "poor" hypnotic subjects. Each subject performed on a hand dynamometer and weight-holding task in four conditions: awake and hypnotized with no special motivation, and awake and hypnotized preceded by several hundred words of motivating instructions.

The results show, first, that all subjects performed better with special motivation, a verification of Orne's finding. Secondly, the poor hypnotic subjects did better throughout than the good subjects. This may be a result of the hypnotic induction technique, which included suggestions of heaviness in the limbs. Certainly these suggestions are likely to influence the good subjects more than the poor ones.

The striking finding is that while hypnosis did not facilitate performance in general, with or without special motivation, there was a significant interaction between hypnotic depth and performance on the weight task. That is, the poor hypnotic subjects performed better in the waking state than in the hypnotic state, while the good subjects did better under hypnosis.

Rosenhan and London (164) speculated that this interaction may result because the good subjects somehow realize that increased performance will be expected of them under hypnosis, and therefore unconsciously depress their waking state performance. The poor subjects, "sensing some threat in the experimental situation," are motivated to work harder initially.

Accordingly, Rosenhan and London (164) compared performances of male subjects without reference to hypnosis, and with both awake and hypnotized "postknowledge." The hypothesis was not borne out. The results indicate that, if anything, the differences between the good and poor subjects are more marked *before* they become aware that hypnosis is to be involved in the experiment, than after such knowledge is acquired. In other respects, the data are generally in line with those of London and Fuhrer (121) with female subjects.

Other Muscular Activity

Helfman, Shor and Orne (93) found that hypnotized subjects experiencing induced emotional states showed more activity of the frontalis muscle of the forehead than they did during waking simulation. However, the same was true for subjects who simulated hypnosis, and the difference between waking and "hypnotic" performance for the latter was larger than for the actual hypnotic subjects. In general, mean activity levels for simulators were higher than for hypnotic subjects. Interpretation is complicated by the fact that subjects were instructed to make facial grimaces, but the nature of the results is strikingly similar to that of Branca and Podolnick (27) with the MMPI. Subjects experiencing hypnotically induced anxiety scored higher on various MMPI scales than in the waking state, but still higher when simulating anxiety in the waking state. This suggests that simulators "overplay" the role, and do not actually produce a true facsimile of the naturally-occurring emotional state.

In an effort to quantify and objectify the responses of subjects to hypnotic suggestion in a free situation, Ferster *et al.* (62) used an operant conditioning situation. They reported characteristic and reproducible changes in the rate of performance of a complex task following such suggestions as "Your hand is getting heavy," and "You are afraid." There is some evidence that the disruption in performance which follows hypnotically induced anxiety in this situation is reduced if the subject is pre-treated with an appropriate ataractic (26).

It has been recently established that eye movements accompany dreaming in normal sleep. A similar finding in hypnotically induced dreaming in a single subject was obtained electromyographically by Schiff, Bunney and Freedman (170).

SENSORY CHANGES

A satisfactory test of sensory alteration should include the following: 1. the criterion measure must transcend the subject's direct verbal report, i.e., it should be involuntary behavior, or behavior or report which the subject cannot connect with the sensory alteration; 2. it must be shown that this behavior cannot be elicited, with appropriate instructions, from at least some of the subjects in the waking state.

Vision

Schwarz *et al.* (171) gave suggestions of blindness to three sub- jects. The pupillary reaction to light was sluggish, and electro- myographic recordings indicated a marked restriction of eye movements when they were instructed to observe a stimulus. The latter phenomenon was observed by Barber (6), though not meas- ured instrumentally. In post-experiment interviews, Barber's sub- jects admitted that they deliberately tried to avoid looking at stimulus objects. This conscious avoidance in a more complicated visual test situation has also been reported by Pattie (150).

Lundholm (126, 127) and Dorcus (46) found that hypnotically blind individuals still give pupillary reflex contraction to strong light, though Lundholm also reported that blinking in response to direct flashing light, and general avoidance reactions to threat to the eye are inhibited.

Ford and Yeager (65) and Lundholm and Lowenbeck (128) report that hypnotic blindness did not alter the EEG alpha rhythm in the expected fashion, but Loomis *et al.* (123) had positive find- ings for this phenomenon.

Improvement in visual acuity through hypnotic suggestion has been reported in single subjects by Weitzenhoffer (197) and Kline (101). Weitzenhoffer carefully compared waking and hyp- notic performances, and found that one of his six subjects showed marked improvement in ability to single out a certain design from other, apparently identical designs, under hypnosis. Kline's sub- ject, performing a similar task, responded no better than chance in the waking state, but significantly better than chance under hypnosis. In both studies, tiny structural variations of the stimulus were cues on which superior performance under hypnosis was based. This consideration has led Crasilneck and Hall (37) to conclude that the increment in visual function under hypnosis is "probably attributable to increased attention focus rather than increased acuity of the receptor organs." Kirkner's review (100) of some of the earlier literature would lead to the same conclusion.

In Erickson's classic study of induced color-blindness (59), six subjects were found to have normal color vision, as measured by the Ishihara test, in the waking state and under neutral hypnosis.

Hypnotic suggestions were apparently effective in producing red, green, red-green, or total color blindness. This study was promptly criticized by Grether (83) on the grounds that the behavioral consequences of various naturally-occurring color vision defects are considerably different from the deficiencies suggested to his subjects by Erickson. Harriman (88) replicated part of Erickson's findings, but felt that the behavior of the subjects reflected a change in attitude toward the stimuli rather than a true sensory alteration. Following up on Harriman's conclusion, Barber and Deeley (11) urged subjects in the waking state to "try as hard as you possibly can to pay no attention to the red (or green). Look carefully at the rest of the (Ishihara) card, but ignore the red (or green)." They found that such instructions were as effective as hypnotic suggestion in eliciting color-blind responses. It should be noted again that studies like those of Harriman and Barber and Deeley demonstrate only that when verbal report is used as the criterion measure, induced color blindness is not specific to the hypnotic state. It is still conceivable that color blindness under hypnosis is sensory, while that induced in the waking state is consciously feigned.

An attempt to distinguish between the two possibilities was made by Goldiamond and Malpass (76). They used an episcotister which produced visual after-images without prior presentation of a color. The results show that the subjects' knowledge of what they could expect to see greatly influenced their verbal responses. This suggests that visual alterations are more likely to be on the verbal, rather than on the sensory, level. It is not clear that the study contributes any novel information, and influences concerning color vision are limited because the experimenters never actually suggested color-blindness to the subjects.

An unusual and confusing set of results were obtained by Barber (7) in another study of color vision. Two of six good hypnotic subjects were able to hallucinate a color under hypnosis, and also hallucinated the appropriate after-image, though both were naive about visual dynamics. These subjects were unable to hallucinate colors in the waking state, but two other subjects in the group were able to hallucinate both color and after-image in the waking state only. One of these admitted knowledge of the principles involved, however. In another group of 11 subjects of unknown hypnotic susceptibility, two were also able to hallucinate both color and after-image in the waking state. Both denied the requisite knowledge. Based on post-experiment interviews, Barber concludes that the good hypnotic subjects who succeeded in hallucinating in the waking state appeared to put themselves in some sort of trance state by their efforts to concentrate on the stimulus background (a white circle). This does not, of course, explain why they could not hallucinate in the hypnotic state, nor why two subjects could hallucinate only in the hypnotic state. Barber's conclusions that "another claim for the hypnotic transcendence of normal functions is not substantiated," but that " 'trance' behavior may be an essential component in 'projecting' or 'hallucinating' color," are both not clearly supported by his findings.

In terms of the response criterion, Weitzenhoffer's and Moore's (199) approach to visual alteration seems promising. The experimenters presented a geometrical illusion to 26 good hypnotic subjects which is perceived only when a specific ground pattern exists. All subjects reported the illusion in the waking state. When it was suggested hypnotically that the requisite ground was not perceived, 12 of the subjects also did not report seeing the illusion.

Audition

Studies of hypnotically-induced deafness often employ a "startle reaction" to sudden, proximate, loud sound as a behavioral criterion. Elimination or retardation of general motoric startle responses in hypnotically induced deafness has been reported by Dynes (49), Erickson (57), Kline et al. (104), and Malmo et al. (133). However, other evidence is conflicting. Dynes, for example, found that three of his subjects admitted afterward that they heard the sound, despite giving no startle reaction. In the investigation of Kline et al., the subject's speech was fed back to him with a quarter-second delay, a procedure which usually results in speech impairment. Such impairment, though apparently markedly reduced compared to the waking state performance, was also found in this subject, though he had not given a startle reaction. The two subjects in the Malmo et al. study manifested eye blink startle reactions as determined by electromyographic recordings.

Pattie (152) utilized a known phenomenon of audition to test hypnotically-induced deafness. After suggesting that one ear was deaf, he presented simultaneously two tones of slightly different frequency, one to each ear. The subject reported hearing a beating sound ,which is the expected effect when *both* ears are functioning normally.

Erickson (58) conditioned hand withdrawal to a buzzer, and reported that hypnotically induced deafness abolished the conditioned response. Fisher (64) reported similar results using the patellar reflex as the conditioned response.

Anesthesia

The effect of hypnotic suggestion on pain is one of the few areas in which clinical reports carry a reasonable weight. Pain is, after all, a highly subjective experience. In the practical situation, the physiology of pain is of theoretical consequence only. If the patient is able to behave as if he experienced less pain or no pain —for example, by significantly reduced frequency of requests for narcotic anodynes, as in the clinical reports of Werbel (203) and Cangello (31)—it hardly matters whether this behavior corresponds to some objective reality.

"Hypnoanesthesia" is, however, an area in which exaggerated clinical claims seem to have been made. The general belief among applied hypnotists, based on a myriad of clinical reports, is that hypnotic anesthesia can be completely substituted for chemical anesthesia in about 10 per cent of general surgical cases. The most recent statements of experienced applied hypnotists (108, 194) suggest that this figure is an overestimate. The survey by Levitt and Hershman (119) disclosed that hypnoanesthesia is employed by surgeons and anesthetists in 15 per cent of surgical patients. Complete elimination of chemical anesthesia was reported in only 13 per cent of these cases. This suggests that the number of all surgical cases in which hypnoanesthesia alone can be successfully used is about two per cent.

The classical experimental studies of hypnotically induced skin anesthesia are those of Levine (117, 118), Sears (174), Dynes (49), and Doupe *et al.* (47). The results are in agreement that hypnoanesthesia can eliminate a number of common pain indicators, like facial flinch, withdrawal, and increased respiration rate and cardiac activity. A point of disagreement concerns the galvanic skin reflex. Levine (117) reported no change in the GSR; Dynes found a slight increase in skin resistance, and Sears, a substantial increase.

The negative findings of Levine are supported by the investigation of Barber and Coules (10) and the clinical study of Brown and Vogel (28). The work of West *et al.* (204) and the recent clinical study by Suzuki *et al.* (182) are in accord with the positive results of Sears.

The conflicting GSR results are not too surprising. The GSR is a notoriously labile measure, easily affected by many extraneous factors, especially the emotional aspects of confrontation by, and impingement of, noxious stimuli. It is doubtful that a reliable evaluation of anesthesia can be based on such a technique.

The study of Doupe *et al.* (47) is, perhaps, more meaningful. They reported that hypnotic anesthesia caused a considerable decrease in peripheral vasoconstriction in response to painful stimuli. An unexpected finding was that the amount of decrease was directly, rather than inversely, related to the severity of the painful stimulation.

A recent clinical report (196) suggests that hypnoanesthesia may be 90 per cent successful in eliminating the use of chemical anesthesia in electroshock therapy. Reynolds (162) reported that the uterine contractions of a single patient in labor under hypnoanesthesia were markedly different from expectancy. The study of Wolff and Goodell (217) showed that hypnoanesthesia raised the pain threshold 40 per cent as measured by the Wolff-Hardy-Goodell thermal stimulator, but placebos also raised the pain threshold by 30 per cent. This finding seems to support Barber's (8) and Conn's (34) contention that hypnoanesthesia functions by distracting the subject from his sensations, and not by an attack on neural mechanisms. Hypnosis and placebos affect the subject similarly, i.e., by exploiting his suggestibility.

For additional discussion of various aspects of hypnotic anesthesia, the reader is referred to Barber's (8) review. And since Barber is a most hard-nosed skeptic concerning hypnotic phenomena, his typically cautious conclusion is worth noting: "In summary, the evidence available at the present time indicates that when the hypnotist properly manipulates the situation *some* "good" hypnotic *Ss* show a mitigated pain response to *some* noxious stimuli, that is: (*a*) they do not show withdrawal or avoidance; (*b*) they report that the stimuli are not painful; (*c*) they do not show discomfort, and (*d*) they do not show physiological responses . . . (p. 449)"

RENAL SYSTEM

Heilig and Hoff (90) reported that hypnotically induced pleasant feelings (e.g. "You are feeling fine") were followed by a reduced renal excretion of water, sodium chloride, and phosphate. Hypnotically induced anxiety, on the other hand, had a diuretic effect and promoted the excretion of chloride and phosphate. These renal changes are the same as those which accompany emotions in the wake state. Marx (138) suggested water intake under hypnosis and reported an increase in urine output, a decrease in specific gravity of the urine, and a decrease in hemoglobin followed by a secondary rise. Control subjects, who were hypnotized but given no suggestion of drinking, showed no renal changes. Hoff and Wermer (96) reported a similar experiment in which the suggestion of drinking water under hypnosis counteracted the antidiuretic effect of pitressin. Recently (16) similar effects on renal function have been reported to follow suggestions of thirst, drinking of water, and work. A remarkable, although uncontrolled, observation is reported by Volgyesi (190). During cystoscopy in a hypnotized subject, unilateral diuresis was observed when the suggestion that a heating pad was applied to the lobar area on that side was made.

Finally, Mohr (141) reported being able to produce glycosuria by anxiety provoking suggestions in an emotionally unstable patient prone to glycosuria.

BLEEDING TENDENCY

The literature abounds with clinical reports of the effectiveness of hypnotic suggestion to reduce bleeding time in dental and medical surgery (51, 107, 152, 166, 181, 184). Experimental studies are rare. In the earlier literature, Kryuntsel (109) reported a reduction in blood clotting time in normal subjects in neutral hypnosis. More recently, Crasilneck and Fogelman (36) attempted a careful study of bleeding and clotting time. The subjects were four normal males and four normal females, ages twenty to thirty-six, who were described as good hypnotic subjects. Blood was drawn from the forearm and ear lobe from each subject under each of four circumstances: I—awake; II—hypnotized, with suggestion that blood letting would be painless; III—same as II with the additional suggestion that blood flow would cease immediately following the puncture; IV—awake, following the hypnotic phases.

Eight measures of clotting time were made, and data were analyzed by means of variance analyses. Crasilneck and Fogelman state that none of the F-tests indicate significant differences among the phases for any of the measures, but if the F values are correctly reported, this conclusion is in error. Actually, F's indicate significant differences among phases for three of the measures: direct platelet count, indirect platelet count, and Lee-White clotting time. Since the platelet counts are usually regarded as poor indices of clotting, while the Lee-White is commonly considered to be the most efficient single measure, inferences might best be based on the latter.

The data are not available in the article to compute t-tests between phases on the Lee-White time, but examination of the means suggests that Phase III (suggestions of anesthesia and immediate clotting) yielded the fastest average clotting time, while Phase II (suggestion of anesthesia only) provided the slowest, with the two waking states in between. These data at least suggest the possibility that bleeding time can be decreased by direct hypnotic suggestion. While the study has methodological weaknesses, it is still probably the most objective investigation in this area.

TEMPERATURE REGULATION

It is a relatively simple task to obtain hypnotically-induced changes in body temperature if the subjective report of the subject is the sole criterion of success. There are also a number of clinical reports (32, 52, 70, 103, 135, 154, 192) which claim success when an objective body or skin temperature measurement is the criterion. There does not appear to be a reasonably definitive, controlled investigation utilizing more than a single subject.

As Polzein (154) points out, reported changes in skin temperature are probably the result of peripheral vasodilation or constriction, which may be a result of an hypnotically-induced emotional state or skin anesthesia. Core temperature variations of the type reported by Eichelberg (52) and by Kline and Guze (103) in single subjects are more difficult to obtain.

CHANGES IN SKIN POTENTIAL

Ravitz (159, 160) describes a technique for measuring differences in electrical potential between the forehead and the palm of the hand in hypnosis. He found that the DC tracings are more regular and the potential difference smaller in hypnosis as compared with the wake state. Ravitz proposed this measure as an index of depth of hypnosis. However, it appears that the same changes accompany relaxation, sleep, and low "arousal" level generally. Contrariwise, decreased regularity and increased voltage accompany emotional states of high "arousal" level such as anxiety.

HYPNOTICALLY INDUCED LESIONS AND PATHOLOGICAL STATES

Blister Formation

One of the most dramatic changes reported to be produced by hypnotic suggestion is the formation of blisters. In 1941, Pattie (151) reviewed the literature on this subject and abstracted 11 cases reported by various investigators between 1886 and 1927. He felt that in 10 of these, reasonably adequate experimental precautions were taken. In some of these studies, rather elaborate precautions were taken, involving multiple observers, histologic verification that a blister had developed, and continuous observation of the subject between the time of the hypnotic suggestion and the appearance of the lesions.

Some more recent, well controlled efforts to produce blisters by hypnotic suggestion (167, 201) report failure. These reports do not clearly contradict the earlier literature, however, since it would be surprising if any but a very few subjects were capable of showing this phenomenon.

Some recent critiques of the reported successes such as that of Barber (9), emphasize that the subjects were all highly neurotic, or had a history of facile skin reactivity (dermatographia, neurotic skin gangrene, hysterical ecchymoses, etc.) and that blisters might be induced in these special subjects with suggestion in the wake state. Of course, this is a possibility, but it would still remain to be seen whether the phenomenon is more easily obtained, or obtainable in a higher percentage of subjects, with hypnosis than without it.

Other Conditions

Related to the production of blisters, are reports of inducing the lesions of herpes simplex by hypnotic suggestion. Heilig and Hoff (92) used three neurotic female patients with a past history of herpes labialis in whom the herpes virus had been isolated from nasal washings prior to the experiment. Several days following a hypnotic session in which anxiety was induced, typical lesions appeared on the lips and the diagnosis was confirmed by inoculation of blister fluid into rabbit cornea. However, the investigators also suggested itching of the lower lip during the hypnotic session, and the subjects may have responded to this in the intervening forty-eight hours with direct mechanical stimulation of the area. Also, controls were not done in the waking state; individuals subject to herpes labialis may develop lesions with emotional upsets of any origin. The investigators did report failure to produce the lesions with emphatic direct suggestion to the effect that blisters would occur.

Ullman (187) reported on a patient who developed multiple herpetic blisters on the lower lip twenty-four hours after the suggestion was made that he was run-down, debilitated, and felt he was catching a cold. No waking state controls were done. Chapman et al. (32) delivered a standard amount of noxious thermal stimulation to the forearm of subjects under hypnosis who were told that the arm was insensitive, numb, and would not hurt. The suggestion was made to other hypnotized subjects that the forearm was tender, painful, and injured by the stimulus. The former group showed less inflammatory reaction and tissue damage than the latter group. The arm in which the suggestion of vulnerability was made also showed more local vasodilation as indicated by changes in finger pulse amplitude and skin temperature. The subcutaneous perfusate from the lesions of this side contained more potent pharmacodynamic substances than the lesion from the other side.

There are a number of more clinical reports of manipulating pathological states by hypnosis. These include the production of hysterical convulsions by hypnotic suggestion, as well as genuine epileptic seizures produced at night by appropriate post-hypnotic suggestions (149). Wittkower and Petow (215) reported the production of asthmatic attacks in an asthmatic patient who was allergic to roses by the hypnotic suggestion that paper roses were real.

MANIPULATION OF PHYSICAL SYMPTOMS

The effects of hypnotic suggestion on lesions or pathological conditions of various sorts imply physiological changes. A very large number of such effects have been reported. A comprehensive survey is not only beyond the scope of this chapter, but would also be of questionable value. Unfortunately, most reports in this category are clinical in nature, lack adequate controls, and do not involve reproducible, objective, or quantitative physiological measurements.

Buell and Biehl (29) took continuous electromyograms on three patients with Parkinson's disease and found markedly diminished or abolished tremor to follow suggestions of improvement. Brady and Drew (25) took continuous electromyograms on a patient with paramyotonia congenita under hypnosis. Myotonia was reduced as evidenced by the EMG tracings when the hand was placed in cold water and a suggestion of relaxation made. Control studies with the hand in cold water but no suggestion of hand relaxation, and controls in which the same suggestion was made in the waking state, produced no changes. Cohen and Cobb (33) report terminating episodes of hysterical hyperventilation in one patient under hypnosis in whom less satisfactory results were obtained with waking suggestion. As would be expected, appropriate changes occurred in the pH and CO_2 of the blood.

Clinical reports of altered physical symptoms and pathological lesions, which suggest marked physiological changes, include the improvement of alopecia (189), of symptoms of multiple sclerosis (1), the removal of warts (134), and the successful treatment of priapism (37), epilepsy (148), sterility in women (157) and objective tinnitus aurium (140).

HYPNOTIC AGE REGRESSION

There are two major, conflicting views of hypnotic age regression among hypnotists. One holds that it is "revivification" of an earlier period in the subject's life, which he relives literally and completely, including the temporary loss of psychological and physiological developments beyond the regressed age. The conflicting view maintains that the adult subject simply dramatizes his concept of himself at the regressed age, perhaps aided by hypnotic hypermnesia, and that adult characteristics and capacities are not actually lost. A compromise viewpoint holds that both explanations are possible, even in the same individual, depending upon situational factors.

Since it does not appear too difficult for an adult to consciously mimic much of the behavior of a child, the weight of evidence lies primarily with physiological phenomena. The cornerstone of the revivification theory is the celebrated demonstration by Gidro-Frank and Bowers-Buch (71). They regressed three subjects to the age of six months and, without any other specific suggestions, succeeded in eliciting a positive Babinski reflex from them on plantar stimulation. Reversal of the age regression resulted in the expected loss of the Babinski and the restoration of plantar flexion. The subjects were unable to produce the Babinski voluntarily. A similar finding was reported earlier by Hakebush et al. (87). LeCron (112) claims to have replicated the Gidro-Frank-Bowers-Buch work with several subjects. He also mentions obtaining an apparent sucking reflex from his subjects.

Kupper (110) regressed a twenty-four-year-old patient with a history of severe convulsive seizures characterized by a diffusely abnormal EEG, dating from age 18. From the 12th to the 18th year, the EEG's were normal, but then became diffusely abnormal. When the patient was regressed to the date of the psychological trauma which had precipitated his first attack, a convulsive seizure resulted.

Ford and Yeager (65) described a patient in whom a right homonymous hemianopsia was cured by neurosurgery. When regressed to a time shortly before surgery, the identical ocular defect could be demonstrated. However, an EEG taken on that occasion was normal. These experimenters also regressed an anxious patient to a "very embarrassing and emotionally tinged episode in his life," which had occurred a year earlier. All EEG alpha activity was then lost, but was restored to normal by removal of the regression. Of course, the EEG alteration may have been due to recall of an emotional experience rather than to "revivification" as such.

A patient described by Erickson (56) showed various physiological signs of unconsciousness when regressed to a period two years earlier, at which time he had been knocked unconscious. There was a marked reduction in respiration and pulse rate, and a loss of patellar and pupillary reflexes. Erickson reported that he was able to reproduce the entire phenomenon a year later.

LeCron (113) reported that regression of an adult to age seven improved vision, while direct suggestion in an unregressed state failed to produce this effect.

Kline (102) indicates, without presentation of data, that regressed subjects do not manifest polygraphic evidence of deliberate faking when "questioned rigorously as to the reality of the regressed state." Deliberate deception in the same subjects is revealed by the polygraph in both waking and hypnotic states.

LeCron (112) conditioned a handwithdrawal response to a buzzer in two subjects. Both subjects lost the conditioned response when regressed to age 10. A similar loss of conditioned response was found for the eyelid reflex in two other subjects. It should be noted that three of LeCron's subjects were themselves experienced hypnotists, and all were aware of the purpose of the study.

McCranie and Crasilneck (130) replicated LeCron's investigation with six subjects. They found that the hand withdrawal was lost in age regression, but the conditioned eyelid reflex was not.

True and Stephenson (185) and McCranie and Crasilneck (129) found no EEG changes accompanying age regression.

SUMMARY

Physiological study has the potential to cast much light upon significant questions concerning the nature and capabilities of the hypnotic state. Despite the heavy volume of physiological investigations, these questions remain largely unanswered.

There is as yet no conclusive evidence from these investigations that the hypnotic state is a discrete entity, with unique, qualitative properties. Many of the physiological alterations which have been reported to accompany neutral hypnosis might very well be a function of muscular relaxation, drowsiness, or other conditions which are by no means indigenous to the hypnotic state.

Marked physiological changes, including the formation of blisters and other lesions, can be induced by hypnotic suggestion in certain individuals, but it has not been clearly established that such conditions cannot also be induced by appropriate suggestions in the waking state.

Emotional states induced by hypnotic suggestion appear *bona fide* in the sense that they are accompanied by physiological changes of the same order and magnitude as those which are manifested in naturally-occurring emotional states. But again, it is not certain that comparable alterations will not follow similar suggestions given in the waking state.

On the basis of physiological criteria, as well as subjective reports, hypnotically induced anesthesia is a valid phenomenon. In other areas, definitive experimentation utilizing proper controls remains to be carried out.

REFERENCES

1. AMBROSE, G.: Multiple sclerosis and treatment by hypnotherapy. *J. Clin. & Exper. Hyp., 3*:203, 1955.

2. ASTRUCK, P.: Über psychische Beeinflussung des vegetativen Nerven-systems in der hypnose. I. Hypnotische Beeinflussung der Herztätigkeit und der Atmund. *Arch. ges. Psychol.,* 95:266, 1923.

3. AUGUST, R. V.: Obstetric hypnoanesthesia. *Am. J. Obst. & Gynec.,* 79:1131, 1960.

4. BARBER, T. X.: "Sleep" and "hypnosis"; a reappraisal. *J. Clin. & Exper. Hyp.,* 4:141, 1956.

5. BARBER, T. X.: Hypnosis as perceptual-cognitive restructuring: II. "Post"-hypnotic behavior. *J. Clin. & Exper. Hyp.,* 6:10, 1958.

6. BARBER, T. X.: Hypnosis as perceptual-cognitive restructuring: IV. "Negative hallucinations." *J. Psychol.,* 46:187, 1958.

7. BARBER, T. X.: The afterimages of "hallucinated" and "imagined" colors. *J. Abn. Soc. Psychol.,* 59:136, 1959.

8. BARBER, T. X.: Toward a theory of pain: relief of chronic pain by prefrontal leucotomy, opiates, placebos, and hypnosis. *Psychol. Bull.,* 56:430, 1959.

9. BARBER, T. X.: Physiological effects of "hypnosis." *Psychol. Bull.,* 58:390, 1961.

10. BARBER, T. X. and COULES, J.: Electrical skin conductance and galvanic skin response during "hypnosis." *Int. J. Clin. & Exper. Hyp.,* 7:79, 1959.

11. BARBER, T. X. and DEELEY, D. C.: Experimental evidence for a theory of hypnotic behavior: I. "Hypnotic color-blindness" without "hypnosis." *Int. J. Clin. & Exper. Hyp.,* 9:79, 1961.

12. BARKER, W. and BURGWIN, S.: Brain wave patterns during hypnosis, hypnotic sleep and normal sleep. *Arch. Neurol. Psychiat.,* 62:412, 1949.

13. BARKER, W. and BURGWIN, S.: Brain wave patterns accompanying changes in sleep and wakefulness during hypnosis. *Psychosom. Med.,* 10:317, 1948.

14. BASS, M. J.: Differentiation of the hypnotic trance from normal sleep. *J. Exper. Psychol.,* 14:382, 1931.

15. BAUMLER: Über die Beeinflussung der Hertztatigkeit in der Hypnose. *Munchen. med. Wchnschr.,* 64:1385, 1917.

16. BELLAND, G.: Experimentelle Untersuchung über die psychische Beeinflussbarket der Nillreufunktion in hypnose. *Zeit. Psychother. med. Psychol.,* 7:109, 1957.

17. BENEDEK, L.: A vegetativ idegrendozer befolyasarol hypnosisban. *Gyógyászat,* 14:1, 1933.

18. BENNETT, L. L. and SCOTT, N. E.: The production of electro-cardiographic abnormalities by suggestion under hypnosis. *Am. Pract.*, *4*:189, 1949.

19. BERG, W., DELIUS, L. and SCHILDGE, E.: Über die Auswirkungen psychischer Erlebuisse wahrend der Hypnose auf den venösen Rückflusz im Kreislauf. *Zeit. Kreislauf.*, *37*:691, 1948.

20. BERMAN, R., SIMONSON, E. and HERON, W.: Electrocardiographic effects associated with hypnotic suggestion in normal and coronary sclerotic individuals. *J. Appl. Physiol.*, *7*:89, 1954.

21. BIER, W.: Beitrag zur Beeinflussung des Kreislaufes durch psychische Vorgange. *Zeit. klin. Med.*, *113*:762, 1930.

22. BIGELOW, N., CAMERON, G. H. and KOROLJOW, S. A.: Two cases of deep hypnotic sleep investigated by the strain gauge plethysmograph. *J. Clin. & Exper. Hyp.*, *4*:160, 1956.

23. BLAKE, H. and GERARD, R. W.: Brain potentials during sleep. *Am. J. Physiol.*, *119*:692, 1937.

24. BOWLES, J. W. and PRONKO, N. H.: Reversibility of stimulus function under hypnosis. *J. Psychol.*, *27*:41, 1949.

25. BRADY, J. P. and DREW, A. L.: Unpublished data.

26. BRADY, J. P. and LEVITT, E. E.: Unpublished data.

27. BRANCA, A. A. and PODOLNICK, E. E.: Normal, hypnotically induced, and feigned anxiety as reflected in and detected by the MMPI. *J. Consult. Psychol.*, *25*:165, 1961.

28. BROWN, R. R. and VOGEL, V. H.: Psychophysiological reactions following painful stimuli under hypnotic analgesia contrasted with gas anesthesia and novocain block. *J. Appl. Psychol.*, *22*:408, 1938.

29. BUELL, F. A. and BIEHL, J. P.: The influence of hypnosis on the tremor of Parkinson's disease. *Dis. Nerv. Sys.*, *10*:20, 1949.

30. BULL, N. and GIDRO-FRANK, L.: Emotions induced and studied in hypnotic subjects. *J. Nerv. & Ment. Dis.*, *112*:97, 1950.

31. CANGELLO, V. W.: The use of hypnotic suggestion for pain relief in malignant disease. *Int. J. Clin. & Exper. Hyp.*, *9*:17, 1961.

32. CHAPMAN, L. F., GOODELL, H. and WOLFF, H.: Changes in tissue vulnerability induced during hypnotic suggestion. *J. Psychosom. Res.*, *4*:99, 1956.

33. COHEN, M. E. and COBB, S.: The use of hypnosis in the study of the acid base balance of the blood in a patient with hysterical hyperventilation. *Res. Publ. Assoc. Res. Nerv. Ment. Dis.*, *19*:318, 1939.

34. CONN, J. H.: Cultural and clinical aspects of hypnosis, placebos, and suggestibility. *Int. J. Clin. & Exper. Hyp.*, 7:175, 1959.

35. CRAMER, H. and WITTKOWER, E.: Affektive Kreislaufveränderungen unter besonderer Berucksichtigung der Herzgrösse. *Klin. Wchnschr.*, 9:1290, 1930.

36. CRASILNECK, H. B. and FOGELMAN, M. J.: The effects of hypnosis on blood coagulation. *Int. J. Clin. & Exper. Hyp.*, 5:132, 1957.

37. CRASILNECK, H. B. and HALL, J. A.: Physiological changes associated with hypnosis: A review of the literature since 1948. *Int. J. Clin. & Exper. Hyp.*, 7:9, 1959.

38. CRASILNECK, H. B. and HALL, J. A.: Blood pressure and pulse rates in neutral hypnosis. *Int. J. Clin. & Exper. Hyp.*, 8:137, 1960.

39. DARROW, C. W., HENRY, C. E., GILL, M., BRENMAN, M. and CONVERSE, M.: Frontal-motor parallelism and motor-occipital in-phase activity in hypnosis, drowsiness and sleep. *EEG Clin. Neurophysiol.*, 2:355, 1950.

40. DARROW, C. W., HENRY, C. E., BRENMAN, M. and GILL, M.: Inter-area electroencephalographic relationships affected by hypnosis: preliminary report. *EEG Clin. Neurophysiol.*, 2:231, 1950.

41. DAVIS, H. and DAVIS, P. A.: The electrical activity of the brain: its relation to physiological states and to states of impaired consciousness. *Res. Publ. Assoc. Res. Nerv. Ment. Dis.*, 19:50, 1939.

42. DAVIS, R. C. and KANTOR, J. R.: Skin resistance during hypnotic states. *J. Gen. Psychol.*, 13:62, 1935.

43. DEMENT, W. and KLEITMAN, N.: Cyclic variations in EEG during sleep and their relation to eye movements, body motility, and dreaming. *EEG Clin. Neurophysiol.*, 9:673, 1957.

44. DEUTSCH, F. and KAUF, E.: Psycho-physische Kreinslaufstudien. II. Mitteilung. Über die Uraschen der Kreislaufstörungen bei den Herzneurosen. *Zeit. Ges. Exper. Med.*, 32:197, 1923.

45. DIAMANT, J., DUFEK, M., HOSKOVEC, J., KRISTOF, M., PEKAREK, V., ROTH, B. and VELEK, M.: An electroencephalographic study of the waking state and hypnosis with particular reference to subclinical manifestations of sleep activity. *Int. J. Clin. & Exper. Hyp.*, 8:199, 1960.

46. DORCUS, R. M.: Modification by suggestion of some vestibular and visual responses. *Am. J. Psychol.*, 49:82, 1937.

47. DOUPE, J., MILLER, W. R. and KELLER, W. K.: Vasomotor reactions in the hypnotic state. *J. Neurol. Neurosurg. & Psychiat.*, 2:97, 1939.

48. DUNCAN, I. W., DRESSLER, R. L., LYON-JAMES, S. and SEARS, A. B.: The search for an index of hypnosis. *J. Clin. & Exper. Hyp.*, 6:1, 1958.

49. DYNES, J. B.: An experimental study in hypnotic anesthesia. *J. Abn. Soc. Psychol.*, 27:79, 1932.

50. DYNES, J. B.: Objective method of distinguishing sleep from the hypnotic trance. *Arch. Neurol. & Psychiat.*, 57:84, 1947.

51. EDEL, J. W.: Nosebleed controlled by hypnosis. *Am. J. Clin. Hyp.*, 2:89, 1959.

52. EICHELBERG: Durch Hypnose erzeugtes "Hysterisches Fieber." *Deutsche Ztschr. Nervenh.*, 68:352, 1921.

53. EICHHORN, R. and TRACKTIR, J.: The effect of hypnosis upon gastric secretion. *Gastroenterology*, 29:417, 1955.

54. EICHHORN, R. and TRACKTIR, J.: The relationship between anxiety, hypnotically induced emotions and gastric secretion. *Gastroenterology*, 29:422, 1955.

55. EICHHORN, R. and TRACKTIR, J.: The effect of hypnotically induced emotions upon gastric secretion. *Gastroenterology*, 29:432, 1955.

56. ERICKSON, M. H.: Development of apparent unconsciousness during hypnotic reliving of a traumatic experience. *Arch. Neurol. & Psychiat.*, 38:1282, 1937.

57. ERICKSON, M. H.: A study of clinical and experimental findings on hypnotic deafness: I. Clinical experimentation and findings. *J. Gen. Psychol.*, 19:127, 1938.

58. ERICKSON, M. H.: A study of clinical and experimental findings on hypnotic deafness: II. Experimental findings with a contioned reflex technique. *J. Gen. Psychol.*, 19:151, 1938.

59. ERICKSON, M. H.: The induction of color blindness by a technique of hypnotic suggestion. *J. Gen. Psychol.*, 20:61, 1939.

60. ESTABROOKS, G. H.: The psychogalvanic reflex in hypnosis. *J. Gen. Psychol.*, 3:150, 1930.

61. EYSENCK, H. J.: An experimental study of the improvement of mental and physical functions in the hypnotic state. *Brit. J. Med. Psychol.*, 18:304, 1941.

62. FERSTER, C. B., LEVITT, E. E., ZIMMERMAN, J. and BRADY, J. P.: The measurement of hypnotic effects by operant-reinforcement techniques. *Psychol. Rec.*, 11:427, 1961.

63. FISHER, S.: An investigation of alleged conditioning phenomena under hypnosis. Unpublished doctoral dissertation, University of North Carolina, 1953.

64. FISHER, V. E.: Hypnotic suggestion and conditioned reflex. *J. Exp. Psychol., 15*:212, 1932.

65. FORD, L. F. and YEAGER, C. L.: Changes in the electroencephalogram in subjects under hypnosis. *Dis. Nerv. Sys., 9*:190, 1948.

66. FOREL, A. H.: *Hypnotism.* 5th ed. New York, Allied Book Co., 1927.

67. FRANCK, B. J.: L'Hypnose et l'EEG. *EEG Clin. Neurophysiol., 11*:107, 1950.

68. FRICK, H. L., SCANTLEBURY, R. E. and PATTERSON, T. L.: The control of gastric hunger contractions in man by hypnotic suggestion. *Am. J. Physiol., 113*:47, 1935.

69. FULDE, E.: Über den Einfluss hypnotischer Erregungszustande auf den Gasaustausch. *Zeit. Ges. Neurol. Psychiat., 159*:761, 1937.

70. GESSLER, H. and HANSEN, K.: Über die suggestive Beeinflussbarket der Warmeregulation in der hypnose. *Deutsche Arch. klin. Med., 156*:352, 1927.

71. GIDRO-FRANK, L. and BOWERS-BUCH, M. K.: A study of the plantar response in hypnotic age regression. *J. Nerv. & Ment. Dis., 107*:443, 1948.

72. GIDRO-FRANK, L. and BULL, N.: Emotions induced and studied in hypnotic subjects: Part I. The method. *J. Nerv. & Ment. Dis., 111*:91, 1950.

73. GIGON, A., AIGNER, E. and BRAUCH, W.: Über den Einfluss der Psyche auf körperliche Vorgänge. Hypnose und Blutzucker. *Schweiz. Med. Wchnschr., 56*:749, 1926.

74. GLASER, F.: Über den klinischen Nachweis psycho-physischer Reaktionen. Die appetitsaft-leucocytosen. *Med. Klin., 20*:535, 1924.

75. GLASER, F.: Psychische Beeinflussung des Blutserumkalkspiegels. *Klin. Wchnschr., 3*:1492, 1924.

76. GOLDIAMOND, I. and MALPASS, L. F.: Locus of hypnotically induced changes in color vision responses. *J. Opt. Soc. Amer., 51*:1117, 1961.

77. GOLDWYN, J.: Effect of hypnosis on basal metabolism. *Arch. Int. Med., 45*:109, 1930.

78. GORTON, B. E.: The physiology of hypnosis. I. A review of the literature. *Psychiat. Quart., 23*:317, 1949.

79. GORTON, B. E.: The physiology of hypnosis. II. A review of the literature. *Psychiat. Quart., 23*:458, 1949.

80. GRAFE, E. and MAYER, L.: Über den Einfluss der affekte auf den Gesamtstoffwechsel. *Zeit. Ges. Neurol. Psychiat., 86*:247, 1923.

81. GRAFE, E. and TRAUMANN: Zur frage des Einflusses Psychischer depressionen und der vorstellung Schwerer Muskelarbeit auf den Stoff-wechsel. (Untersuchungen in der hypnose.) *Zeit. Ges. Neurol. Psychiat., 62*:237, 1920.

82. GRASSHEIM, K. and WITTKOWER, E.: Suggestive modifications of the specific dynamic action of protein. *Deutsche Med. Wchnschr., 57*:141, 1931.

83. GRETHER, W. F.: A comment on "the induction of color blindness by a technique of hypnotic suggestion." *J. Gen. Psychol., 23*: 207, 1940.

84. GROSZ, H. J.: The relation of serum ascorbic acid level to adreno-cortical secretion during experimentally induced emotional stress in human subjects. *J. Psychosom. Res., 5*:253, 1961.

85. GUZE, H.: Hypnosis as a physiological state. In Bowers, M. K.: *Introductory Lectures in Medical Hypnosis.* New York, Institute for Research in Hypnosis, 1958.

86. GWARTNEY, R. H. and KRIKES, N.: Hypnosis in suppression of cough reflex. *New Eng. J. Med., 253*:561, 1955.

87. HAKEBUSH, BLINKOWSKI and FOUNDILLERE, R.: An attempt at a study of development of personality with the aid of hypnosis. *Trud. Inst. Psikhonevr., Kiev, 2*:236, 1930.

88. HARRIMAN, P. L.: Hypnotic induction of color vision anomalies: I. The use of the Ishihara and the Jensen tests to verify the acceptance of suggested color blindness. *J. Gen. Psychol., 27*:289, 1942.

89. HEILIG, R. and HOFF, H.: Beiträge zur hypnotischen Beeinflussung der Magenfunktion. *Med. Klin., 21*:162, 1925.

90. HEILIG, R. and HOFF, H.: Über hypnotische Beeinflussung der Nierenfunktion. *Deutsche Med. Wchnschr., 51*:1615, 1925.

91. HEILIG, R. and HOFF, H.: Psychische Beeinflussung von Organfunktionen insbesondere in der Hypnose. *Allg. Artz. Zeit. Psychotherap. Psych. Hyg., 1*:262, 1928.

92. HEILIG, R. and HOFF, H.: Über psychogene Entstehung des Herpes Labialis. *Med. Klin., 24*:1472, 1928.

93. HELFMAN, E., SHOR, R. E. and ORNE, M. T.: Physiological effects during hypnotically-requested emotions. Paper read before the American Psychological Association, Chicago, 1960.

94. HEYER, G.: Die Magensekretion beim Menschen. *Arch. Verdkrank.*, 27:226, 1921; 29:11, 1922.

95. HEYER, G.: Psychische Einflüsse auf die Motilität von Magen und Darm; zugleich ein Beitrag zur Gastroptosenfrage. *Klin. Wchnschr.*, 2:2274, 1923.

96. HOFF, H. and WERMER, P.: Untersuchungen über den Mechanismus der Diuresehemmung durch Pituitrin am Menschen. *Arch. Exper. Path. Pharmakol.*, 119:153, 1926.

97. HULL, C. L.: *Hypnosis and Suggestibility*. New York, Appleton-Century, 1933.

98. IKEMI, Y., AKAGI, M., MAEDA, J., FUKUMOTO, T., KAWATE, K., HIRAKAWA, K., GONDO, S., NAKAGAWA, T., HONDA, T., SAKAMOTO, A. and KUMAGAI, M.: Hypnotic experiments on the psychosomatic aspects of gastrointestinal disorders. *Int. J. Clin. & Exper. Hyp.*, 7:139, 1959.

99. JENNESS, A. and WIBLE, C. L.: Respiration and heart action in sleep and hypnosis. *J. Gen. Psychol.*, 16:197, 1937.

100. KIRKNER, F. J.: Control of sensory and perceptive functions by hypnosis. In Dorcus, R. M.: *Hypnosis and Its Therapeutic Applications*. New York, McGraw-Hill, 1956.

101. KLINE, M. V.: The transcendence of waking visual discrimination capacity with hypnosis: a preliminary case report. *Brit. J. Med. Hyp.*, 4:32, 1953.

102. KLINE, M. V.: Hypnotic age regression. *Dis. Nerv. Sys.*, 22:1961.

103. KLINE, M. V. and GUZE, H.: The alteration of oral temperature through hypnotic techniques: 1. Pilot experimentation. *J. Clin. & Exper. Hyp.*, 2:233, 1954.

104. KLINE, M. V., GUZE, H. and HAGGERTY, A. D.: An experimental study of the nature of hypnotic deafness: effects of delayed speech feedback. *J. Clin. & Exper. Hyp.*, 2:145, 1954.

105. KOSTER, S.: Experimental investigation of the character of hypnosis. *J. Clin. & Exper. Hyp.*, 2:42, 1954.

106. KRETSCHMER, M. and KRÜRER, R.: Über die Beeinflussung des Serumkalkgehaltes in der Hypnose. *Klin. Wchnschr.*, 6:695, 1927.

107. KROGER, W. S.: Hypnosis in obstetrics and gynecology. In Schneck, J. M.: *Hypnosis in Modern Medicine*, 2nd ed. Springfield, Thomas, 1959.

108. KROGER, W. S.: Hypnoanesthesia in surgery. *West. J. Surg. Obstet. Gyn., 68*:25, 1960.

109. KRYUNTSEL, A. A.: Effect of hypnotic suggestion on blood coagulation. *Klin. Med., 10*:842, 1932.

110. KUPPER, H. I.: Psychic concomitants in wartime injuries. *Psychosom. Med., 7*:15, 1945.

111. LANE, A. and RUSKIN, A.: Failure in labile essential hypertension. *Texas Rep. Biol. Med., 8*:66, 1950.

112. LECRON, L. M.: The loss during hypnotic age regression of an established conditioned reflex. *Psychiat. Quart., 26*:657, 1952.

113. LECRON, L. M.: A study of age regression under hypnosis. In LeCron, L. M.: *Experimental Hypnosis*. New York, Macmillan, 1952.

114. LEUBA, C.: Images as conditioned sensations. *J. Exper. Psychol., 26*:345, 1940.

115. LEUBA, C.: The use of hypnosis for controlling variables in psychological experiments. *J. Abn. Soc. Psychol., 36*:271, 1941.

116. LEVIN, S. and EGOLINSKY, I. A.: The effect of cortical function upon energy changes in basal metabolism. *Fiziol. Zhur., 20*: 979, 1936.

117. LEVINE, M.: Electrical skin resistance during hypnosis. *Arch. Neurol. & Psychiat., 24*:937, 1930.

118. LEVINE, M.: Psychogalvanic reaction to painful stimuli in hypnotic and hysterical anesthesia. *Bull. Johns Hopkins Hosp., 46*:331, 1930.

119. LEVITT, E. E. and HERSHMAN, S.: The clinical practice of hypnosis in the United States: a survey. Paper read at the XIV International Congress of Applied Psychology, Copenhagen, 1961.

120. LEVITT, E. E. and PERSKY, H.: Relation of Rorschach factors and plasma hydrocortisone level in hypnotically induced anxiety. *Psychosom. Med., 22*:218, 1960.

121. LONDON, P. and FUHRER, M.: Hypnosis, motivation and performance. *J. Pers., 29*:321, 1961.

122. LOOMIS, A. L., HARVEY, E. N. and HOBART, G.: Brain potentials during hypnosis. *Science, 83*:239, 1936.

123. LOOMIS, A. L., HARVEY, E. N. and HOBART, G.: Electrical potentials of the human brain. *J. Exp. Psychol., 19*:249, 1936.

124. LOVETT DOUST, J. W.: Studies on the physiology of awareness: oxiometric analysis of emotion and the differential planes of consciousness seen in hypnosis. *J. Clin. & Exper. Psychopathol., 14*:113, 1953.

125. LUCKHARDT, A. B. and JOHNSTON, R. L.: Studies in gastric secretion: 1. The psychic secretion of gastric juice under hypnosis. *Am. J. Physiol.*, *70*:174, 1924.

126. LUNDHOLM, H.: An experimental study of functional anesthesia as induced by suggestion in hypnosis. *J. Abn. Soc. Psychol.*, *23*:338, 1928.

127. LUNDHOLM, H.: A new laboratory neurosis. *Charact. Pers.*, *9*:11, 1940.

128. LUNDHOLM, H. and LÖWENBACH, H.: Hypnosis and the alpha activity of the electroencephalogram. *Charact. Pers.*, *11*:145, 1942.

129. McCRANIE, E. J. and CRASILNECK, H. B.: The electroencephalogram in hypnotic age regression. *Psychiat. Quart.*, *29*:85, 1955.

130. McCRANIE, E. J. and CRASILNECK, H. B.: The conditioned reflex in hypnotic age regression. *J. Clin. & Exper. Psychopath.*, *16*:120, 1955.

131. McDOWELL, M.: Juvenile warts removed with the use of hypnotic suggestion. *Bull. Menninger Clin.*, *13*:124, 1949.

132. McDOWELL, M.: Hypnosis in dermatology. In Schneck, J. M.: *Hypnosis in Modern Medicine*, 2nd ed. Springfield, Thomas, 1959.

133. MALMO, R. B., BOAG, T. J. and RAGINSKY, B. B.: Electromyographic study of hypnotic deafness. *J. Clin. & Exper. Hyp.*, *2*:305, 1954.

134. MANZER, C. W.: The effect of verbal suggestion on output and variability of muscular work. *Psychol. Clin.*, *22*:248, 1934.

135. MARCHAND, H.: Die Suggestion der Warme in Oberbauch und ihr Einfluss auf Blutzucker und Leukozyten. *Psychother.*, *1*: 154, 1958.

136. MARCUS, H. and SAHLGREN, E.: Untersuchungen über die Einwirkung der hypnotischen Suggestion auf die Funktion des Vegetativen Systems. I. Mitteilung. *München Med. Wchnschr.*, *72*:381, 1925.

137. MARINESCO, G., SAGER, O. and KREINDLER, A.: Etudes electroencephalographiques. Le sommeil natural et le sommeil hypnotique. *Bull. Acad. Med.*, *117*:273, 1937.

138. MARX, H.: Untersuchungen über den Wasserhaushalt. II. Mitteilung. Die Psychische Beeinflussung des Wasserhaushaltes. *Klin. Wchnschr.*, *5*:92, 1926.

139. MEAD, S. and ROUSH, E. S.: A study of the effect of hypnotic suggestion on physiologic performance. *Arch. Phys. Med., 30*: 700, 1949.

140. MIHALYKA, E. E. and WHANGER, A. D.: Objective tinnitus aurium hypnotically treated. *Am. J. Clin. Hyp., 2*:85, 1959.

141. MOHR, F.: *Psychophysische Behandlungsmethoden.* Leipzig, Hirzel, 1925.

142. MOSS, A. A.: Hypnodontics. In LeCron, L. M.: *Experimental Hypnosis.* New York, Macmillan, 1952.

143. NICHOLSON, N. C.: Notes on muscular work during hypnosis. *Bull. Johns Hopkins Hosp., 31*:89, 1920.

144. NIELSEN, O. J. and GEERT-JORGENSEN, E.: Untersuchungen über die Einwirkung der hypnotischen Suggestion auf den Blutzucker bei Nichtdiabetikern. *Klin. Wchnschr., 7*:1457, 1928.

145. NEMTZOVA, O. L. and SCHATTENSTEIN, D. I.: The effect of the central nervous system upon some physiological processes during work. *Fiziol. Zhur., 20*:581, 1936.

146. NORRIS, A. and HUSTON, P.: Raynaud's disease studied by hypnosis. *Dis. Nerv. Sys., 17*:163, 1956.

147. ORNE, M. T.: The nature of hypnosis: artifact and essence. *J. Abn. Soc. Psychol., 58*:277, 1959.

148. OWEN-FLOOD, A.: Hypnotism in epilepsy. *Brit. J. Med. Hyp., 3*: 49, 1952.

149. PASQUARELLI, B. and BELLAK, L.: A case of co-existence of idiopathic, epileptic, and psychogenic convulsions. *Psychosom. Med., 9*:137, 1947.

150. PATTIE, F. A.: A report of attempts to produce uniocular blindness by hypnotic suggestion. *Brit. J. Med. Psychol., 15*:230, 1935.

151. PATTIE, F. A.: The production of blisters by hypnotic suggestion: a review. *J. Abn. Soc. Psychol., 36*:62, 1941.

152. PATTIE, F. A.: The genuineness of unilateral deafness produced by hypnosis. *Am. J. Psychol., 63*:84, 1950.

153. PERSKY, H., GROSZ, H. J., NORTON, J. A. and McMURTRY, M.: Effect of hypnotically-induced anxiety on the plasma hydrocortisone level of normal subjects. *J. Clin. Endocrinol. Metab., 19*:700, 1959.

154. POLZIEN, P.: Die Anderung der Temperaturregulation bei der Gesamtumschaltung durch das autogene Training. Ein physikalischer Nackweis des hypnotischen Zustands. *Zeit. Ges. Exp. Med., 125*:469, 1955.

155. POVORINSKIJ, J. A. and FINNE, W. N.: Der Wechsel des Zucker-gehaltes des Blutes unter dem Einfluss einer Hypnotisch Sug-gerierten Vorstellung. *Zeit. Ges. Neurol. Psychiat., 129*:135, 1930.

156. PRONKO, N. H. and HILL, H.: A study of differential stimulus function in hypnosis. *J. Psychol., 27*:49, 1949.

157. RAGINSKY, B. B.: The use of hypnosis in the treatment of medical and surgical conditions. In Bowers, M. K.: *Introductory Lectures in Medical Hypnosis.* New York, The Institute for Research in Hypnosis, 1958.

158. RAGINSKY, B. B.: Temporary cardiac arrest induced under hyp-nosis. *Int. J. Clin. & Exper. Hyp., 7*:53, 1959.

159. RAVITZ, L. J.: Electrometric correlates of the hypnotic state. *Science, 112*:341, 1950.

160. RAVITZ, L. J.: Standing potential correlates of hypnosis and nar-cosis. *Arch. Neurol. Psychiat., 65*:413, 1951.

161. REITER, P. J.: The influence of hypnosis on somatic fields of function. In LeCron, L. M.: *Experimental Hypnosis.* New York, Macmillan, 1952.

162. REYNOLDS, S. R. M.: Uterine contractility and cervical dilatation. *Proc. Roy. Soc. Med., 44*:695, 1951.

163. ROHMER, F. and ISRAEL, L.: L'electroencephalogramme dans le training autogene. *Rev. Neurolog., 96*:559, 1957.

164. ROSENHAN, D. and LONDON, P.: Hypnosis: expectation, suscepti-bility and performance. *J. Abn. Soc. Psychol.,* 1962. In Press.

165. ROUSH, E. S.: Strength and endurance in the waking and hyp-notic state. *J. Appl. Physiol., 3*:404, 1951.

166. SAMPIMON, R. L. H. and WOODRUFF, M. F.: Some observations concerning the use of hypnosis as a substitute for anesthesia. *Med. J. Australia, 1*:393, 1946.

167. SARBIN, T. R.: Physiological effects of hypnotic stimulation. In Dorcus, R. M.: *Hypnosis and Its Therapeutic Applications.* New York, McGraw-Hill, 1956.

168. SCANTLEBURY, R. E.: The effect of psychic phenomena on the movements of the empty stomach of man. *Grad. Stud. Monogr. Sci. Wayne Univ., 1*:32, 1940.

169. SCHAZILLO, B. A. and ABRAMOV, N. P.: Über die Wirkung der Hypnose auf das Verhaltnis der K-und Ca-Elektrolyte im Blutserum. *Zeit. Ges. Neurol. Psychiat., 112*:54, 1928.

170. SCHIFF, S. K., BUNNEY, W. E. and FREEDMAN, D. X.: A study of ocular movements in hypnotically induced dreams. *J. Nerv. & Ment. Dis., 133*:59, 1961.

171. SCHWARZ, B. E., BICKFORD, R. G. and RASMUSSEN, W. C.: Hypnotic phenomena including hypnotically activated seizures, studied with the electroencephalogram. *J. Nerv. & Ment. Dis., 122*:564, 1955.

172. SCOTT, H. D.: Hypnosis and the conditioned reflex. *J. Gen. Psychol., 4*:113, 1930.

173. SEARS, A. B. and BEATTY, J. M.: A comparison of the galvanic skin response in the hypnotic and waking state. *J. Clin. & Exper. Hyp., 4*:49, 1956.

174. SEARS, R. R.: Experimental study of hypnotic anesthesia. *J. Exper. Psychol., 15*:1, 1932.

175. SECTER, I. I.: Some notes on controlling the exaggerated gag reflex. *Am. J. Clin. Hyp., 2*:150, 1960.

176. SIRNA, A. J.: An electroencephalographic study of the hypnotic dream. *J. Psychol., 20*:109, 1945.

177. SOLOVEY, G. and MILECHNIN, A.: Concerning the nature of hypnotic phenomena. *J. Clin. & Exper. Hyp., 5*:67, 1957.

178. STEIN, T.: Über die Hypnotische Beeinflussung des Blutzuckers, des Natrium und Chlorgehaltes des Blutes. Inaug. Diss. Basel, 1929.

179. STERN, J. A., WINOKUR, G., GRAHAM, D. T. and GRAHAM, F. K.: Alterations in physiological measures during experimentally induced attitudes. *J. Psychosom. Res., 5*:73, 1961.

180. STOKVIS, B.: Der Einfluss der Hypnose auf den Puls. *Schweiz. Med. Wchnschr., 19*:764, 1938.

181. STOLZENBERG, J.: Clinical application of hypnosis in producing hypno-anesthesia control of hemorrhage and salivation during surgery: a case report. *J. Clin. & Exper. Hyp., 3*:24, 1955.

182. SUZUKI, Y., IWATSUKI, K., SATO, I., HARIU, T. and KIKUCHI, T.: Application of hypnosis and suggestion in anesthesiology. *Tohuku Psychol. Folia, 20*:35, 1961.

183. TALBERT, G. A., READY, F. L. and KUHLMAN, F. W.: Plethysomographic and pneumographic observations made in hypnosis. *Am. J. Physiol., 68*:113, 1924.

184. THOMAS, A. T. G.: Hypnotherapy in medical treatment. *E. African Med. J., 32*:345, 1955.

185. TRUE, R. M. and STEPHENSON, C. W.: Controlled experiments

correlating electroencephalogram, pulse, and plantar reflexes with hypnotic age regression and induced emotional states. *Pers., 1*:252, 1951.

186. ULETT, G., STERN, J. A., EDMONDSTON, W. E. and LEVITSKY, A.: The GSR in experimental amnesia. Paper read before the American Society of Clinical Hypnosis, 1961.

187. ULLMAN, M.: Herpes simplex and second degree burn induced under hypnosis. *Am. J. Psychiat., 103*:828, 1947.

188. VAN PELT, S. J.: The control of the heart rate by hypnotic suggestion. In LeCron, L. M.: *Experimental Hypnosis*. New York, Macmillan, 1952.

189. VAN PELT, S. J.: Hypnosis and baldness. *Brit. J. Med. Hyp., 7*:14, 1956.

190. VOLGYESI, F. A.: *Hypnosetherapie und Psychosomatische Problems*. Stuttgart, Hippokrates, 1950.

191. VON EIFF, A. W.: Über die Moglichkeit einer Grundumsatzenkung durch Psychische Beeinflussung. *Artzl. Forsch., 4*:611, 1950.

192. VON EIFF, A. W.: Der Einfluss der Hypnose auf Temperaturempfindung und Warmeregulation. *Zeit. Ges. Experimentelle Med., 117*:261, 1951.

193. WALDEN, E. C.: A plethysmographic study of the vascular conditions during hypnotic sleep. *Am. J. Physiol., 4*:124, 1900.

194. WALLACE, G. and COPPOLINO, C. A.: Hypnosis in anesthesiology. *New York State J. Med., 60*:3258, 1960.

195. WALLIS, G. G.: Metabolic rate, hypnosis and thiopentone. *J. Roy. Nav. Med. Serv., 37*:48, 1951.

196. WEINBERG, A., CAMMER, L. and DELL'ARIA, S.: A preliminary report on hypnosis as an anesthetic agent in electroconvulsive therapy with succinyl choline. *J. Neuropsychiat., 2*:178, 1961.

197. WEITZENHOFFER, A. M.: The discriminatory recognition of visual patterns under hypnosis. *J. Abn. Soc. Psychol., 46*:388, 1951.

198. WEITZENHOFFER, A. M. and HILGARD, E. R.: *Stanford Hypnotic Susceptibility Scale*. Palo Alto, Consulting Psychologists Press, 1959.

199. WEITZENHOFFER, A. M. and MOORE, R. K.: Influence of certain hypnotic suggestions upon a type of visual illusion: preliminary report. *Psychol. Rep., 11*:137, 1960.

200. WELLER, C., LINDNER, M., NULAND, W. and KLINE, M. V.: The effects of hypnotically-induced emotions on continuous, un-

interrupted blood glucose measurements. *Psychosomatics, 2*: 1, 1961.

201. WELLS, W. R.: The hypnotic treatment of the major symptoms of hysteria: a case study. *J. Psychol., 77*:269, 1944.

202. WELLS, W. R.: Expectancy versus performance in hypnosis. *J. Gen. Psychol., 35*:99, 1947.

203. WERBEL, E. W.: Experiences with frequent use of hypnosis in a general surgical practice. *West. J. Surg., Obst. & Gynec., 68*: 190, 1960.

204. WEST, L. J., NIELL, K. C. and HARDY, J. D.: Effects of hypnotic suggestion on pain perception and galvanic skin response. *Arch. Neurol. & Psychiat., 68*:549, 1952.

205. WHEELER, W. M., LITTLE, K., DORCUS, R. M., CLEMENS, T. L., STERNBERG, T. H. and ZIMMERMAN, M. C.: The effects of psychological stress as measured by a decrease in the number of circulating eosinophiles. *J. Clin. & Exper. Hyp., 2*:130, 1954.

206. WHITE, M. M.: Blood pressure and palmar galvanic changes in normal and hypnotic states. *Psychol. Bull., 37*:577, 1940.

207. WHITEHORN, J. C.: Physiological changes in emotional states. *Res. Pub. Assoc. Res. Nerv. & Ment. Dis., 19*:1939.

208. WHITEHORN, J. C., LUNDHOLM, H. and GARDNER, G. E.: Metabolic rate in emotional moods induced by suggestion in hypnosis. *Am. J. Psychiat., 9*:661, 1929.

209. WHITEHORN, J. C., LUNDHOLM, H., FOX, E. L. and BENEDICT, F. G.: Metabolic rate in "hypnotic sleep." *New Eng. J. Med., 206*: 777, 1932.

210. WIBLE, C. L. and JENNESS, A.: Electrocardiograms during sleep and hypnosis. *J. Psychol., 1*:235, 1936.

211. WILLIAMS, G. W.: The effect of hypnosis on muscular fatigue. *J. Abn. Soc. Psychol., 24*:318, 1929.

212. WILLIAMS, G. W.: A comparative study of voluntary and hypnotic catalepsy. *Am. J. Psychol., 42*:83, 1930.

213. WITTKOWER, E.: Über den Einfluss der Affekte auf den Gallefluss. *Klin. Wchnschr., 7*:2193, 1928.

214. WITTKOWER, E.: Über Affektiv-Somatische Veranderungen. II. Mitteilung: Die Affektleu-kozytose. *Klin. Wchnschr., 8*: 1082, 1929.

215. WITTKOWER, E. and PETOW, H.: Beiträge zur Klinik des Asthma Bronchiale und Verwandter Zustände. V. Zur Psychogenese des Asthma Bronchiale. *Zeit. klin. Med., 119*:293, 1931.

216. WOLBERG, L. R.: *Medical Hypnosis.* New York, Grune and Stratton, 1948.
217. WOLFF, H. G. and GOODELL, H.: The relation of attitude and suggestion to the perception of and reaction to pain. *Res. Publ. Assoc. Res. Nerv. & Ment. Dis., 22*:434, 1943.
218. YOUNG, P. C.: An experimental study of mental and physical functions in the normal and hypnotic states. *Am. J. Psychol., 36*:214, 1925.
219. YOUNG, P. C.: An experimental study of mental and physical functions in the normal and hypnotic states: additional results. *Am. J. Psychol., 37*:345, 1926.
220. ZIKMUND, V.: Príspevok k liecbe alkoholizmu hypnózou. *Bratislavske Lekárs, 36*:267, 1956.
221. ZYNKIN, A. M.: Blood pressure in hypnosis. *Psikotherapia, 123*: 141, 1930.

11

PSYCHODYNAMICS OF HYPNOTIC INDUCTION AND TERMINATION

JOHN G. WATKINS, M.S., PH.D.

The more intensely one becomes involved in the study of hypnosis the more one is drawn to the view that the response of entering an hypnotic state, deepening and terminating the condition is intimately related to the inter-personal communications between hypnotist and subject and to the motivational needs of both. The amateur tends to think of hypnosis as simply a state entered by the subject in reaction to certain passes or other cues provided by the hypnotist. Such a beginner often shows the greatest interest in reading and memorizing "techniques" completely oblivious to the fact that it is the meaning of the inter-personal interaction implied in a so-called "technique" and not the simple stimulus value of certain words which is of most significance in determining the kind and extent of the hypnotic response.

DEFINITION OF PSYCHODYNAMICS

That psychological sub-science which deals with the complex of unconscious motivational patterns in the determination of behavior has been termed *psychodynamics* (55). It considers presumed cause and effect relationships in psychic life. Thus, the origin of a type of behavior may lie far from the actual response, so far that neither the subject nor nearby observers suspect its true cause. Like the music in a popular song of some years ago: "You push the first valve down. The music goes round and around, and it comes out here." Psychodynamics is the study of the "round and round."

Let us consider a simple, illustrative example. The promiscuous, Don Juan-type lover has been renowned in literature and opera. At superficial glance he seems to be quite a man. After all, he has possessed many women. One might think that he would be very proud of his masculinity. However, it turns out from the psychodynamic viewpoint that quite the opposite prevails. The Don Juan is a very insecure male, doubting his potency, uncertain of his masculinity, and at unconscious levels defending himself against latent feminine or homosexual drives. His seductive behavior is necessary as a constant proof to himself that he really is masculine. Each conquest temporarily allays this inner anxiety but does not last long. He is driven to seek a new conquest to quell the small inner voice which whispers that he is really not a man. Only from such a psychodynamic point of view can we understand his behavior, deal with it rationally, and help him with an appropriate treatment strategy which will restore to him a sense of confidence that he is truly what he was structurally born to be—a man. Once he has acquired this new understanding, genuine hetero-sexual love becomes possible. A meaningful relationship with a woman replaces his promiscuity.

Similarly, the hypnotic subject reacts in an inter-personal relationship situation to the hypnotist via the communications received during what is called "induction." He enters trance. He does not enter trance. Or he does so, but only lightly. Through the study of psychodynamics we are trying to understand the complex of inner and outer motivations which cause him to make the response he does—and to learn to control these more effectively with the aim of increasing the likelihood that he will respond with an hypnotic state deep enough for the effective application of various beneficial hypnotherapeutic techniques (9, 10).

HYPNOSIS AS A STATE OF REGRESSION

Various writers (Kline 29, 30, Gill and Brenman 22, Meares 35) have emphasized that hypnosis may be viewed both as a state and as a relationship. As a state it has a number of specific characteristics such as lowered criticality, diminished intellectual control, less emotional inhibition, and a return to childish patterns of behavior. This return can be described as a regression (3).

During sleep, illness, psychosis and psychoneurosis we "regress," hence, return to earlier and simpler patterns of response. Sometimes this regression is forced upon an individual. He is confronted with environmental demands which overwhelm his ego, and he is unable to cope with them. His ego suffers a devastating annihilation. Psychosis results. However, in most cases the ego, like the good military commander, knows enough to withdraw from the scene of battle when faced with superior forces. It pulls back, shortens its lines of responsibility, and by conserving its energies within a simpler existence prevents its total destruction. In choosing to do this, such as in normal sleep, the ego rests and awaits the time when with renewed srtength and vigor it can venture back to the arena of human struggle. This is called "regression in the service of the ego" (23).

Gill and Brenman (21, 22) have described hypnosis as a kind of regression in the service of the ego. It must be considered first as happening because of the existence of certain psychic pressures within the hypnotic relationship, and second as representing a return to a more primitive form of psychic functioning characterized by the behavior found in the child or in primitive peoples. Meares (35) has termed this "atavistic regression."

FACTORS INFLUENCING HYPNOTIC REGRESSION

Therefore, when inducing and deepening hypnotic trance we are very much concerned with understanding the factors which will initiate regressive trends in our patient, how these can be stimulated, and how controlled. It will be noted that all the methods of trance induction represent techniques for initiating psychic regression. Gill and Brenman (22) classify these under two headings: 1. By sensorimotor-ideational deprivation, or, 2. By the stimulation of an archaic (hence transference) relationship to the hypnotist. Putting it another way, we regress when we do not receive adequate stimulation from the environment to cause us to live in the reality of the external present; and we regress when we are in intimate inter-personal contact with one who through transference represents early authoritative figures toward whom we have established primitive and childish patterns of response. The psychodynamic approach to hypnotic induction will, of course, concern itself with both avenues, but it is in the second where it is prepared to make its greatest contribution to our understanding and therapeutic skill.

Let us compare the induction of the regression of sleep with the induction of the regression of hypnosis (1, 33). In order to sleep we restrict our sensori-motor input. The room is darkened. We lie still. We are made warm by covers and when possible protected from undue skin stimuli by smooth, non-scratchy sheets. We do not talk, and we do not want to listen to the sounds of others. In this absence of stimuli the ego withdraws its energies from the sensory organs and nearly eliminates its communication with the outside world.

Within, conscious thoughts fade and are gradually replaced by those bits of more archaic mental material called dreams in which the logic (or rather psychologic) proceeds according to the rules which govern unconscious or primary-process thinking. The dream becomes like the psychosis, irrational, concretistic, illogical, yet still subject to various ego defensive maneuvers. The ego vacillates between the external world which demands social-reality behavior, and the inner world of primitive drives, which the psychoanalysts call the Id. At this stage the state of the regression is not unlike that which obtains during deep hypnosis. In fact, there have been many studies comparing ordinary dreaming with hypnotic dreaming (6, 16, 20, 27, 38, 46, 52).

As the ego energies (cathexes) are further withdrawn from the dreamer's ego, mental activity becomes less and less, and may finally approach a deep state of coma in which only the continuation of minimal, vital organic functions indicate that the individual still exists. Erickson (14) has described such a state of "plenary trance" which he has induced through prolonged induction procedures in a few subjects.

These various stages also appear as the ego is regressed chemically through the anesthetization of its functions on the surgical operating table. And studies on sensori-deprivation (4) have shown that the individual so deprived experiences hallucinations and similar mental phenomena, even as the sleeper dreams, and the hypnotized subject vivifies or hallucinates inner past or suggested experiences.

In the hypnotic induction we facilitate this regression by telling our patient to do such things as stare at a fixed point (restricting his sources of visual stimulation), asking that he attend to the relaxation in his muscles (lowering his motor activities), calling his attention to involuntary actions such as eye-closure or hand levitation, hence, demonstrating to him that increasing parts of his body are becoming de-egotized and are no longer subject to voluntary control. We suggest his falling during a standing, body-sway approach (dis-orienting his kinesthetic and equilibratory sense contacts with reality). Or we ask him to preoccupy himself with a soothing inner fantasy which stresses comfort, rest and peace—again pushing away the outer world. In so doing, the hypnotist tips the balance between the intellectual controls of the ego and the inner press of more primitive needs. The patient regresses. He relaxes. His eyes usually close. He relinquishes to a considerable extent direction of his mental processes by his own ego and permits increased activity to be initiated by sources outside of his ego, e.g., suggestions of the hypnotist, and the unegotized impulses of his unconscious self, or their related derivatives. The hypnotized person is not exactly child, nor psychotic, nor just dreaming, but he demonstrates behavior which is closely related to all of these.

His hypnotic productions often appear like the reactions of a dissociated person such as are found in the multiple personality or fugue state. It is not surprising that most multiple personalities have been studied through hypno-analytic procedures (5, 36) since in the hypnotic state it is so easy to induce the various personalities to appear or disappear.

We often forget that the induction procedure is a communication between two parties, and it is the *meaning*, the essential inner significance of each communicative act which determines our subject's response, not the fact of the administration of the technique. To close the eyes means to one person that he is to rest, to another, that he is to ignore the outer world, to a third, that something is to be "put over" on him without his control, to another, to die, to another to pretend or to imagine, etc. Not only may each hypnotic subject interpret the meaning of each suggestion differently, but a single subject may interpret the suggestion one way when given by hypnotist A, who is viewed as a helper, and another way when the same suggestion is administered by hypnotist B, who is viewed as an exploiter. These two different attitudes may have been determined by differences in the real behavior of the two hypnotists, or by the inner, personal (transference) attitudes stimulated within the subject by two different people who possess different physical and psychological characteristics.

HYPNOTIC INDUCTION AS A METHOD OF EVALUATING THE PATIENT

A subject may react to a standardized procedure differently from time to time because of a change in ego state. A young woman being treated hypnoanalytically had been trained to respond with a medium-deep trance in about five minutes of suggestions involving eye-fixation, relaxation and the dropping of her arm. At one session she reported late, much disturbed because the newspapers had been carrying the account of a sadistic murder in which a young woman had been killed, her body cut into pieces and strewn about the community. The patient reacted to the usual trance induction with great anxiety, fidgeting, and resistance. Very slowly she involved herself in the hypnotic regression. Toward the end of the induction procedure the hypnotist had usually lifted her arm by the wrist, suggested that at the count of twelve, when he dropped her hand, that as it fell into her lap she would "fall" into a profoundly deep state. This time as he touched her wrist, she shrieked and shrunk away.

No further attempts were made to deepen the trance until she had been asked about her fears. She indicated that today she perceived her therapist as a potential, sadistic murderer, not as a helper. She was frightened. Following the full airing of this feeling under the light trance state she relaxed. A deeper state could be induced, and it proved to be one which was fruitful with the production of much significant material. On emerging, she stated that when coming to the therapeutic office she had seen a child's

shoe lying beside the walk and immediately felt frightened, perceiv-
ing it as an amputated foot. Had the hypnotist failed to be sensitive
to her changed reaction and proceeded mechanically with the
usual suggestions there might have been an overwhelming, traumatic fear response, perhaps even a termination of treatment. By
interrupting the induction to inquire into this source of anxiety,
not only was it possible to resolve the matter and induce a productive hypnotic state, but also much of value was learned regarding
her own psychodynamic needs as they were being transferred (projected) onto the hypnoanalyst and the hypno-analytic situation.

We shall not concern ourselves here with the full meaning of
this reaction to the sadistic news event and its significance within
her own neurosis, but rather with its impact on the process of trance
induction. What started as a resistance to the hour's work became
a valuable source of new understanding and progress.

Thus, we see that the psychodynamic situation in the hypnotic
relationship varies from subject to subject, from hypnotist to hypnotist, and within a given hypnotist-subject gestalt from time to
time. The mechanical application of any induction procedure,
however initially effective, loses much of its therapeutic efficacy
when the therapist fails to be sensitive to the subtle psychodynamic
inter-play within the regressive, hypnotic relationship.

SPECIAL MEANINGS OF THE HYPNOTIC STATE TO THE PATIENT (11, 13, 15, 19, 58)

Let us move to consideration of some of the special personal
meanings which hypnosis can have for various patients. To relax,
either in chair or on couch, to relinquish defensive postures, and
to give one's self over to the suggestions of another can mean to
involve one's self in a state of submission. This same meaning may
arise in the patient undergoing relaxation on the psychoanalytic
couch. Both submissive needs and fears are stimulated. However,
two different people, both of whom equate being hypnotized to
submitting one's self to another, may still react to it quite differently. To one, this is an enjoyable experience wherein he is no
longer held accountable for his actions or fantasies. He is freed
of any guilt. The hypnotist must take the blame for whatever

transpires. Such a person welcomes the hypnotic experience and may sink rapidly into a very deep trance.

However, to another, who has devoted his life to the struggle for independence, to whom dependence on another or submission to another constitutes a real threat (one could be taken advantage of), the induction becomes the signal for a battle of "wills." He must show the doctor that he is resolute and cannot be imposed upon. Unconsciously he views himself as the Rock of Gibraltar, impregnable in the face of an assault on the integrity of his ego which is perceived as dangerous and malevolent. He is resistant, and either unhypnotizable, or hypnotizable only with great difficulty. His resistance must be recognized, and either by-passed through appropriate technique and manner, over-powered through superior skill and the mobilization of stronger motivations, or analyzed and worked-through to reduce its efficacy in the prevention of the hypnotic state.

The recognition of the fact of this resistance should be possible for all experienced hypnotherapists; the understanding of its significance to the patient and the initiation of measures for dealing with it constructively can often be handled by any sensitive therapist. However, the approach to it through analysis and "working-through" is generally a job for the analytically-trained psychotherapist.

HYPNOSIS AS AN EROTIC FANTASY EXPERIENCE (48, 50, 58)

Some subjects may welcome the hypnotic state as a situation in which one is free to enjoy pleasurable fantasies, often erotic. During a regression the later-formed psychic structures tend to be eliminated first, hence, the super-ego (conscience) controls may be lessened, then the ego defenses, leaving infantile and erotic impulses more free to gain fantasy expression. This lowering of inhibition is characteristic of hypnosis. Sometimes the temptation to enter a trance state becomes so pleasurable that the patient undergoes either spontaneous inductions, or inductions on the slightest provocation. This is similar to the tendency in the schizoid or pre-schizophrenic person who finds indulging in fantasy life more pleasant than real existence. Such a tendency in an hypnotic subject is probably not healthy and would be a contra-indication for continued use of hypnosis. In this case the regression is no longer temporary and in the service of the ego but is a tendency toward a permanent, pathological state.

Often the patient interprets the hypnotic induction as either a prelude to sexual seduction, or as itself a symbolic seduction. This mobilizes both wishes and fears. Whether the subject who perceives it thus enters the hypnotic state or not will depend on the relative balance between the wish to be seduced and the fear of being seduced. Once such a patient has received adequate reassurances of protection from that which he fears, his unconscious erotic wish serves as a strong motivating agent facilitating the inductive process.

FEARS OF DEATH

The fear of death is universal. Few people are able to master this fear. Federn (17) has stated that the ego cannot accept or face its own non-existence. The problems inherent in conflicts over approaching death have had some, but inadequate, attention from psychotherapists (12, 45, 47, 49). Death is equated with the loss of ego, stillness, immovability and the end of volition. Accordingly, it is not surprising that some subjects view the hypnotic state as if it were a condition of non-existence. As their fears of death are mobilized their resistance to induction increases. Some people are afraid to sleep because they think they may die during their sleep. Ordinarily though, when hypnosis is equated with sleep it becomes acceptable, because all people have experienced sleep, and it is considered normal in the average person.

Since the trance state is meaningful in itself there lies imbedded within the patient both the nucleus of resistance and the acceptance of welcome involvement depending on this inner significance. We should note that while it is advantageous for the practitioner to be aware as much as possible of the psychodynamic significance of the hypnotic state to his patient, it is not usually desirable that this "insight" be transmitted to the patient. Meares (35) has warned against the stimulation of intellectual and critical modes of thinking during the induction process. It is precisely the elimination of such (mature and recently-formed) observant mental attitudes which are essential for the adequate regression of the ego to the state of more archaic functioning called hypnosis. Immediately following an induction, however, it is sometimes helpful to inquire indirectly of the patient as to his feelings and reactions during the induction stage, and as to those communications from the therapist which most facilitated or impeded his deeper involvement in the hypnotic state.

HYPNOSIS AS RELATIONSHIP (10, 18, 19, 22, 53, 58)

Not only the *state* of hypnosis, but also, the *hypnotic relationship* and any interactive communications between doctor and patient have certain inner and special meanings. In any interpersonal relationship situation, but especially the psychotherapeutic ones, the patient perceives "the other" through the eyes of the past. The hypnotherapist is endowed with characteristics, good or bad, which the patient has experienced as inherent in authority figures. Mother was gentle. Father was harsh. Mother persuaded. Father commanded. One obeyed mother through affection. One obeyed father through fear. Or, perhaps, one overtly obeyed, but inwardly rebelled, and ultimately sabotaged father's wishes through a cleverly ineffectual passivity. Whatever patterns or attitudes were developed by the individual toward earlier significant figures in his life become easily mobilized in the form of transference reactions and made active in the hypnotherapeutic relationship. The doctor is father. If he, like father, thunders his suggestions in commanding voice, he must be obeyed, but he will be feared. The hypnotherapist becomes the heir to the resources and to the obstacles which previously had influenced the parent-child relationships. Hypnotizing through love or fear has been termed by Ferenczi (18) as "mother hypnosis" and "father hypnosis."

Hypnosis is a complex response, and one whose roots we are often unable to comprehend. Even the most sensitive, well-trained and experienced hypnotic practitioner, like the good analyst, will capture and understand only a small part of the infinitely rich meanings which permeate his patient's reactions. The patient resists. We say he is not hypnotizable; but we do not know why. Sometimes the patient can tell us why. He may reveal his motivations through the many postural, gestural and inflective cues by which the sensitive psychotherapist receives subtle communications from his patient. At times, through our knowledge of personality theories and commonly expected psychodynamics we may be able to determine intuitively what is the disturbing factor and to make appropriate adjustment to it.

FEAR OF THE HYPNOTIC RELATIONSHIP

A middle-aged, unmarried woman presented herself for hypnotherapeutic treatment because of a speech difficulty. She was highly motivated to undertake hypnotherapy. Yet, during three attempts at induction, there was much resistance. She relaxed only into a very light state. Material from projective psychological tests, associations, and dreams indicated strong sexual frustrations in the face of a moralistic conscience which made her feel guilty and depressed at even permitting erotic thoughts. Suspecting that her anxiety was the manifestation of a resistance against erotic feelings being mobilized toward the hypoanalyst, induction was attempted by the postural-sway method (56) with the deliberate attempt to so mobilize this conflict that it would become more manifest and subject to resolution.

In the postural-sway induction method the patient stands with eyes closed while the practitioner stimulates minor swaying movements through suggestions that the patient is "falling forwards, falling backwards," etc. As the patient increasingly loses equilibrium the ego is unseated. He will often fall backwards or collapse into a deep trance state necessitating a pair of strong arms to ease him back into a waiting chair. Such a situation may stimulate erotic fantasies in the patient (if she falls, a man will catch her). In this case the patient's tension increased greatly, as did the amplitude of the swaying arc, until she lost her balance and had to be helped back into the chair. She also reported that after reclining in the chair she experienced unusual sensations about her mouth and lips. These were described as "tingling."

The therapist's manner at this point became most gentle. As he accepted and recognized her fears there was a flood of tears. Feelings burst to the surface. Tensions were released. Following this outburst the patient became more relaxed and secure. For the first time she and her therapist were able to begin a frank discussion of her loneliness, her desires for a man of her own, and her sexual frustrations.

During the induction the following *unverbalized* communications had passed between the doctor and the patient. The patient transmitted, "I am afraid of you. I am attracted to you. I want to be kissed (tingling—lip erotism). I might lose control of myself. You could take advantage of me, and then I would feel terribly guilty. I must keep firm control of this situation. I can no longer keep control. I cannot stand up *straight*. I might *fall*" (*Straight* and *fall* have primary-process double meanings relating simultaneously to physical and to moral posture).

After the patient had lost control of her equilibrium and had "fallen" the doctor by his manner said, "I like you. I respect you. I want to help you. I understand your fear. I will not take advantage of you. You need not fight and resist." Her tears communicated a release of many different feelings simultaneously: joy that fears would not be realized, guilt that they existed, shame that she felt sexual strivings, and sorrow in the realization that she could not have that which she wished for—to possess the therapist as hers. All these feelings were communicated in the unverbalization of tears. In the understanding and acceptance of these communications the therapeutic relationship moved into new and more rewarding ground.

The induction technique had been used as a situational stimulus to initiate and bring to focus a transference conflict about the person of the therapist which, until this session, had blocked trust, communication and confidence. Genuine therapy had begun. Of course, at this point no attempt was made to interpret to the patient the more specific meaning of the therapist as a father surrogate— a point made more obvious by projective and other material—one to whom she had been so tied as to prevent her from marrying. Deeper understandings would come later. Here we are concerned only with removing a block to the use of hypnosis. However, it should never be forgotten that our final goal is to help our patient, not just to hypnotize him. The hypnotic relationship is not an end in itself. Its induction is valuable only in so far as it gives us more therapeutic leverage in the accomplishment of our treatment mission.

It will be noted that the patient expressed her desire to be kissed by "tingling" sensations in her lips. Patients during hypnosis will often experience small movements of various parts of the body, or sensations in different bodily areas to express wishes or impulses. These somatic communications (51) are of great significance, and the sensitive psychotherapist maintains an alert attitude toward them (2, 7, 8, 42).

One frequent problem here is that he recognizes these as some type of communication, but he does not "read" this response. What could the twitching represent? What does that sudden anxiety mean? Why does the patient suddenly sense a pain in his abdomen? It is of help to ask one's self the question, "What does that part of the body do?" In the case above, we might think of eating, talking or kissing—the last being more meaningful in the light of our knowledge about the frustrations of this patient's love life.

THE AFFECT BRIDGE

A technique which is of value, both in the induction and in hypno-analytic therapy in general, for ascertaining the meaning of a symptom is one which has been termed by this writer, the "affect bridge." Attention is focused on the symptom, and it is intensified. Other elements of the present experience are suppressed. For example, a patient reported that the previous day, when applying for a job, he had, in the presence of his potential new boss, suddenly experienced a wave of anxiety accompanied by trembling in the lips. He was hypnotized, regressed to the previous day, and instructed as follows: "You are standing before this employer. All you can experience is a great anxiety and a trembling of your lips." The experience was vivified by further description and the patient soon became a seething mass of fear.

Next, the present situation was ablated except for the affect of anxiety. "Now the image of this boss is fading. You are no longer in his office. There is only a great confusion, and the whole world seems to be filled with anxiety and trembling. You are forgetting where you are, how old you are, what year this is. You are going back, back, back along a railroad track in time—a track consisting only of anxiety and trembling. Time is changing, and only your anxiety is constant. You are going back to some time when you experienced these same feelings. How old are you? Where are you?"

The patient then reported that he was thirteen years old and facing an angry father who was raging at him for breaking a window. The same fear had been initiated the day before during the employment interview because in transference he felt that the boss, like his father, would be angry at him for his fantasied or actual, destructive mis-deeds. By association to the past over the "affect bridge" we can understand his present anxiety.

When utilizing this technique any affect, lust, rage, tenderness, etc. may be used as the vehicle between the present situation and the earlier experiences. We select for such investigation those affects which seem to be inappropriate in the present situation, and hence, are probably transferred from earlier experiences. The "affect bridge" is a kind of semi-free association except that the common element which connects experience A in the present with experience B in the past is an affect or feeling, not a thought or intellectual mental content. The analytic work moves along trains of *feeling* rather than trains of *ideas*.

SPONTANEOUS CHANGES IN THE HYPNOTIC
RELATIONSHIP (2, 7, 8, 18)

Fluctuations so often seen in the depth of the hypnotic state may be related to alterations in the transference situation between patient and doctor (31, 43, 44, 53). Slight changes in the clinician's behavior may provoke new feelings in the patient which impel him deeper into hypnosis or immediately lighten, or even terminate, his present hypnotic state. In this respect it might be hypothesized that the need for anxiety reduction plays a significant role. Reinforcement learning theory (24) emphasizes the tendency of an organism to move toward and to repeat responses which through the lowering of tension afford pleasureable relief. In moving from the wide-awake, alert and conscious state to the deepest trance there is a gradual withdrawal of cathectic energy from the ego and a corresponding relative increase in activity of unconscious and repressed elements (when the ego's away the id will play). During the light to medium stages the repressed material begins to make increasing manifestation as the defenses are lessened. When increasingly-energized, unacceptable material comes into closer contact with the less well defended and weaker ego, anxiety can be expected to increase. If this reaches a point of intolerability the patient can defend himself by coming out of hypnosis, hence, re-energizing the ego and re-repressing the unintegrated and threatening material. Or, he can salvage the ego by withdrawing it almost entirely into deep hypnosis, so that it is no longer in recognizable contact with that which it cannot tolerate. Similarly, the upset child may go to sleep, or the pain-ridden soldier may black-out. It is possible that there are certain points of high anxiety on the scale of hypnotic depth from which the ego will tend to move either way—into deeper trance or into lighter trance.

CHANGING TRANSFERENCE ROLES TO FACILITATE INDUCTION

It may also be that different transference roles stimulate or inhibit the induction process differently in its early and in its later stages. Watkins (53) describes a case in which three different roles were required to initiate hypnosis in a subject and carry her into a deep state. At first, the hypnotist was non-directive and permissive. After entering a light trance the subject indicated difficulty in going deeper, whereupon a sweet and seductive, persuasive manner was employed. The subject entered a medium deep state. Further suggestions delivered in this manner did not carry her any deeper until in a commanding voice she was ordered to "go deep." A somnambulistic trance then appeared. It would seem that the need to be independent, the need to be seductively lulled, and the need to be overpowered lay at different levels of unconsciousness. By an appropriate change in the role of the hypnotist, and hence, in his relationship with the subject, it was possible to take a subject who previously could only enter a light trance and induce a deep state.

COUNTER-TRANSFERENCE IN THE HYPNOTIC RELATIONSHIP

One factor often overlooked in hypnotherapy is the motivation and need of the hypnotist—his counter-transference. Hypnosis is a bi-polar human experience. There are two parties to it. And the needs of the hypnotist are a significant part of the interaction. Consciously or unconsciously he will transmit them to his subject thus initiating affective and other behavioral reactions which adjust to or oppose the communicated needs of the hypnotist. The following example can illustrate this point:

The patient, a middle aged woman, who had been a secretary at the teaching hospital on the staff of which the therapist had served, developed a breast carcinoma, which in spite of surgery metastasized. Her case became terminal. Having been familiar with the therapist's work, and also knowing him personally, she requested that he administer hypnotherapy to alleviate her pain. The first session, devoted primarily to orientation, suggestibility tests and preparation was rather uneventful. During the second session a serious attempt to induce hypnosis was made. After an hour of intensive work it still was unsuccessful. The patient was discouraged, and the therapist left the session feeling very much a failure. That night the therapist had two dreams. In the first, a university man said to him, "You are insufferable." In the second, he was killing an ugly man.

It occurred to him that his most immediate problem was his failure to hypnotize and to help this woman whose need for pain alleviation was great and who was both a personal friend and an employee of his own hospital. Perhaps these dreams threw some light on this matter. The habit of examining one's self when one is failing in a therapeutic situation is desirable. It is often one's own blocks and not the patient's that are impairing progress. The successful resolution of these in the therapist is a pre-requisite for the resumption of constructive and meaningful treatment.

The therapist's associations to the first dream ran somewhat as follows: "University man—teacher, scholar, professor; my father was a teacher, a source of intellectual integrity and respect. Furthermore, our hospital is a teaching hospital; we are connected with the medical school. This must condense both the ideas of the place, our teaching hospital, and the pressures from my super-ego (conscience), my teacher, my father. And these say, "You are insufferable." You do not suffer. You do not co-suffer. You are oblivious of the suffering of others. You are concerned only with your satisfactions, your own triumphs. What a triumph you were expecting in hypnotizing this patient and relieving her pain when others had failed. Your colleagues in the hospital, those who have been so skeptical of your work in hypnotherapy, would have to sit up and take notice. It would be quite a feather in your cap. Yes, you are not concerned with this woman's suffering—only your own triumph. What an ugly person you are."

And then the second dream. "You are slaying an ugly man. It must be telling you what you must do about yourself, just as the first dream told you what you really are. You must kill the ugly man, abolish the ugliness in yourself, approach this patient in true humility and with only the motivation to be helpful. You must eliminate the ugly drive for self glory. Otherwise you cannot be successful."

The next evening the patient was again seen. The therapist approached her with much greater equanimity of mind. It was really not important that this be a triumph. Even if his colleagues in the hospital never heard of his success it made no difference. It was only important to try to relieve this poor woman's pain if at all possible. The trance induction was successful. A medium state was reached in about forty-five minutes. At sub-liminal levels the communication in this relationship had been changed. No longer was the patient receiving unconscious cues that the doctor's interest in her was primarily selfish. Now, she sensed that he was for her a true and dedicated ally. She gave of her self. She responded. She let him be the therapeutic father. She hypnotically regressed and became his child.

Suggestions were administered to the effect that she would ignore unpleasant sensations coming to her from below her shoulders. She would enjoy her friends, conversation, books, music, radio, television. Intellectually her existence would be rich and meaningful.

During the next few days the administration of morphine was no longer necessary. She seemed more radiant. In three days it was necessary to repeat the induction and the suggestions. During the following five weeks she was seen twice a week and the procedure repeated. She slept well. Her days were relatively free of pain and disquiet. Six weeks later she died.

It is not always so important what we *do* to our patient as what we *are* to him that counts. Within the sensitive interpersonal relationship of hypnosis, communications of the meaning of our own and of his existence are highly intensified. It is because of this that therapeutic transactions within the state of hypnosis have something to add to those in the ordinary non-hypnotic psychotherapeutic situation. For successful hypnotic induction and therapy the self of the therapist cannot be ignored.

EGO CATHEXIS AND HYPNOSIS

Paul Federn, whose writings have been compiled and amplified by Weiss (17, 54, 55), has posited the existence of an ego energy or cathexis. When a mental or physical element is invested with this cathexis it is incorporated within the boundaries of the ego and becomes part of the "I." It is the investment of some of this energy into any part of the body such as the foot which makes one experience this as "my" foot or within the body ego. Likewise, the ego cathexis of a mental content permits me to experience it as "my" idea, hence, within my mental ego. If such an idea enters consciousness without the investment of ego cathexis it is experienced as a hallucination and attributed as coming from outside one's self. Judgments as to whether phenomena are real (objective, in the outside world) or within (subjective, created within the person) are made as stimulations from these strike a well-cathected boundary separating ego from non-ego. As the boundary is more highly invested with ego cathexis it distinguishes ego-alien from ego-syntonic material more keenly. When the heart of the ego is more highly invested with this ego-energy the self is felt as living more richly and meaningfully.

Viewed from the standpoint of Federn's Ego Psychology hypnotic induction is the process of withdrawing ego cathexis from mental contents until they become un-egotized and subject to primary mental process, such as is found in the child and the psychotic—hence, the regressed one. When we de-hypnotize, we re-egotize these mental contents. We again extend "selfness" over them. Hypnosis thus becomes a method for manipulating ego cathexis in the interests of inducing a therapeutic regression.

Psychodynamics studies the economics and strategies of displacements of ego cathexis, the interchange of mental energies which from our present focus involves the initiating of the hypnotic state, its deepening and termination. Some of the methods of induction involve the manipulation of subject-object relationships by directing ego cathexis displacements (32). For example, we ask our subject to imagine that he is driving his car to our office. We picture to him the passing scene, the road, the other cars, the stores, the houses. He parks his car near our office. He turns off the key, opens the door and gets out of the car. In all of this he feels himself as the focus of the activity, the hero of the drama. There is no doubt as to where the "I" is. It is that to whom all these things are happening, and who is reacting.

Next, we suggest that he see himself close the car door. He is standing behind "that man" getting out of the car, the man who looks like him and who is dressed like him, the man whose features resemble what he sees when he looks into the mirror. This man proceeds along the walk and enters the waiting room. Soon he is called into the consultation room by the practitioner.

"You watch him as he sits down in the easy chair, that man who looks like you. You notice his eyes becoming heavy. You watch them close. You see his hand becoming lighter and approaching the man's face. You know that he is entering a deep and profound state."

Here, we have a manipulation of subject-object. The observing ego is detached from the body ego. The body is de-egotized and becomes object—it. In this type of induction the patient may become quite insensitive to painful stimuli since the outside observing ego cannot feel what "that man over there" is experiencing. Obstetricians have used this method to initiate painless childbirth (34). The patient mentally sits in a chair at the side of the room and observes "that woman over there on the delivery table" having a baby. Such phenomena become more understandable in the light of Federn's theory of the investment and withdrawal of ego cathexis into mental and bodily contents.

IDENTIFICATION AND MASS HYPNOSIS

Identification becomes a process whereby the perceptual image of another is invested with ego cathexis, thus making it part of the "I." In some cases the patient identifies with the hypnotist and thereby participates in his presumed omnipotence. He mentally "joins" him and enjoys hypnotizing his own body, which is viewed as an "other" or outside person. This loss of self is sometimes a great need for many people, especially those who despise and reject their selves (26). They identify themselves with other people or causes by investing their ego energies into the mental representations of these causes (25). Thus, millions of people in Germany were induced to identify with Hitler, to participate in his omnipotence, to lose their own despised selves in fusion with the great "wave of the future." When there is such a withdrawal of ego cathexis by members of a group from their own egos in order to invest it into an outside source (group identification) we have the experience of group hypnosis. It was truly said that Hitler was a great mass hypnotist. The Nazi movement started in a mass induction. The same principles were applied nationally as are found in the interactions of the hypnotic induction within the one-to-one psychotherapeutic, interpersonal relationship. Psychological and sociological studies can supplement each other in the understanding of hypnotic induction.

FANTASIES AND INDUCTION (28)

Day-dreaming is closely akin to light hypnosis. The schizoid individual constantly revels in such imaginations. But even the normal person occasionally indulges. One of the more sophisticated approaches to hypnotic induction involves the use of fantasy. The patient is asked to imagine a scene and progressively to "live" within it. This may then be moved time-wise to secure regression to some earlier age level. The fantasy becomes the experienced reality of the moment.

It is always easier to involve one's self in a fantasy experience if this "dream" includes pleasureable stimuli—thus, it lets us enjoy highly satisfying, personal situations. Especially potent in inducing an hypnotic state are those fantasied situations which appeal to immature and childish cravings. For example, skin eroticism has been considered ontogenetically as preceding genital eroticism. Thus, when the hypnotist pictures for the patient the soothing touch of a soft, grassy slope on which he is reclining, or the smooth, velvet sensation about his body when floating on a cloud, he is invoking tactile, erotic fantasies reminiscent of the maternal touch in earliest childhood. It is not surprising that the regression of the patient is encouraged.

A common unconscious fantasy is the desire to return to the womb, to an early, warm, environmentally perfect existence. Rank (37) insists that the process of violent detachment from that environment which once met all needs represents the greatest trauma of life. We need not concur with his conclusion to understand when the hypnotist talks about "a soft, warm space with the most beautiful feelings of comfort and peace," that he is trying to encourage the hypnotic regression through re-vivification as far as possible of the patient's unconscious somatic memories of the pre-birth period.

Sometimes the hypnotist suggests that in entering hypnosis the subject will experience great feelings of omnipotence. Thus, the child in the dental chair is asked to close his eyes, to picture a TV screen, and to imagine he is watching "Mighty Mouse"—that little midget who is so successful in over-powering the great cat, dog, or other animal representation of parent figures. The little patient's fantasy wish-life is stimulated to aid him to regress into an hypnotic state wherein sensations from the dental drill are ignored.

In the initiation of such fantasies the pictorial descriptive powers of the hypnotist are fully utilized. Vivid description, attention to minute details within the images, the allowance of time for involvement, and the willingness to modify the fantasy as directed by the patient, all enhance the induction or deepening process (32).

The more the hypnotist understands the motivational needs of his patient, the more skillful he becomes in flexibly adapting his induction techniques to different subjects. In some cases, such as our little dental patient, we may expect that his needs for omnipotence and his desire to best his elders, represent some part of his fantasy life—this is characteristic of almost every child. Often though, we must rely on our own knowledge derived from interview (or psychological testing) contacts with the patient, and the degree of sensitiveness to less obvious communications to which we have conditioned our own "third ear" (39).

TERMINATION OF HYPNOSIS (40, 57)

If hypnosis is indeed a regression, then its termination means a return to the reality and maturity demands of the present. Just as the physicist must be aware of both centrifugal and centripetal forces, so must the good hypnotherapist consider both the regressive and the progressive needs of his patient. In one sense the termination of each trance is a return to maturity, a re-birth. The regression has truly been "in the service of the ego," not a permanent state. Some patients need reassurance on this. They fear that maybe they "won't come out of it." The therapist stands on the side of the ego, of reality and of mature adjustment. His excursions into the hypnotic regression are limited, purposeful, only for the benefit of his patient, and always to be concluded at some point. He will do well to see that his patient understands this, whether this is communicated directly or by implication.

But in bringing the patient back from the hypnotic state the therapist is a respecter of his subject's regressive needs. He will take time, and not require that the patient make instant response to the de-hypnotizing suggestions. The sudden return of ego awareness to the deeply hypnotized patient can in some cases be traumatic. The patient may not be ready to re-face the world, and perhaps some of the unconscious material about which he was communicating in the hypnotic state. We must protect his ego and not submit it to the sudden battery again of external stimuli (or emerging internal material) until it is ready.

The patient, himself, sometimes telegraphs his reluctance to leave the comfortable, regressed state to return to the unpleasant realities. He stays in hypnosis or may temporarily even go deeper (41) in spite of suggestions to the contrary. The hypnotist does not panic. He merely conveys to his patient that he understands the patient's enjoyment of his present condition and his wish to remain. He either permits the patient to emerge "when you are ready and at your own speed," or he kindly suggests that the patient may return to this state "the next time" when he can re-experience and understand better his present sensations. Under no circumstances should the therapist react as if this were a challenge—which it may so represent. If such a "challenge" continues it may become necessary for him to seek to understand and interpret its meaning to the patient. However, this is seldom necessary. If told that he will awaken when he is ready, and then left to himself, the patient usually soon becomes alert.

It is important to see that the hypnotic state has been fully terminated, and a full state of ego awareness has been established before releasing the patient to drive home. Accordingly, a few minutes should be permitted at the end of the hypnotic period for interactions in the conscious state.

THE VALIDITY OF PSYCHODYNAMICS

The reader might gather from this brief discussion of the psychodynamics of induction that we are dealing with an exact science. The writer wishes to leave no such impression. Through psychodynamic understanding we can increase our percentage of success, and if we are doing psychotherapy we can with greater likelihood induce that kind of hypnotic state and relationship which is most conducive to therapeutic intervention. But at best we can only aim at increasing our sensitivity in communication and our flexibility in technique. There will be many times when we are at a total loss to understand what is happening within our patient and why he seems so completely unresponsive to our induction attempts.

Psychodynamics is far from an exact science. However, the practitioner who views his hypnotherapeutic work with a continuous consideration of his patient's conscious and unconscious motivational needs, and with studied attention to his own feelings and his relationship with his patient, will develop his sensitivity to these experiences. He finds his reward through an increased therapeutic effectiveness in the practice of hypnotherapy.

REFERENCES

1. BARBER, T. X.: Sleep and hypnosis, a reappraisal. *J. Clin. & Exper. Hyp.*, *4*:144, 1956.
2. BARTEMEIER, L.: Discussion of "Alterations in the state of the ego in hypnosis." *Bull. Menninger Clin.*, *11*:66, 1947.
3. BELLAK, L.: An ego-psychological theory of hypnosis. *Int. J. Psycho-Anal.*, *36*: Part 6, 1955.
4. BEXTON, W., HERON, W. and SCOTT, T.: Effects of decreased variation in the sensory environment. *Canadian J. Psychol.*, *8*:70, 1954.
5. BOWERS, M. K. and BRECHER, S.: The emergence of multiple personalities in the course of hypnotic investigation. *J. Clin. & Exper. Hyp.*, *3*:188, 1955.
6. BRENMAN, M.: Dreams and hypnosis. *Psychoanal. Quart.*, *18*:455, 1949.
7. BRENMAN, M., GILL, M. and HACKER, F. J.: Alterations in the state of the ego in hypnosis. *Bull. Menninger Clin.*, *11*:60, 1947.
8. BRENMAN, M., GILL, M. and KNIGHT, R. P.: Spontaneous fluctuations in the depth of hypnosis and their implications for ego-function. *Int. J. Psychoanal.*, *33*:22, 1952.
9. CHRISTENSON, J. A., JR.: Dynamics in hypnotic induction. In LeCron, L. M.: *Experimental Hypnosis*. New York, Macmillan, 1952.
10. CONN, J. H.: Hypnosis as dynamic psychotherapy. *Sinai Hosp. J.*, *5*:14, 1956.
11. EHRENREICH, G. A.: The influence of unconscious factors on hypnotizability: a case report. *Bull. Menninger Clin.*, *15*:45, 1951.

12. Eissler, Kurt R.: *The Psychiatrist and the Dying Patient.* New York, Int. Univ. Press, 1955.

13. Ellis, A.: Reactions of psychotherapy patients who resist hypnosis. *J. Clin. & Exper. Hyp., 1*:12; 2:261, 1954.

14. Erickson, M. H.: Deep hypnosis and its induction. In LeCron, L. M.: *Experimental Hypnosis.* New York, Macmillan, 1952.

15. Erickson, M. H. and Hill, L. B.: Unconscious mental activity in hypnosis—psychoanalytic implications. *Psychoanal. Quart., 13*: 60, 1944.

16. Farber, L. H. and Fisher, C.: An experimental approach to dream psychology through the use of hypnosis. *Psychoanal. Quart., 12*:202, 1943.

17. Federn, P. (Edoardo Weiss, Editor): *Ego Psychology and the Psychoses.* New York, Basic Books, 1952.

18. Ferenczi, S.: *Sex and Psychoanalysis.* New York, Basic Books, 1950.

19. Fisher, C.: Studies on the nature of suggestion. Part II, The transference meaning of giving suggestions. *J. Am. Psychoanal. A., 1*:406, 1953.

20. Fisher, C.: Studies on the nature of suggestion. Part I, Experimental induction of dreams by direct suggestion. *J. Am. Psychoanal. A., 1*:333, 1953.

21. Gill, M. M.: Spontaneous regression on the induction of hypnosis. *Bull. Menninger Clin., 12*:41, 1948.

22. Gill, M. M. and Brenman, M.: *Hypnosis and Related States.* New York, Int. Univ. Press, 1959.

23. Hartmann, H.: *Ego Psychology and the Problem of Adaptation.* New York, Int. Univ. Press, 1958.

24. Hilgard, E. R.: *Theories of Learning,* 2d. ed. New York, Appleton-Century-Crofts, 1956.

25. Hoffer, E.: *The True Believer.* New York, Harper, 1951.

26. Horney, K.: *Neurosis and Human Growth.* New York, Norton, 1950.

27. Kanzer, M.: The metapsychology of the hypnotic dream. *Int. J. Psychoanal., 34*:288, 1953.

28. Klemperer, E.: Social anxiety, early sexual and agressive theories as revealed through hypnoanalysis. *Psychoanal. Rev., 44*:81, 1957.

29. Kline, M.: *Freud and Hypnosis.* New York, Julian Press and Institute for Research in Hypnosis, 1958.

30. KLINE, M.: *Hypnodynamic Psychology*. New York, Julian Press, 1955.

31. KLINE, M.: Toward a theoretical understanding of the nature of resistance to the induction of hypnosis and depth hypnosis. *J. Clin. & Exper. Hyp., 1*:32, 1953.

32. KLINE, M.: A visual imagery technique for the induction of hypnosis in certain refractory subjects. *J. Psychol., 35*:227, 1953.

33. KOSTER, S.: Experimental investigation of the character of hypnosis. *J. Clin. & Exper. Hyp., 1*:16, 1953.

34. KROGER, WILLIAM S.: *Childbirth with Hypnosis* (Edited by Jules Steinberg). New York, Doubleday, 1961.

35. MEARES, A.: *A System of Medical Hypnosis*. Philadelphia, Saunders, 1961.

36. PRINCE, M.: *The Dissociation of a Personality*. New York, Meridian Books, 1957 (Reprinted).

37. RANK, O.: *The Trauma of Birth*. New York, Robert Brunner, 1952 (Reprinted).

38. REGARDIE, F. I.: Experimentally induced dreams as psychotherapeutic aids. *Am. J. Psychotherap., 4*:643, 1950.

39. REIK, T.: *Listening with the Third Ear*. New York, Farrar, 1948.

40. ROSEN, H.: Dehypnosis and its problems. *Brit. J. Med. Hyp., 5*:18, 1954.

41. SCHNECK, J. M.: Depth reversal during termination of the hypnotic state. *Psychoanal. Rev., 43*:506, 1956.

42. SCHNECK, J. M.: Spontaneous sensory and motor phenomena with related imagery during hypnosis. *Psychiat. Quart. Supp.*, Part 1, 1956.

43. SCHNECK, J. M.: Transference and hypnotic behavior. *J. Clin. & Exper. Hyp., 3*:132, 1955.

44. SCHNECK, J. M.: Hypnoanalytic elucidation of motivation and goal in relation to psychotherapy. *Dis. Nerv. Syst., 16*:173, 1955.

45. SCHNECK, J. M.: Hypnosis-death and hypnosis-rebirth concepts in relation to hypnosis theory. *J. Clin. & Exper. Hyp., 3*:40, 1955.

46. SCHNECK, J. M.: Dreams in self-hypnosis. *Psychoanal. Rev., 41*:1, 1954.

47. SCHNECK, J. M.: The unconscious relationship between hypnosis and death. *Psychoanalyt. Rev., 38*:271, 1951.

48. SCHNECK, J. M.: Some aspects of homosexuality in relation to hypnosis. *Psychoanalyt. Rev., 37*:351, 1950.

49. SCHNECK, J. M.: Hypnoanalytic elucidation of the hypnosis-death concept. *Psychiat. Quart. Suppl., 24*:286, Part 2, 1950.

50. SCHNECK, J. M.: Notes on the homosexual component of the hypnotic transference. *Brit. J. M. Hyp., 1*:24, 1950.

51. SCHNECK, J. M.: Psychosomatic reactions to the induction of hypnosis. *Dis. Nerv. Syst., 11*:118, 1950.

52. SWEETLAND, A. and QUAY, H.: An experimental investigation of the hypnotic dream. *J. Abn. Soc. Psychol., 47*:678, 1952.

53. WATKINS, J. G.: Trance and transference. *J. Clin. & Exper. Hyp., 2*:284, 1954.

54. WEISS, E.: *Structure and Dynamics of the Human Mind.* New York, Grune and Stratton, 1960.

55. WEISS, E.: *Principles of Psychodynamics.* New York, Grune and Stratton, 1950.

56. WEITZENHOFFER, A.: *General Techniques of Hypnotism.* New York, Grune and Stratton, 1957.

57. WILLIAMS, G. W.: Difficulty in dehypnotizing. *J. Clin. & Exper. Hyp., 1*:3, 1953.

58. WOLBERG, L. R.: *Hypnoanalysis.* New York, Grune and Stratton, 1945.

12

THEORIES OF HYPNOSIS

Ainslie Meares, M.D., B.Agr.Sc., D.P.M.

The First Edition of this work did not deal with the theories of hypnosis. This may seem a strange omission. But when the book was first published in 1953, although there were a great number of theories, at that time it was clear that none of them adequately explained all the phenomena of hypnosis. However, since then our knowledge of these matters has advanced, and two new theories have been put forward which are of themselves not mutually incompatible (1), and which at present appear to explain all the varied phenomena of hypnosis. These are the primitive psychophysiological theory of Schneck (2), and the atavistic theory of Meares (3, 4). Both theories regard the basic element of hypnosis as a regression to a primitive mode of functioning.

If, as at present seems possible, these theories do come to provide a rational and generally acceptable explanation of hypnosis, then the reader may well wonder why we should concern ourselves with other theories which have proved to be inadequate. However, it is more than just historical interest that leads us to discuss these past theories. Each of them emphasises some particular aspect of hypnosis. By studying them, the clinician gains much information that is of value in his daily round of treating patients.

ANIMAL MAGNETISM

What can we learn from Mesmer's theory of Animal Magnetism which he offered to the flamboyant society in the days before the French revolution? Even this theory, which nowadays seems almost ridiculous, can show us much. It shows us that the act of making a pass with the hands carries with it very powerful suggestion. More than this, it serves to alert us to the very important fact that the non-verbal communication of suggestion is often more effective than the statement of the same idea in words. Furthermore, from a study of the way in which Mesmer treated his patients we come to realize that the hypnotized subject to a great extent behaves in the way in which he believes that a hypnotized subject does behave. Thus Mesmer's patients believed that the animal magnetism would throw them into a convulsion; so when they took hold of the handles of his famous baquet which they believed contained specially magnetized iron, they felt the animal magnetism working on them, and they were in fact thrown into a convulsion. Perhaps there is one further point that Mesmer's theory shows us. The various theories of hypnosis are all closely related to the philosophical, religious and scientific sophistication of the times. We can see how well the theory of animal magnetism fits in with the pseudo-science and sensation seeking of the period.

Those who followed Mesmer became known as "Mesmerists" or "Magnetizers." They came to emphasize the strength of their own will in overcoming the patient. This element of the theory of animal magnetism has some reference to present day practice. Many patients come to consultation with the deeply ingrained belief that the induction of hypnosis involves them in being overpowered by the strength of will of the therapist. This heritage of the days of the "Magnetizers" is so widespread that it is well to be quite sure with each individual patient that he does not feel this way about hypnosis. Otherwise a passive induction with such a patient will be extremely difficult.

SUGGESTION

The theory of animal magnetism was disproved by James Braid in 1841 (5) when he showed that the trance state could be induced without the aid of any Mesmeric passes. Nevertheless, many adherents to the theory of animal magnetism persisted in their claims, and Magnetizers continued to practice for a half a century after Braid's experiment.

In 1866, Liébeault, a French general practitioner, was the

first to clearly state that the phenomena of hypnosis were due to the operation of the mechanism of suggestion. He became associated with Professor Bernheim of Nancy, who widely publicized the suggestive theory of hypnosis, but who at the same time always acknowledged his debt to Liébeault.

In our everyday clinical practice there is no doubt that the increased suggestibility is the most conspicuous feature of the hypnotized patient. We offer the suggestion; the patient carries it out. There is no need to evoke esoteric concepts such as animal magnetism. We can see that many of the complex phenomena of hypnosis such as the amnesia and the regression can be produced in direct response to suggestion. The wide acceptance of Liébeault's theory can be easily demonstrated by merely asking a few medical colleagues what is hypnosis. The majority will quickly answer that hypnosis is a state of increased suggestibility.

However, if we examine the matter more closely, we realize that the theory gives no explanation as to what causes the increased suggestibility. In other words, Liébeault's theory is no more than a statement of the most conspicuous clinical feature of hypnosis. Nevertheless, we must not underestimate the great importance of this theory to medical and psychological thinking. His great contribution lies in the fact of offering a psychological as opposed to an organic explanation. In an indirect way he thus came to pave the way for the acceptance of the psychological and psychosomatic concepts of the next half century.

Liébeault's suggestive theory really included another important concept. He emphasized the idea of levels of hypnosis. In different patients the process of suggestion may operate to varying degrees, thus producing different levels of the hypnotic state. This was a further advance in the theory of hypnosis, and this concept has been reiterated in various forms by most authorities to the present day. However, the important thing for the clinician to understand is that, with changed circumstances, the concept of levels of hypnosis is no longer valid. In the days of Liébeault and Bernheim, hypnosis was induced by an authoritative and rigid approach. As long as one adheres to a single method of induction the concept of levels of hypnosis remains valid. But if the technique of induction is modified according to the various defences of the patient, then levels of hypnosis are no longer demonstrated. In fact, in some areas of mental activity, the patient may be functioning at a very deep level, and at the same time in other areas he may be quite light. Thus, some patients are deep enough to go into deep hypnotic sleep, but at the same time are not deep enough to paint in hypnosis; while others are so deep that they disclose deeply repressed material in painting, but at the same time are not sufficiently deep to go into hypnotic sleep. With our increased knowledge of psychodynamics, Liébeault's once useful concept of levels of hypnosis must now be discarded.

HYPNOSIS AS A FORM OF HYSTERIA

Charcot, the great neurologist of Salpêtrière hospital believed that hypnosis was a form of hysteria which could be induced in certain constitutionally predisposed persons. This was essentially an organically orientated theory as opposed to the psychological theory that hypnosis was purely the result of suggestion which was put forward by Liébeault and Bernheim. Thus, there arose the famous controversy between the schools of Salpêtrière and Nancy, in which Charcot's enormous prestige in medicine did much to delay the acceptance of the more scientific views of the Nancy school.

We now know that almost any normal person can be hypnotized if he really wishes it. Yet Charcot's idea of constitutional predisposition is not entirely irrelevant to our present day work. We are familiar with those constitutionally ill-endowed persons who come into the psychiatric classification of personality defect or inadequate personality. These persons are particularly easy to hypnotize by the authoritative approach which was used by Charcot.

Then again, in holding that hypnosis is a form of hysteria, Charcot drew attention to the very important hysterical phenomena which are so frequently observed in the hypnotized patient. We now know that these hysterical manifestations are either hysterical psychological defences or hysterical modes of communication, and are not the basic factor of hypnosis, although they are often the most conspicuous feature of the behaviour of the hypnotized subject.

The theory that hypnosis is a form of hysteria still has its influence on modern hypnotherapy in the way in which patients are referred to us. There is a general belief in the medical world that hypnosis is much more useful in the the treatment of hysteria than it is in the other psychoneuroses and psychosomatic conditions. This erroneous belief results in our colleagues referring for hypnosis a disproportionate number of hysterics, many of whom are in fact not particularly suitable for hypnotherapy.

DISSOCIATION

Like Charcot, Janet (6) also noted the similarity between hypnosis and hysteria. He felt that dissociation was an important factor in both conditions, and that dissociation was in fact the basis of hypnosis. According to this theory, some functions of the mind become dissociated or split off, as it were, from the main personality and come to act independently of the main personality. The process is seen in extreme form in the development of multiple personalities which may occur both in hysteria and in hypnosis. This theory, which is also associated with the name of Morton Prince, accounts very easily for the dissociative phenomena of hypnosis which can be demonstrated so easily in such procedures as automatic writing and hypnography. However, dissociation by itself cannot adequately account for the increased suggestibility which is clinically the most conspicuous feature of hypnosis, and the theory of dissociation has few adherents in the present day.

HYPNOSIS AS A CONDITIONED RESPONSE

Pavlov (7) came to apply the idea of the conditioned reflex as an explanation of hypnosis. According to this theory the phenomena of hypnosis result from the process of conditioning. A word, or gesture, or some aspect of the behaviour of the therapist becomes the conditioned stimulus. He held that hypnosis is due to a radiation of cerebral inhibitions which followed monotonous stimulation.

The idea of cerebral inhibition is analogous to his theory of sleep. It explains very well the tendency for the hypnotized patient to fall asleep, and the cerebral inhibition can likewise explain the complete or partial failure of repression in hypnosis which makes hypnoanalysis possible. However, a number of electroencephalographic studies has shown that from the point of view of cerebral function, hypnosis is related to the waking state rather than sleep.

The concept of conditioning is a useful one to keep in mind during the process of induction by suggestions of relaxation. The presentation of carefully graded suggestions to the patient has the effect of enabling him to accept progressively more difficult suggestions. This in fact is the basis of our most commonly used technique of induction. The theory also brings the spontaneous pseudo-trance states, such as "highway" hypnosis, into line with the general theory of hypnosis. However, the conditioned response theory does not explain the spontaneous regression which is often a feature of hypnosis, nor does it account for the importance of the affective relationship between subject and hypnotist. It appears that at the present time the conditioned response theory of hypnosis is widely held in Russia, but has few adherents elsewhere.

THE IDEO-MOTOR THEORY

The ideo-motor theory is based on the fact that the thought of an act tends to produce small contractions in the muscles which would be used to carry out the act. The physician is familiar with this response from the way in which some patients respond when we ask them to relax their limbs. When we are about to elicit the tendon reflexes or induce hypnosis by suggestions of relaxation we sometimes feel an increased tension in the muscles, so that the patient may involuntarily lift his arm off the couch. By ideo-motor activity the thought of the movement has produced tension in the muscles which would carry out the movement.

This concept accounts very well for some of the phenomena of hypnosis, particularly the motor phenomena. Thus it explains hypnotic induction by arm levitation and the various cataleptic phenomena of hypnosis. On the other hand, it is at a loss in accounting for the psychic phenomena of hypnosis, such as age regression and the ventilation of repressed material.

HYPNOSIS AS A LOVE RELATIONSHIP

Freud considered hypnosis as analogous to falling in love—an erotic relationship in which the overtly sexual elements were repressed. He considered that it took place in a transference relationship, and that all the mechanisms of transference were active. (8)

The theory explains very well the positive affective relationship between subject and hypnotist, and the various aspects of hypnotic rapport. It explains the motivation of the subject when he is so eager to carry out the suggestions of the hypnotist, and in this way accounts for his suggestibility.

It was formerly believed that women are easier to hypnotize than men. This would seem to fit in with Freud's theory. But the belief that women are more easily hypnotized than men arose at a time when hypnosis was induced by an authoritative approach. As long as an authoritative approach is maintained women are in fact more easily hypnotized than men, but if we change our technique according to the patient's particular defenses, we find that men are just as easily to hypnotize as women. This in itself would lead one to doubt Freud's theory. However, the theory that hypnosis is a kind of distorted love relationship falls down completely in relation to hypnosis by mechanical means, such as the metronome and hypnodisc, nor can it adequately explain the phenomena of autohypnosis.

In describing the past theories of hypnosis we have made an attempt to discuss aspects of these theories which may be of value to the present-day clinician in dealing with his patients. From Freud's theory we learn the very great importance of our emotional relationship with the patient. But there is another truth to be learned of even greater significance. In reading Freud's papers we cannot help but be dismayed by the incredible prejudice and hostility with which he was received when he dared to challenge the orthodox concepts of the day. However, the time has now come when Freud's own views represent the orthodox concepts of the present day. It is interesting to note that those who would enquire into and challenge the validity of some of Freud's views, in many quarters meet the same prejudice and hostility which Freud himself encountered when he came to challenge that which was orthodox in his day.

HYPNOSIS AS A CHILD-PARENT RELATIONSHIP

In his psychoanalytical investigations of hypnosis, Ferenczi (9) concluded that it was a state of regression to a child-parent relationship. In this theory the patient is considered to be as a child in the face of the parent, and he carries out the latter's wishes without question.

This theory accounts very well for many of the phenomena of hypnosis. The tendency to regression in hypnosis is fully explained. So is the rapport between subject and hypnotist. An explanation is offered for the readiness with which the hypnotist's suggestions are carried out. However, like Freud's theory, the theory of hypnosis as a regression to a child-parent relationship falls down completely on the matter of hypnosis by mechanical means, and gives no adequate explanation of autohypnosis.

Although his theory is not a complete explanation for the phenomena of hypnosis, Ferenczi made a very valuable contribution indeed. The idea of regression as a basic factor was a move in the right direction, and his concept of paternal or maternal hypnosis according to which parent becomes the subject of identification has great clinical significance in our practical dealing with patients. Thus, if we wish to bring about a paternal identification, we present ourself as the powerful and authoritative father, but if we aim for a maternal identification, we present ourself as a loving, passive, soothing figure. We thus come to have an explanation of the two different clinical approaches to induction—the authoritative approach and the passive approach.

Following Ferenczi's lead, in more recent years Solovey and Milechnin (10) have written of hypnosis as a retrogression to the emphatically induced emotional state of the infant during psychological mothering. They point out that in this emotional state the infant is freed of psychological and physiological tensions. They thus come to give an explanation of the important fact that the induction of hypnosis often has a therapeutic effect, irrespective of verbal and non-verbal suggestive mechanisms.

HYPNOSIS AS GOAL-DIRECTED STRIVING

R. W. White (11) in 1941 published a paper in which he described hypnosis as "meaningful, goal-directed striving, its most general goal being to behave like a hypnotized person as this is continually defined by the operator and understood by the subject."

On first consideration, this statement seems to give a very adequate explanation of the behaviour of the hypnotized subject. We give suggestions which in fact define what we expect of the patient: and motivated by his rapport with us he strives to act in the manner which we have indicated. However, the theory fails to explain hypnosis by mechanical means in the absence of any instructions or clues from the therapist, nor does it explain the hypnosis of a subject against his will with him actively resisting, nor are the spontaneous phenomena experienced in hypnoanalysis adequately explained by this theory.

HYPNOSIS AS ROLE-TAKING BEHAVIOUR

This theory put forward by Sarbin (12) brings us back to our earlier consideration of hypnosis as a form of hysteria. According to this theory the subject acts the role of a hypnotized person. This is a much more pronounced form of the way in which we all play roles in our ordinary life. The theory explains very well the tendency for the hypnotized subject to behave in the way in which he believes a hypnotized person to behave, and the theory is consistent with the obvious hysterical manifestations which are so often a feature of hypnosis.

The theory gives us at least one important clinical hint. When we see a patient very obviously playing a role, it is very easy to get the impression that the patient is not properly hypnotized, that he is consciously fooling us. This need not be so. I have suspected this on a number of occasions, only to find out from other tests that the patient was in fact deeply hypnotized. However, the role-taking theory does not explain the spontaneous ventilation of repressed material or the altered physiology which can be obtained in hypnosis.

HYPNOSIS AS LOSS OF EGO BOUNDARIES

Kubie and Margolin (13) have advanced a theory in which it is considered that in the induction of hypnosis there is a progressive elimination of all channels of communication between the subject and the outside world, with the exception of the hypnotist. As a result of this, the hypnotist becomes the subject's sole contact with the outside world. This phase of the induction resembles the sensori-motor relationships of the infant to the outside world with the hypnotist playing a role similar to the parents. The onset of the hypnotic state consists of a partial sleep, and an obliteration of ego boundaries which leads to a psychological fusion between hypnotist and subject.

This aspect of the theory explains very well both the suggestibility and the rapport of hypnosis. However, Kubie and Margolin continue by stating that this same restriction of sensori-motor relationships makes possible a state of hypnagogic reverie in which vivid sensory memories are released, which in turn lead the way to buried memories. This aspect of the theory is less convincing than a theory which can more directly account for the failure of repression in hypnosis.

From the psychological point of view they regard hypnosis as an extension of the process of normal attention with the creation in the central nervous system of a focus of excitation with surrounding areas of inhibition. They regard this as physiologically dependent upon relative immobilization of the head or eye, and the influence of monotony. The immobilization is related to work on animals. In evaluating these ideas it is clear that immobilization and monotony are important aids in the technique of hypnosis, but they are not always essential, even with subjects who have not previously been hypnotized.

Kubie and Margolin consider that in full hypnosis there is a partial re-expansion of the ego boundaries, and the incorporation of a fragmentary image of the hypnotist which comes to act as the subject's temporary ego. This phase is analogous to the development of the infant's ego in which its boundaries gradually expand, with the retention of the parental image as an unconscious incorporated component of the developing ego.

The aspects of this theory which are of most value to the practicing clinician are the concepts of dissolution of ego boundaries and the temporary introjection of the image of the hypnotist in an analogous way to that in which it is believed the image of the parent was incorporated in childhood.

HYPNOSIS AS HOMOACTION, HETEROACTION AND DISSOCIATION

Weitzenhoffer (14) has advanced a theory in which he attempts to explain hypnosis through the operation of three mechanisms, homoaction, heteroaction and dissociation.

Homoaction is the process by which the acceptance of one suggestion facilitates the later acceptance of a suggestion of the same kind. This is related to well known psychological principles, and is observed in our everyday experience of hypnotizing patients by graded suggestions.

Heteroaction is the process by which the acceptance of one suggestion modifies the response to suggestions of a different kind. The clinician is familiar with this process from his everyday experience. These two processes, together with dissociation are regarded as accounting for the phenomena of hypnosis.

HYPNOSIS AS AN INTERPERSONAL RELATIONSHIP

Barber (15) in 1958 offered the theory that hypnosis was essentially an interpersonal relationship which is characterized by a number of overlapping processes. Taking the subject as the frame of reference, there is the process of becoming concerned only with the words of the hypnotist and those aspects of his self and his surroundings to which the hypnotist specifically directs his attention. There is the process of becoming ready and willing to carry out the instructions of the hypnotist, and the process of coming to believe that the hypnotist's words are true statements.

This theory accounts for the rapport of hypnosis and the desire of the subject to carry out the hypnotist's wishes. But the theory is clearly too superficial, and it fails to explain autohypnosis, or hypnosis by mechanical means, nor does it relate hypnosis to the pseudo-trance states.

HYPNOSIS AS PRIMITIVE PSYCHOPHYSIOLOGICAL FUNCTIONING

In 1953, Schneck (2) offered a new theory as to the nature of hypnosis. He feels that the basic fallacy of other theories has been that they have focussed attention on the induction of hypnosis or the phenomena attainable in hypnosis, rather than on the hypnotic state itself. In the author's opinion this would seem a very valid criticism. The phenomena of sleep, suggestion, hysterical mechanisms, ideo-motor activity, dissociation, goal-directed striving and role-playing all occur to a significant extent in hypnosis, but it is clear that none is the basic phenomenon. Schneck feels that the basic ingredient of hypnosis is a state which is far removed from both waking consciousness and natural sleep. This state exists in its most pure form when conscious thinking is eliminated, so that contact with the environment is reduced, and differentiation of the self from the environment is at a minimum. This is the most primitive level of psychophysiological functioning when the first awareness of the individual's differentiation from the environment occurs. This state is the basic ingredient of hypnosis, and Schneck does not limit it to the human species.

In offering this theory Schneck has ignored the attraction of the obvious and dramatic elements of hypnosis which have waylaid investigation in this field for more than a century. He has attempted to formulate the basic ingredient of hypnosis. All who work with hypnosis must become aware that it involves certain very primitive features. The theory of primitive psychophysiological functioning accounts very well for this important aspect of the hypnotic state.

Schneck summarizes his theory with the statement, "This theory of hypnosis proposes then, that the hypnotic state, in terms of its basic ingredient, is that condition represented by the most primitive form of psychophysiological awareness of individual-environmental differentiation attainable among living organisms."

While accepting Schneck's theory as an important contribution, the author would offer criticism on the grounds that it lacks clarity, and that there is no attempt to relate it more specifically to the suggestibility and rapport of hypnosis.

THE ATAVISTIC THEORY OF HYPNOSIS

Meares (3, 4) in 1957 offered a theory which has some aspects in common with Schneck's theory, in that both regard the essential element in hypnosis as something primitive.

In the atavistic theory the process of suggestion is regarded as an archaic mental function. The ability of logical thought is believed to be a recently acquired function of the mind. In primitive man, before the evolution of logical processes, simple ideas must have been accepted by some other more primitive mechanism. Suggestion seems to be the process which fulfilled this function. In other words, suggestion is believed to be a primitive mental process which acted to determine the acceptance of ideas in the evolutionary period prior to man's acquisition of the ability of logical thought. This concept is supported by the greater activity of suggestion in childhood, in primitive man and in sub-human animal species.

The atavistic theory regards the basic element of hypnosis as a regression to this type of primitive mental functioning in which ideas are accepted by suggestion. It is emphasized that this type of regression differs from simple age regression which is commonly observed in psychiatry and in which the individual returns to childhood or infantile patterns of behaviour. The atavistic regression involves a regression to a primitive mode of mental function. This is regarded as the basis of hypnosis. On this primitive basis there is an overlay of the common psychological mechanisms of which hysteric defences, identification, introjection, dissociation and hysteroid communications are conspicuous. This overlay of psychological mechanisms accounts for the more obvious aspects of the behaviour of the hypnotized subject.

In applying the atavistic theory to the induction of hypnosis it is seen that the great number of apparently unrelated techniques of induction readily fall into three groups of procedures, each of which facilitates atavistic regression.

a) Procedures which dull the recently acquired logical functions and so allow the primitive function of suggestion to operate: Intellectual activity is dulled by giving the suggestions in a monotonous voice, by the repetition of the suggestions, and by the sensory fatigue of Braid's method. Keeping the room warm, and the exclusion of extraneous stimuli act similarly; so does the use of drugs and the various mechanical aids, such as the metronome, revolving discs, and flashing lights. In the passive induction of hypnosis, the patient is encouraged voluntarily to let himself drift into hypnosis. By the process of abandoning himself, of letting his mind go blank, he voluntarily quietens the critical faculties of the intellect, and so allows the suggestive mechanisms to come into play. Similarly, in autohypnosis, the activity of the intellect is dulled on the subject's own initiative.

b) Procedures which activate the latent process of suggestion: The latent suggestive function of the mind is reactivated by subjecting the patient to a series of very simple suggestions. The acceptance of one suggestion seems to activate the suggestive mechanism, so that the acceptance of further suggestions is facilitated. This process is, of course, the basis of the techniques commonly used in medical practice for the induction of hypnosis.

c) Procedures which encourage behavioural regression and so facilitate the basic atavistic regression: In the authoritative approach the assumption of prestige and paternal authority forces the subject to regress into the role of a child. In the passive approach the soothing, loving and permissive atmosphere similarly encourages regression with the therapist identified as a maternal figure. This behavioural regression activates the regressive process and facilitates the basic atavistic regression.

The atavistic theory seemingly accounts for all the phenomena of hypnosis. The suggestibility is explained as the return to the primitive mode of mental functioning. The tendency to regression is similarly explained. Amnesia may occur either as a response to suggestion or as a defence as a part of the overlay of psychological mechanisms. The apparent somnolence which we know is not true sleep is explained by the absence of intellectual activity as a result of the atavistic regression. The rapport of hypnosis is explained on the grounds that in the primitive state it would be a biological necessity for the individual to accept ideas from those kindly disposed toward him, that is, those with whom he had rapport, and not from those who might be ill-disposed towards him and with whom he had no positive affective relationship. The bizarre behaviour is explained in terms of hysteric defences and hysteroid communication. The tendency for the ventilation of repressed material is due to failure of the repressive mechanism which is a recently acquired function of the mind and is consequently impaired or lost in atavistic regression.

The theory explains autohypnosis, hypnosis by mechanical means, and also brings the pseudo-trance states into line with the general concept of hypnosis. In light hypnosis the atavistic regression is not so complete as in deep hypnosis, and the difference in phenomena observed by different workers in different circumstances is explained by the relative activity of the overlay of psychological mechanisms.

REFERENCES

1. SCHNECK, J. M.: Comment on a theory of hypnosis. *Int. J. Clin. & Exper. Hyp., 8*:231, 1960.
2. SCHNECK, J. M.: A theory of hypnosis. *J. Clin. & Exper. Hyp., 1*: 16, 1953.
3. MEARES, A.: A working hypothesis as to the nature of hypnosis. *A.M.A. Arch. Neur. Psychiat., 77*:54, 1957.
4. MEARES, A.: *A System of Medical Hypnosis.* Philadelphia, Saunders, 1960.
5. BRAID, J.: *Neurypnology, or the Rationale of Nervous Sleep Considered in Relation with Animal Magnetism.* London, 1843.
6. JANET, P.: *Major Symptoms of Hysteria.* New York, Macmillan, 1920.
7. PAVLOV, I. P.: *Conditioned Reflexes.* New York, Oxford University Press, 1934.
8. FREUD, S.: *Group Psychology and the Analysis of the Ego.* Authorized Translation by James Strachey. London, Hogarth Press, 1948.

9. FERENCZI, S.: *Further Contributions to Theory and Technique of Psychoanalysis.* Translated by James Suttie, International Psychoanalytical Library No. 11. London, Hogarth Press, 1952.

10. SOLOVEY, G. and MILECHNIN, A.: Concerning the theory of hypnosis. *J. Clin. & Exper. Hyp.,* 4:37, 1956.

11. WHITE, R. W.: A preface to a theory of hypnotism. *J. Abn. Soc. Psychol., 36*:477, 1941.

12. SARBIN, T. R.: Contributions to role-taking theory. *Psychol. Rev., 57*:255, 1950.

13. KUBIE, L. S. and MARGOLIN, S.: The process of hypnotism and the nature of the hypnotic state. *Am. J. Psychiat., 100*:5, 1944.

14. WEITZENHOFFER, A. M.: *Hypnotism.* New York, Wiley, 1953.

15. BARBER, T. X.: The concept of hypnosis. *J. Psychol., 45*:115, 1958.

13

HISTORY OF MEDICAL HYPNOSIS: ADDITIONS AND ELABORATIONS

JEROME M. SCHNECK, A.B., M.D.

George Rosen, in an earlier chapter, traced the significant developments in hypnosis from the late eighteenth to the late nineteenth centuries. His starting point was the work of Mesmer, and properly so because his efforts are essentially the main beginnings of a trend toward the eventual blossoming of medical and scientific hypnosis. It should be realized that the mesmeric "crises" and trance experiences of some form existed long before Mesmer, and there is little doubt that in some way they played a role in happenings among ancient man during the era of paleomedicine, perhaps similar to the trance rites and rituals encountered in contemporary times among primitive tribes. In these surroundings concepts of disease involve the influence of spirits and the power of offended gods. Trance states are incorporated into magico-religious medicine and its bond with supernaturalism. Curiously, the holistic view of man and disease, the concern of medicine today, is in its unitary aspect a predominant element in primitive medicine (1).

The Siberian shaman is an example of the possessed medicineman. In his possession, he enters a trance state while participating in tribal rites (2). He is the healer and trance experience is a fundamental part of his magico-religious activity. Frazer described trance states among primitive peoples (3). He noted that some trance states were death-like. For some groups, such states are hardly distinguished from death. This is not too remote. Recently the identification of hypnosis and death on an unconscious level has been described for some patients in clinical settings (Schneck, 4). Hyp-

nosis and re-birth may also be equated (Schneck, 5). Others have
noted also the utilization of trance among primitive groups and
the specific hypnosis-death identification too (6). But the trance
state need not be involved for the death theme. The Dyak medicineman, for example, may simply lie down and pretend to be dead.
His return to life is intended to benefit the ill person in his recovery.
The medicine man among the Loango of French Equatorial Africa
may enter a trance at night with the result that his soul leaves him
in order to consult ancestral spirits. When it returns, the diviner is
informed about the cause of the patient's illness (3). In such primitive settings, magic, religion, and medicine are one (7).

Although clear, specific data are generally not available, it is
assumed that trance experience and the use of hypnosis for healing
purposes have a continuous history dating from the early days of
man, through ancient times, the Middle Ages, and the Renaissance.
References in this respect are often made in cursory fashion to
ancient China, India and Egypt. Thus, Hull writes of "phenomena
more or less resembling those of the hypnotic trance" (8) "especially
among Oriental peoples" (9). Another writer is willing to claim,
"On the zodiac in the arched vault of the Temple at Denderah,
Isis is depicted holding a child by the hand, while she passes her
other hand in front of him in the attitude of a magnetizer." Also,
"In India, mythology represents Vishnu with flames issuing from
his finger-ends" (10). Most references of this type are, however, difficult to evaluate, including interpretations placed on some aspects
of the Temple sleep among the Greeks. Then, because of the early
association of magnets with mesmeric practice, there are allusions,
in historical accounts of hypnosis, to the activities of Cardan, and
Paracelsus among others.

Much more is known about the Mesmeric period, and there is
a feeling of being on firmer ground (11). Yet the essence of Mesmer
himself seems difficult to evaluate, and opinions about him differ
so very much. For some he was a man of stature and ability, for
others a charlatan, perhaps a plagiarist as well and lacking scholar-
ship (12). Although Mesmer's views, including the 27 propositions
of his *Mémoire sur la découverte du magnétisme animal,* are usually
thought of today as extreme and unscientific, George Rosen has

already indicated that the themes and theoretical concepts were common to the eighteenth century medical world. It would seem too that there are points among these propositions reflecting ingredients of thought that were to develop afterwards into some concrete conceptions of suggestion in its many aspects, and complex issues of transference relationships too (Schneck, 13). Even now this is probably not fully appreciated although Mesmer's work is so often referred to as the beginnings of modern psychotherapy.

There is perhaps a special point of interest in connection with Mesmer's technique of eliciting convulsive movements or crises, a goal that frequently evoked negative professional reactions. When Mesmer was involved in this work, electrotherapy was already on the medical scene, and the clinical demonstrations of psychiatric patients by William Battie in England initiated, some believe, psychiatry as a specialty there (14). More attention was given now to "nervous disorders," an area to which Mesmer himself called attention. Not only was he calling attention to it, but a number of his patients were undoubtedly helped. Electrotherapy was administered by individual physicians and in hospital settings.

Now a careful examination of Mesmer's propositions reveals reference to electricity in numbers twenty-one and twenty-two. "This system will furnish fresh explanations as to the nature of Fire and Light, as well as the theory of attraction, ebb and flow, the magnet and electricity." "It will make known that the magnet and artifical electricity only have, as regards illnesses, properties which they share with several other agents provided by Nature, and that if useful effects have been derived from the use of the latter, they are due to Animal Magnetism." Here it is implied that the therapeutic effect of magnets and electricity is related essentially to the same forces that promote the operation of animal magnetism. In this historical interpretation, the issue of Mesmer's theory must be set aside in favor of his clinical observations. Again, disregarding his theoretical concerns, it appears to be the doctor-patient relationship with all its psychological implications, and the complex facets of suggestion in its dynamic aspects, that play a role in the eventual outcome of treatment. Furthermore, it must be noted that Mesmer's statements are consistent with present day observations regarding the psychological elements that share a place in electrotherapeutic techniques and outcome. As a matter of fact, the psychological aspects of therapeutic results with electrotherapy have attracted attention for some time (16, 17).

Electrical measures elicit convulsive reactions to varying degree depending on therapeutic settings and the intent of the physician. Mesmer elicited convulsive reactions of varying form as "crises" which he believed to be therapeutically significant, and his techniques were essentially psychological. In terms of the dynamics of the illness, these reactions must have been of considerable importance to the patients in the same way that electroconvulsive therapy must have its psychodynamic implications for the patient in relation to underlying psychopathology. The parallel timing of the magnetic convulsive crises and the electrotherapeutic efforts during the late eighteenth century probably cannot be ignored when viewed historically, and this is reenforced by Mesmer's propositions quoted above and by his later statement, "It will be seen from the facts, in accordance with the practical rules I shall draw up, that this principle can cure nervous disorders directly and other disorders indirectly" (Schneck, 13, 15). In the historical development of scientific ideas, the correlation between Mesmer's animal magnetism and the history of electrotherapy with their allied psychodynamic themes is surely deserving of recognition. Mesmer has been called a typical rationalist and speculative systematist of the eighteenth century (1). Whether or not it is agreed that he falls into this category or some other, the influences he set in motion developed significant ramifications (Schneck, 13).

The memory of Mesmer's work invariably gives rise to associated thoughts about investigating commissions. The best known is probably that of 1784 which had a devastating effect on Mesmerism. But there were others. References may be found, for example, to the Husson Commission of 1831. Henri-Marie Husson (1772-1853) was actually a member not of one, but of two commissions. That of 1831 was the second (Schneck, 18). Both commissions stemmed from the interest of Pierre Foissac in animal magnetism and in attempts to reevaluate it. The first commission was a study group that presented its report to the Section of Medicine of the

Royal Academy of Medicine on December 13, 1825. It concluded that magnetism should be reexamined. Animated discussions extended into the following year when a special commission (the second) was appointed February 28, 1826. It reported on June 21 and 28, 1831. Husson had been appointed to it only after Laennec became ill and had to leave Paris (19). A few years after the Husson report was issued, another commission was on the scene, again in France, in 1837. It rendered an unfavorable report on animal magnetism. The point to be made about all of these commissions is that they are of historical importance because they influenced strongly the general attitudes assumed toward the subject investigated. It is of interest that this applies less to the influence of the appointing bodies regarding the conclusions reached in the reports. The appointing groups were inclined usually to accept unfavorable decisions and to reject favorable findings. This is of interest in connection with what the present writer chooses to refer to as the history of scientific attitudes.

In his chapter, George Rosen describes the British mesmeric movement. He takes up the work of James Esdaile among others. During the past decade, important advances have been made in hypnotic anesthesia. Prior to this, there had been sporadic interest in it. James Esdaile's contributions loom large in this aspect of the history of hypnosis because of his extensive activities with mesmeric anesthesia accompanying his surgical procedures. This work was done in the mid-nineteenth century. One may note in examining Esdaile's work, *Mesmerism In India,* a small section pertaining to mesmeric dream material (20). It is of interest for historical correlation with current activities in hypnotherapy, hypnoanalysis, and some aspects of experimental hypnosis (Schneck, 21). Esdaile was interested in dreams that involved planning, problem solving, sudden insight, and creative experience. "I see no reason," he wrote, "to doubt that the mental organs can be isolated and exalted by the mesmeric influence under the direction of a skillful leader and suggester, and can readily believe that the mind, by this artificial stimulus, may be excited into more vigorous activity than when acted upon by the usual conditions of life." His remarks in general bear the imprint, of course, of the hypnotic practice and theory of his time, but he was aware of many potentialities of hypnotic subjects. Regarding these interests, Esdaile said, "My psychological experiments have been very limited, partly because I fear to bewilder myself at the outset, and also from want of proper subjects to try them on. The mental range of my patients is so circumscribed, that the topics of food, drink and clothing almost exhaust it, and with most of them I have no common language. But I have done enough to show me how the higher grades of somnambulism may be reached; and with more highly organised and intellectual natures, I should have good hopes of doing so." Esdaile worked mostly with natives in India. Perhaps his failure to capitalize on his observations along psychological channels was based on lack of knowledge about any system of psychology that would have given them more meaning. His comments, however, perhaps warrant a small place for him in the history of the psychological areas of hypnotic practice and research (Schneck, 21).

The nineteenth century witnessed also a popularization of mesmerism and hypnosis resulting in their inclusion in works of fiction among others. Some of the writings and their authors achieved considerable fame. In the earlier historical chapter there is brief reference to the writings of Edgar Allan Poe and Henry James. A more complete evaluation of the latter's novel, *The Bostonians* was presented by the present writer (Schneck, 22), and among several points of interest it was shown that the hypnotic theme in it supplies several parallels to George du Maurier's *Trilby* which is probably the best remembered work centering on a hypnotic relationship. Du Maurier's book is an especially interesting work for study, and several themes from it have been presented under headings of induction of hypnosis, the hypnotized person as a sexual object, the masochism of Svengali, the psychology of the amateur hypnotist, the suggestibility of Trilby and the comments on her death, the dual representation of Svengali, the naiveté of Trilby in relation to hypnotic experience, the role of hypnosis in Trilby's achievement, the hypnosis-death concept, and Du Maurier, Carry of Malines and mesmerism (Schneck, 23).

The present writer has evaluated also those writings of Poe that touch on hypnotic themes and his contributions have been described in detail (Schneck, 24). Poe wrote *Mesmeric Revelation* and *The Facts in the Case of M. Valdemar*. He was quite taken by certain links between hypnosis and death. Robert Browning was interested in mesmerism too, and he wrote a poem by that name. In a study of Browning with reference to mesmerism, the present writer was able to show that his special interests and psychological orientations probably established the foundation for impressions, feelings, and thoughts from which the shape of this poetic work was crystalized. In addition, it is to be noted that Elizabeth Barrett Browning was interested in mesmerism and had evidently considered it as treatment for herself at one time. Furthermore, she had friends who were involved with this subject and were attentive to the work of John Elliotson. This too may well have been part of the background of Robert Browning's concern with the subject (Schneck, 25).

It has been demonstrated that fantasies of hypnotic time obliteration may be discovered not only in clinical settings but in literary productions and fairy tales. For example, the writer has demonstrated a version of this theme in the classic novel, *Looking Backward,* by Edward Bellamy. It is illustrated too in the tale of Briar Rose (Schneck, 26, 27).

While the developments in scientific aspects of hypnosis during the first part of the nineteenth century were making themselves felt on the literary scene, there were happenings continuing into the second part of the century of which the Nancy-Paris controversy is outstanding. It has been possible to show that while these factions were on the scene, a third but lesser known group was in existence. It has been called the School of the Hospital de la Charité (28). To understand it, the views of Liébeault and Bernheim of the Nancy School and those of Charcot and his co-workers of the Paris or Salpêtrière School had best be summarized first. The opinions and conclusions of Charcot have since been largely discounted. He incorrectly saw hypnosis as a psychopathological phenomenon. The lethargic, cataleptic and somnambulistic stages of hypnosis as he described them are not inherent to it, nor are the methods by which they can be presumably brought about. The Paris faction stressed hypnotic production of muscle "contractures" and skin anesthesias elicited by pressure on areas of peripheral nerve distribution. These observations proved to be inaccurate. Charcot was mistaken in his belief about intimate connections between metals and magnets and their influence on the hypnotic state. With his co-workers he stressed experimental studies. They used a few, select, grossly hysterical patients. Unlike Charcot and his assistants, Liébeault and Bernheim appreciated the broad range of hypnotizability in the general population, the less dramatic manifestations of hypnotic reaction and behavior, and broad therapeutic possibilities in clinical experience. Hypnotizability was stressed as an expression of normal behavior, whereas for Charcot hypnosis was essentially an experimental neurosis (Schneck, 29). Yet Charcot's name is important in the history of hypnosis and indelibly associated with it because his authority and popularity stirred considerable interest in it. He is often said to have made hypnosis respectable (30).

In a recent biography of Charcot, Guillain (31) made claims about his hypnotic activities that the present writer regards as questionable (Schneck, 32). For example, he said Charcot never personally hypnotized a single patient. He said Charcot never checked the experiments of his co-workers, thus accounting for errors that resulted. Both points have been examined in detail and appear to be discounted on the basis of facts supplied by Binet and Féré in their classic volume, *Le magnetisme animal* (33). They are among the best known of Charcot's co-workers, particularly in the field of hypnosis. Neither is mentioned by Guillain in this connection, nor is the aforementioned book.

The operations of the School of the Hospital de la Charité were described by one of its representatives, Foveau de Courmelles (10). It has been possible to organize his views and to correlate them with the concurrent activities in Paris and Nancy (Schneck, 28). This School had a three-fold orientation—hypnotism, magnetism, and suggestion. Its experimental and physicalist approach paralleled the Salpêtrière School. The suggestion and therapeutic concepts were consistent with the Nancy School. It seemed to lean more toward the Salpêtrière faction. It appears to have retained post-Mesmeric fluidist concepts. J. Luys (34), the distinguished neurologist and neuroanatomist, was the chief investigator of the

Charité group. His revolving mirror for use in hypnosis is still remembered. His studies on motor attitudes and emotions in hypnosis have been forgotten although some of the issues reappear on the current scene without direct reference to his work. His concern with hypnotic behavior in relation to ingredients of sealed tubes has been dismissed. Bottey, Regnier, and de Grandchamps were his co-workers.

Sigmund Freud, disappointed in the therapeutic possibilities of electrotherapy, explored other horizons. He spent time in Paris with Charcot in 1885. He observed the work of Bernheim and Liébeault in 1889. He was impressed with Bernheim's experiments and saw the possible existence of strong forces at work within patients while hidden from consciousness (35). In the meantime, Josef Breuer, conducting a general practice in Vienna, had been interested in hypnosis. Of particular concern were his findings pertaining to the cathartic method involving spontaneous verbalizations by patients and the discharge of emotions during the hypnotic state. The collaboration between Breuer and Freud was fruitful, and in it lay the origins of psychoanalysis. Their co-authored paper on the mechanisms of hysterical phenomena appeared in 1893 and their classic volume, *Studies on Hysteria,* in 1895 (36). The issue of priorities is often of interest, provided it is not stressed unduly, and an example of such interest is the early work with the cathartic method. Recently attention has been given to activities in this area by Bourru and Burot at the time Breuer and Freud were also exploring its possibilities (37). As for the origin of psychoanalysis, Breuer deferred pointedly to Freud. In his own autobiography, Breuer wrote, "In 1880 I had observed a patient suffering from a severe hysteria, who in the course of her illness displayed such peculiar symptoms as to convince me that here a glimpse was being offered into deeper layers of psychopathological processes. The insights then gained were presented by S. Freud and myself, first in a short preliminary study and later in the *Studies On Hysteria* by Breuer and Freud. This book, which was rather unfavorably received at first, went into its fourth edition last year. It is the seed from which psychoanalysis was developed by Freud" (38).

Freud believed he found it necessary eventually to give up

hypnosis on clinical grounds. Points involved in this move included claims regarding difficulties in adequate hypnotizability of many patients and in effecting meaningful and sustained results. Both issues are no longer tenable as a result of more extensive clinical observations and activities and reevaluations with deeper understandings of personality functioning plus therapeutic maneuvers to cope with such functioning. Of special interest is the fact that to a great extent these strides stem from new knowledge gleaned from psychoanalytic insights introduced by Freud. However, the reasons he offered for relinquishing hypnosis appear to be questionable for his time on clinical grounds alone. Certain aspects of the "objective or scientific" reasons in Freud's discontinuing the use of hypnosis have been delineated and discussed (39). Additional features pertain to Freud's personal and emotional involvements influencing this move and the theme has been highlighted with special reference to his countertransference reactions (Schneck, 40). At that stage of his clinical and self-knowledge he may have been unable to deal with problems of his hypnotherapeutic encounters that he might possibly have managed well at a later date. It has also been said of him that the rejection of hypnosis related perhaps to a reaction formation connected with his own fantasies of omnipotence (41). Regardless of these issues, the fact is that the step was a turning point in the history of hypnosis and of psychoanalysis. Emotional allegiances to Freud and his work followed, and intense identifications with him obscured potential scientific horizons and blocked legitimate evaluations of theory and technique by those otherwise capable of pursuing these goals (40).

While these activities were in progress, attention was given to hypnosis to greater or lesser degree by a number of clinicians and experimenters. Only a few need be mentioned because of their meaningful contributions at the time or their lasting fame. Some published notable books. These investigators are Moll (42), Forel (43), Bramwell (44), Janet (45), Prince (46) and Sidis (47). It would be a mistake for students now to believe that Moll's book, for example, has no significance because it was published at the end of the last century. It has not only historical merit, but is a mine of important observations that still deserve attention and consideration.

Pierre Janet was a meticulous psychopathologist, much interested in problems of hysteria. Although some historians feel he was unable to overcome the view of hysteria as degenerative, he is credited, on the other hand, with initiating the trend toward bringing clinical and academic psychology together in the development of meaningful concepts. Janet's special influence on Morton Prince has been pointed out by Boring (48). Prince was interested much in the issue of co-conscious and multiple personalities and his work with hypnosis is of particular merit in this connection. For a time, after he supplied detailed contributions in this field, it was given less attention by others. More recently there has been an activation of concern with the subject not only for essential clinical therapeutic purposes, but for the light that can be shed on personality functioning in general. In a further attempt to bring together the fields of clinical and academic psychology, Prince founded the Harvard Psychological Clinic. The dissociation concept of Janet still carries an imprint on some current investigations and publications. Significant influences of his work on the ideas advanced by Freud are generally denied although Janet himself and his scientific contributions have strong supporters. As for Prince, it is usually agreed that he did not accept the implications of the unconscious in a Freudian sense, and the opinion has been offered that in his views he was influenced by ideas such as those put forward by von Hartmann (13).

Developments in the first half of the twentieth century included varying levels of involvement with hypnosis from clinical and experimental approaches. Occasional investigators, by virtue of their personalities, directions, or specific contributions, stand above the rest. For example, Paul Schilder's studies continue to hold interest. He brought to bear on his work a broad range of thought and interests and a number of his propositions show the influence of psychoanalytic concepts (49). Clark Hull engaged in a series of studies on hypnosis and suggestibility, producing with his assistants a large body of work highlighting the laboratory approach to hypnosis investigations. Bringing to the subject the academic atmosphere and setting had, despite its limitations, the advantage of encouraging additional interest of psychologists who might otherwise have bypassed the field (9).

Combinations of abreactive techniques and varying degrees of reeducational work have been attempted from time to time and in this connection the term "hypno-analysis" had been employed for such efforts during the first World War. As a matter of fact, this term has been used for differing therapeutic maneuvers, a number of which seek to uncover problems and others which may have no specific relation to "analysis" in terms of psychoanalytic theory and method. The combining of hypnotic theory and method and psychoanalytic theory and technique has been achieved in a number of ways and lends itself to some flexibility. One example, though not typical of the work others have done, is the contribution of Robert Lindner (51).

A view of the history of hypnosis reflects periodic revival and recession of interest in it. Both World Wars have been accompanied by revival of interest that has not been sustained, and these revivals probably stemmed considerably from pressure for brief psychotherapy. This is reasonable up to a point in that possibilities for many good results are present when dealing with acute traumatic circumstances, but there has been a concurrent lack of appreciation for longer term clinical and research possibilities. Hypnotherapy was used during the Second World War but not as extensively as some imagine and it probably did not meet the role of narcoanalysis and narcosynthesis which gained passing prominence. Physicians had to be trained rapidly in psychiatric techniques and they were more accustomed to mechanical injection methods and employment of drugs than with heavy emphasis on verbal psychological measures, the latter also requiring more new training than the former. After the War there was not a significant, persistent development of any interest in hypnosis by most of the people who may have previously considered it for emergency expedients. Occasional workers, who had not been necessarily directly involved in military activities, published their findings as had always been the case.

A turning point in this state of affairs was the founding of The Society for Clinical and Experimental Hypnosis in 1949, a scientific organization that elevated the stature of clinical and experimental investigations in this field. It promoted work of high calibre, stimulated significant publications, encouraged qualified participants, reactivated the interest of earlier workers whose productivity had diminished, attempted to check extravagant claims, furthered meaningful instruction, and stimulated worthwhile activity on an international front. Other organizations in general or specialized areas had existed before and were formed afterwards, but this Society has continued to be representative of scientific activities of high standard. It has fostered the integration of dynamic psychological and psychiatric concepts with continuing developments of hypnosis in all medical and scientific areas. With these developments, once again in keeping with a historic heritage, special committees and commissions have come into view. Members of the organization were called on for consultation by the American Medical Association which eventually rendered a favorable report on hypnosis in 1958 after the British Medical Association had issued its statement in 1955. Should careful clinical and experimental operations continue, extravagant and unwarranted claims be tempered and inaccurate and unjustified criticisms be set aside, the future appears to be favorable for continued growth in this area.

REFERENCES

1. ACKERKNECHT, E. H.: *A Short History of Medicine.* New York, Ronald Press, 1955.
2. ACKERKNECHT, E. H.: "Mesmerism" in primitive societies. *Ciba Symp., 9*:826, 1948.
3. FRAZER, J. G.: *The Golden Bough.* New York, Macmillan, 1922.
4. SCHNECK, J. M.: The hypnotic trance, magico-religious medicine, and primitive initiation rites. *Psychoanal. Rev., 41*:182, 1954.
5. SCHNECK, J. M.: Hypnosis—death and hypnosis—rebirth concepts in relation to hypnosis theory. *J. Clin. & Exper. Hyp., 3*:40, 1955.
6. ROSE, R.: Psi and Australian aboriginals. *J. Am. Soc. Psychical Res., 46*:17, 1952.
7. SIGERIST, H. E.: *A History of Medicine,* Vol. 1. New York, Oxford University Press, 1951.
8. HULL, C. L.: Hypnotism in scientific perspective. *Sc. Monthly, 29*: 154, 1929.

9. HULL, C. L.: *Hypnosis and Suggestibility*. New York, D. Appleton-Century, 1933.

10. FOVEAU DE COURMELLES, F. V.: *Hypnotism*. London, George Routledge and Sons, 1891.

11. MESMER, F. A.: *Mesmerism, by Doctor Mesmer* (1779), *Being the first translation of Mesmer's historic "Memoire sur la découverte du magnétisme animal" to appear in English*, trans. by V. R. Myers with an introductory monograph by Gilbert Frankau. London, Macdonald, 1948.

12. PATTIE, F. A.: Mesmer's medical dissertation and its debt to Mead's *De Imperio Solis ac Lunae. J. Hist. Med. & Allied Sc., 11*:275, 1956.

13. SCHNECK, J. M.: *A History of Psychiatry*. Springfield, Thomas, 1960.

14. HUNTER, R. A.: A brief review of the use of electricity in psychiatry. *Brit. J. Physical Med., 20*:98, 1957.

15. SCHNECK, J. M.: The history of electrotherapy and its correlation with Mesmer's animal magnetism. *Am. J. Psychiat., 116*:463, 1959.

16. STAINBROOK, E.: Shock therapy: psychologic theory and research. *Psychol. Bull., 43*:21, 1946.

17. STAINBROOK, E.: The use of electricity in psychiatric treatment during the nineteenth century. *Bull. Hist. Med., 22*:156, 1948.

18. SCHNECK, J. M.: The first and second Husson commissions for the study of animal magnetism. *Bull. Hist. Med., 27*:269, 1953.

19. POYEN ST. SAUVEUR, C.: *Report On The Magnetical Experiments Made By The Commission Of The Royal Academy Of Medicine, Of Paris*. Read in the Meetings of June 21 and 28, 1831, by Mr. Husson the Reporter. Translated from the French and Preceded by an Introduction. Boston, D. K. Hitchcock, 1836.

20. ESDAILE, J.: *Mesmerism in India and Its Application in Surgery and Medicine*. Chicago, Psychic Research Company, 1902.

21. SCHNECK, J. M.: James Esdaile, hypnotic dreams, and hypnoanalysis. *J. Hist. Med. & Allied Sc., 6*:491, 1951.

22. SCHNECK, J. M.: Mesmerism in Henry James' *The Bostonians*. In Schneck, J. M.: *Studies in Scientific Hypnosis*. Baltimore, Williams and Wilkins, 1954.

23. SCHNECK, J. M.: Du Maurier's *Trilby* and modern hypnosis. In Schneck, J. M.: *Studies in Scientific Hypnosis*. Baltimore, Williams and Wilkins, 1954.

24. SCHNECK, J. M.: A medical hypnotherapeutic addendum to the case of M. Valdemar. *Bull. Med. Lib. A., 41*:144, 1953.

25. SCHNECK, J. M.: Robert Browning and Mesmerism. *Bull. Med. Lib. A., 44*:443, 1956.

26. SCHNECK, J. M.: The fantasy of hypnotic time obliteration with related literary allusions. *J. Clin. & Exper. Hyp., 5*:172, 1957.

27. SCHNECK, J. M.: The hypnotic state and the psychology of time. *Psychoanal. Rev., 44*:323, 1957.

28. SCHNECK, J. M.: The School of the Hospital de la Charité in the history of hypnosis. *J. Hist. Med. & Allied Sc., 7*:271, 1952.

29. SCHNECK, J. M.: Charcot and hypnosis (letter). *J.A.M.A., 176*:73, April 8, 1961.

30. WECHSLER, I.: Jean-Martin Charcot. In Haymaker, W.: *Founders of Neurology.* Springfield, Thomas, 1953.

31. GUILLAIN, G.: *J.-M. Charcot 1825-1893, Sa Vie-Son Oeuvre.* Paris, Masson et Cie, Libraires de l'Academie de Médecine, 1955 (English trans. by Pearce Bailey, New York, Paul B. Hoeber, 1959).

32. SCHNECK, J. M.: Jean-Martin Charcot and the history of experimental hypnosis. *J. Hist. Med. & Allied. Sc., 16*:297, 1961.

33. BINET, A. and FÉRÉ, C.: *Le Magnétisme Animal.* Paris, 1887. (English trans., New York, D. Appleton and Company, 1888.)

34. KRIEG, W. J. S.: Jules Bernard Luys (1828-1897). In Haymaker, W.: *The Founders of Neurology.* Springfield, Thomas, 1953.

35. FREUD, S.: *An Autobiographical Study.* New York, W. W. Norton, 1952.

36. BREUER, J. and FREUD, S.: *Studies on Hysteria.* New York, Basic Books, 1957.

37. CHERTOK, L.: On the discovery of the cathartic method. *Int. J. Psycho-Anal., 42*:284, 1961.

38. OBERNDORF, C. P.: Autobiography of Josef Breuer. *Int. J. Psycho-Anal., 34,* Part 1, 1953.

39. KLINE, M. V.: Freud and hypnosis: II: further observations on resistance and acceptance. *J. Clin. & Exper. Hyp., 3*:124, 1955.

40. SCHNECK, J. M.: Countertransference in Freud's rejection of hypnosis. *Am. J. Psychiat., 110*:928, 1954.

41. EHRENWALD, J.: History of psychoanalysis. In *Science and Psychoanalysis.* New York, Grune and Stratton, 1958.

42. MOLL, A.: *Hypnotism.* London, Walter Scott, 1890.

43. FOREL, A.: *Hypnotism.* New York, Rebman, 1907.

44. BRAMWELL, J. M.: *Hypnotism*. London, Grant Richards, 1903.
45. JANET, P.: *The Major Symptoms of Hysteria*. New York, Macmillan, 1907.
46. PRINCE, M.: *The Dissociation of a Personality*. New York, Longmans, Green, 1908.
47. SIDIS, B.: *The Psychology of Suggestion*. New York, D. Appleton, 1898.
48. BORING, E. G.: *A History of Experimental Psychology*. New York, Appleton-Century-Crofts, 1950.
49. SCHILDER, P. and KAUDERS, O.: *Hypnosis*. New York, Nervous and Mental Disease Monograph Series, 1927.
50. HADFIELD, J. A.: Treatment by suggestion and hypno-analysis. In Miller, E.: *Neuroses in War*. New York, Macmillan, 1940.
51. LINDNER, R. M.: *Rebel Without A Cause*. New York, Grune and Stratton, 1944.

NAME INDEX

A

Abramov, N. P., 328, 358
Abramson, H. A., 63, 92
Abramson, M., 167
Abt, L., 311
Ackerknecht, E. H., 418
Adams, A. J., 285, 313
Adler, A., 263
Aigner, E., 352
Akagi, M., 354
Alexander, F., 46, 60, 63, 74, 92, 93
Alexander, I. E., 95
Alvarez, W. C., 92
Ambrose, Gordon, 84, 92, 204, 228, 347
Ament, P., 261, 262, 277
Arluck, E. W., 289, 290, 309
Arnold, H. L., 140
Astruck, P., 326, 348
Atterbury, R. A., 279
Auerback, A., 92
August, Ralph V., 143, 167, 348
Azam, 23, 25

B

Bailey, Pearce, 420
Balinsky, B., 289, 290, 309
Ball, T. L., 167
Balk, 279
Barber, T. X., 314, 319, 320, 335, 336, 337, 339, 343, 348, 386, 400, 405
Barker, W., 317, 318, 319, 348
Barnes, R. H., 203
Barnett, S., 268, 278
Baron, J. H., 106, 120
Bartemeier, L., 386
Barth, Joseph, 6
Bass, M. J., 320, 321, 348
Battie, William, 408
Baumler, 348
Beatty, J. M., 319, 320, 359

Beaunis, 24
Beecham, C. T., 168
Beecher, H. K., 104, 120
Bell, 14
Bellak, L., 284, 309, 357, 386
Bellamy, Edward, 412
Belland, G., 348
Benedek, L., 348
Benedict, F. G., 328, 361
Benjamin, J. E., 93
Bennett, L. L., 322, 349
Berg, W., 349
Berger, 13
Bergler, 97
Bergman, M. S., 286, 309
Bérillon, E., 225, 228
Berjot, A., 25
Berkowitz, B., 169, 201
Berman, R., 322, 323, 349
Berna, 22
Bernheim, Hippolyte, 13, 24, 25, 26, 280, 392, 393, 412, 413, 414
Bernoulli, 26
Bernstein, G., Jr., 96, 279
Bersot, Ernest, 26
Bertrand, Jacques-Francois-Alexander, 21
Betcher, A. M., 119
Bexton, W., 386
Bick, J. W., 67, 93
Bicker, George, 9
Bickford, R. G., 319, 321, 335, 359
Biehl, J. P., 344, 349
Bier, W., 321, 349
Bigelow, N., 321, 349
Binet, A., 413, 420
Binger, C. A., 61, 92
Bjornstrom, Friederich, 26
Blackwell, Elizabeth, 13, 14
Blake, H., 318, 349
Blinkowski, 345, 353

SUBJECT INDEX